International Library of Ethics, Law, and the New Medicine

Volume 59

The book series *International Library of Ethics, Law and the New Medicine* comprises volumes with an international and interdisciplinary focus. The aim of the Series is to publish books on foundational issues in (bio) ethics, law, international health care and medicine. The 28 volumes that have already appeared in this series address aspects of aging, mental health, AIDS, preventive medicine, bioethics and many other current topics.

This Series was conceived against the background of increasing globalization and interdependency of the world's cultures and governments, with mutual influencing occurring throughout the world in all fields, most surely in health care and its delivery. By means of this Series we aim to contribute and cooperate to meet the challenge of our time: how to aim human technology to good human ends, how to deal with changed values in the areas of religion, society, culture and the self-definition of human persons, and how to formulate a new way of thinking, a new ethic.

We welcome book proposals representing the broad interest of the interdisciplinary and international focus of the series. We especially welcome proposals that address aspects of 'new medicine', meaning advances in research and clinical health care, with an emphasis on those interventions and alterations that force us to reexamine foundational issues.

More information about this series at http://www.springer.com/series/6224

Ralf J. Jox • Galia Assadi
Georg Marckmann
Editors

Organ Transplantation in Times of Donor Shortage

Challenges and Solutions

Springer

Editors
Ralf J. Jox
Galia Assadi
Georg Marckmann

Institute of Ethics, History
and Theory of Medicine
Ludwig-Maximilians-University Munich
Munich
Germany

ISSN 1567-8008 ISSN 2351-955X (electronic)
International Library of Ethics, Law, and the New Medicine
ISBN 978-3-319-16440-3 ISBN 978-3-319-16441-0 (eBook)
DOI 10.1007/978-3-319-16441-0

Library of Congress Control Number: 2015943746

Springer Cham Heidelberg New York Dordrecht London

Printed on acid-free paper

Springer is part of Springer Science+Business Media (www.springer.com)

Contents

Chapter 1
Organ Transplantation in Times of Donor Shortage. An Introduction

Galia Assadi, Ralf J. Jox and Georg Marckmann

Organ transplantation is an exceptional success story of modern medicine. From 1954, when Joseph E. Murray conducted the first living kidney donation among twins, to 2013, when 6866 transplants[1] were conducted within the Eurotransplant[2] region, the new discipline of transplantation medicine has been confronted with a long list of different challenges and obstacles. In the beginning, medical difficulties were in the foreground, e.g. tissue typing or the matching of donors and suitable recipients. One of the major problems, the allogeneic rejection caused by antigen differences, was able to be solved in the course of the 1950s. Due to the groundbreaking discovery of the French hematologist Jean Dausset, who in 1958 discovered that Human Leukocyte Antigens (HLA) function as body markers indicating whether a tissue is own or foreign, it became possible to develop immunosuppressive drugs which counteract rejection. Based on the development of more specific and effective immunosuppressants, transplantation technology could expand. Thereby the 1960s became the decade of transplantation success with the first post-mortem kidney transplantation in 1962, the first liver and lung transplantations in 1963, followed by the first pancreas and the first heart transplantations in 1966 and 1967, respectively.

[1] Eurotransplant, http://www.eurotransplant.org/cms/.

[2] Eurotransplant, a collaboration of eight European countries cooperating to heighten the amount of available organs and optimizing the allocation process, was founded in 1967.

R. J. Jox (✉) G. Marckmann
Institute for Ethics, History and Theory of Medicine, Ludwig-Maximilians-University Munich, Munich, Germany
e-mail: ralf.jox@med.uni-muenchen.de

G. Assadi
Munich, Germany
e-mail: galia.assadi@web.de

G. Marckmann
e-mail: georg.marckmann@med.uni-muenchen.de

R. J. Jox et al. (eds.), *Organ Transplantation in Times of Donor Shortage*,
International Library of Ethics, Law, and the New Medicine 59,
DOI 10.1007/978-3-319-16441-0_1

While the major medical obstacles to transplantation could be overcome by pioneer scientists and physicians, the emerging discipline faced another challenge that is still unresolved today. Due to the growing effectiveness of transplantation and the increase of organ failure in aging societies, the problem of organ shortage became prominent. In order to close the gap between an accelerating demand and a rather staggering supply, many responses have been conceptually invented and practically tested. Yet, despite all the efforts that are being undertaken to resolve the problem, every year thousands of potentially curable patients die while waiting for an organ transplant. Health authorities, medical professionals and bioethicists worldwide point to the urgent problem of organ shortage, which will be further intensified due to increasing life expectancy, particularly in newly industrialized, emerging countries with huge populations. Even though the practical problem seems to be well known, the search for suitable solutions is often constrained by disciplinary and national borders. In addition, organ transplantation is surrounded by numerous ethical and emotional problems that stir public discussions, e.g. brain death, consent for post-mortem and living organ donation, organ allocation, and implantation of animal organs in humans—just to name a few.

This book approaches the relevant ethical questions of organ transplantation by investigating and critically rethinking the moral and ethical foundations of current solutions. Taking these as a starting point, the contributions engage in the development of new approaches, which can be viewed as fruitful concepts to inform the public discourse. As the topic of organ transplantation has come to the fore of the broader public, due to scandals happening e.g. in Germany, a public debate is needed in order to gain new orientation and restore trust in the transplantation system. Contributing to this debate was the aim of an international conference that brought together young scholars and experts in spring 2013 at the University of Munich, Germany, funded by the German Ministry for Education and Research. The presentations and ensuing discussions at this conference laid the basis for the articles collected in this volume, refined by several rounds of peer review.

The goal of this book is twofold. First, it analyzes and critically reviews the currently established solutions to alleviate the problem of organ shortage (e.g. consent procedures, moral obligation of donating organs, organ procurement practices). Second, it presents innovative, creative and applicable solutions for the problem of organ shortage (e.g. financial incentive schemes, living advocates for organ donation, organizational innovations, xenotransplantation). In order to achieve these aims, we split the publication into four different sections that will be summarized by us.

The diversity of contributions presented in this volume can be interpreted as a sign for the diverse, controversial, enthralling discussions surrounding the ethics, politics and legal regulation of organ donation worldwide. We consider the international plurality of reflections undertaken, solutions practiced and experiences gained to be a fruitful humus of ideas and a permanent inspiration for improvement, and we are therefore grateful to be able to enrich this international endeavor.

Many people have helped us bring this book into existence. In order to make their contribution explicit and visible, we want to thank Dorothee Wagner von Hoff for providing competent language and translation support and Carolin Lorenz and Johannes Pömsl for their engaged assistance with formatting and correspondence. Furthermore, we want to express our gratitude to the German Ministry for Education and Research that rendered the whole publication possible in the first place and to our kind and patient editor at Springer, Christopher Wilby, and to Prasad Pramod for organizing a smooth production of this book. We also thank all authors and reviewers for their intellectual contributions and their sustained patience during the production of this book.

Ralf J. Jox is a medical ethicist, neurologist and palliative care specialist working as Assistant Professor at the Institute of Ethics, History and Theory of Medicine at the University of Munich, Germany. His research activities focus on transplantation ethics, neuroethics, end-of-life care ethics, and clinical ethics consultation. He has published extensively in leading journals in medical ethics and clinical medicine, such as J Med Ethics and The Lancet Neurology. He is also the principle editor of an international book on the Vegetative State. Dr. Jox received multiple awards, among them the Young Investigator Awards of the European Association for Palliative Care (2011) and the German Academy of Ethics in Medicine (2004). In 2012, he was Caroline Miles Visiting Fellow at the Ethox Centre, University of Oxford.

Galia Assadi studied Social Work at the University of Applied Sciences Munich and mastered in Sociology at the LMU. Subsequently, she completed her PhD in Philosophy at the LMU. Her main research interests lie on the intersection of sociology, philosophy and politics. Her focus is on the critical reflection on normative orders of modern society and feminist theory. Following the works of Michel Foucault, she is currently investigating the connection between modern economical, philosophical, political and psychiatric thinking.

Georg Marckmann studied medicine and philosophy at the University of Tübingen (Germany) and received a master's degree in Public Health from Harvard School of Public Health (Boston, MA). He was a scholar in the Postgraduate College "Ethics in the Sciences and Humanities" in Tübingen from 1992 to 1995. He received a doctoral degree in medicine in 1997. From 1998 to 2010, he was Assistant Professor at the Institute of Ethics and History of Medicine at the University of Tübingen and since 2003 served as vice director of the institute. Since 2010, he is full professor of medical ethics and director of the Institute of Ethics, History, and Theory of Medicine at the Ludwig-Maximilians-University of Munich. His main research interests include ethical issues of end-of-life care, distributive justice in health care, ethical issues in organ transplantation and public health ethics.

Part I
The Ethics of Organ Donation: Foundations and Challenges

The contributions of the first Part raise the question of actual and potential ethical foundations of organ transplantation both on a theoretical and an empirical level. Starting with a critical investigation of the ethical obstacles that need to be overcome in order to increase the amount of organs available, the contributions not only develop a critique but go on to provide a variety of innovative – and sometimes controversial – perspectives on the ethics of organ donation.

Tobias Eichinger's contribution broaches the intensely debated issue of brain death in an innovative way. Instead of arguing in favor or against brain death as a matter of law, he shifts the question and reframes the whole discussion by conceptualizing a third category between life and death – a category that puts humans in a new and ambiguous realm *between* life and death, in accordance with the requirements of the transplantation practice and with fundamental moral commitments. Thus, brain-dead patients whose bodies – or relevant parts of their bodies – retain good functions, but whose brains are irreversibly damaged would be considered neither *still living* nor *already dead*, but rather seen as *both* already dead *and* still living at the same time. By presenting philosophical reflections on the necessity and possibility of a third category and adding some considerations about the interplay of film and societal issues, Eichinger approaches the topic in an innovative way. In order to illustrate the philosophical and societal potential of films, he argues that the metaphorical figure of the zombie could help to raise awareness of emotional abysses and personal fears, which are evoked by brain death and post-mortem organ donation.

Adrian Viens critically investigates the role of the physical integrity of the body in individual decision making as well as for policies and collective practices. He explicates ideas of bodily integrity in decisions regarding organ transplantation and explores some of the potential problems related to the endeavor to increase the supply of high-quality organs for transplantation. He first provides an overview of the concept of bodily integrity itself and how ideas about the importance of the physical integrity of the body come into play in the context of organ donation. Second, he examines the extent to which the beliefs and attitudes of individuals and their families about bodily integrity act as an empirical barrier to their willingness to be involved in organ donation. Third, he raises some issues with respect to the extent to which bodily integrity should also be seen as a normative barrier for different practices and policies surrounding organ donation. He concludes by arguing that the idea of bodily integrity admits different conceptions and interpretations.

Investigating the influence of body concepts on the willingness for organ donation, *Sabine Wöhlke, Julia Inthorn and Silke Schicktanz* present the results of an empirical survey conducted among students of medicine and economics. The authors start with the puzzling observation that various opinion polls suggest that the majority of German citizens are in favor of organ transplantation, but the number of citizens that possess an organ donor card is very low compared to other Western countries. By switching the commonplace perspective and questioning the impact of (hidden) cultural factors such as body image, concepts of death, and personal identity on attitudes towards organ transplantation, they make an important contribution to a yet scarcely investigated area. By focusing on the role of body concepts and the impact of attitudes towards brain death on the acceptance of organ donation, they prove the ethical relevance of lay anthropologies that are often neglected by the academic, legal, and ethical discourse, especially in the analytical and liberal tradition. They argue that philosophical or anthropological considerations are a necessary condition to develop consistent bioethical theories without comprehensively reflecting the positions represented in society. Therefore, public bioethics and policies, which aim to develop ethically justified models based on democratic norms, should not only consider consequentialist arguments to increase *social benefit* by increasing the number of available organs, but should also consider citizens' rights to have particular concepts about death and about their bodies. They conclude by encouraging the development of better ethical models of consent and donation by considering more concretely how to deal with plurality and moral uncertainty over such difficult issues.

Katherine Mendis' article focuses on developing an ethical foundation of a duty to donate organs based on the Kantian theory as well as the social contract theory. She argues that inventing an alternative ethical foundation could help to avoid the controversy and denial evoked by proposals designed to increase the supply of cadaveric organs (e.g. confiscation of organs, an "opt-out" system, and various methods of compensation). The view that people are not obligated to make their organs available after death is based on Kantian respect for autonomy and a notion of rights derived from social contract theory. Mendis looks to both Kant and contractarian views of free-riding to argue instead that making one's own organs available for donation after death is in fact a moral duty. According to the Kantian concept of a duty of mutual aid, we have a duty to respond to the true needs of rational beings when fulfilling such needs places little burden on us. In addition, a refusal to donate organs entails the kind of indifference to interdependency that characterizes morally problematic free-riding. Mendis concludes by showing that accepting cadaveric organ explantation as morally obligatory avoids the concerns that other proposals, such as confiscation, an opt-out system, or some sort of donor or family compensation systems, have – namely that they violate rights or fail to respect autonomy. It also avoids the criticism that these more *aggressive* policies would disadvantage vulnerable populations.

Taking a different approach to the problem of the ethical foundation of a duty to donate organs, *Diana Aurenque* examines to what extent altruism arguments are likely to increase willingness to donate organs. Her working hypothesis is that altruistic arguments are unsuitable for this purpose. In order to demonstrate this, Aurenque first elaborates the concept of altruism. In a second step, she investigates the motivational nature of altruistic actions and presents this as a problem in the face of organ shortage. Due to the ethical and political challenge to tackle organ shortage – in order to enhance the survival of seriously ill patients or to improve their quality of life – she points to the urgent need for binding measures. In a third step, she suggests that solidarity instead of altruism is the key to promoting organ donation. For that purpose, Aurenque argues that a model based on the values of solidarity and responsibility is suitable to justify other policy interventions that might increase donation rates. Finally, she draws attention to the meaning of justice (as fairness) for the success of these actions.

Instead of searching for a different ethical foundation of voluntary organ donation, *Christoph Schmidt-Petri* investigates the ethical legitimacy of organ confiscation as a radical way to resolve the problem of organ shortage. His argumentation is based on an analogy: if inheritance taxes and mandatory autopsies are legitimate, then so is organ confiscation. Therefore, he starts by exposing that neither the widely accepted practice of inheritance taxes nor the practice of mandatory autopsies requires prior consent of the dead. Both are typically performed in order to benefit other citizens, and autopsies also involve opening the body of the deceased. Therefore, he argues, these practices do not really differ from transferring body parts. Subsequently, he discusses objections against this proposal based on concerns about the brain death criterion. He concludes by arguing that, given the legitimacy of inheritance taxes and autopsies, routine salvaging of organs is also legitimate; or, to put it more cautiously, if inheritance taxes and mandatory autopsies are (considered) legitimate, then so should routine post-mortem salvaging of organs.

Investigating organ transplantation under a theological-ethical perspective, *Konrad Hilpert* discusses the theological challenges arising from organ donation against the background of the German situation, where an opt-in system is practiced and fraudulent manipulations of the waiting list for liver transplantations have recently agitated the public. Hilpert sketches three tasks that appear to be necessary for pastors and theologians: first, accepting that the donor is not just a vehicle for salvaging valuable human material and respecting the legacy of an individual whose dignity is to be appreciated after death; second, remaining honest and humble, not only by contextualizing the success of the greater spectrum of possibilities and power within high-tech medicine, but also by recognizing boundaries, fears, dependencies, and the possibility of failing; third, providing spiritual guidance for the donor's relatives as well as the organ recipient, who will have numerous questions both before and after the transplant.

Barbro Fröding and *Martin Peterson* switch the perspective and expand the range of the ethical discussion surrounding organ transplantation by focusing on the ethical obligations of the recipient. Their chapter discusses to what extent organ recipients ought to be held morally accountable for lifestyle choices that may jeopardize the function of their new organ. They sketch some key elements of Aristotelian virtue ethics, focusing on the doctrine of the mean as relevant to our moral attitude towards transplanted organs. Their main point is that, from a virtue-ethical perspective, the donation of a biological organ is a gift made for a good cause by the donor (or by the family of the deceased donor), and as a consequence a set of special obligations for the recipient arises. This includes the obligation to take good care of that gift. Thus, they show that we have good reasons to accept what they call enforced medium-level lifestyle infringements. By this they mean reasonable limitations on the range of lifestyle choices made available to recipients of transplant organs. They conclude by addressing four objections to their analysis and briefly discuss some practical implications of their conclusion.

Chapter 2
Brain Death, Justified Killing and the Zombification of Humans – Does the Transplantation Dilemma Require New Ways of Conceptualizing Life and Death?

Tobias Eichinger

2.1 Introduction

Medicine has not only saved the life of ethics, as Stephen Toulmin stated 30 years ago, but has also rejuvenated an old field of philosophy. As Toulmin claimed, it was clinical medicine with its growing ethical problems and new types of conflict situations that obliged philosophers to once again address "substantive ethical questions" (Toulmin 1982/1997, p. 101) by applying "principles to particular situations" (Toulmin 1982/1997, p. 107) instead of just practicing metaethics. The topic of organ transplantation is a very good example of what the reanimation of ethics by medicine could resemble. It is not only a current and controversial subject of applied ethics, namely medical ethics, but is also concerned with a subject from the heart of philosophy, which has been rejuvenated by the possibilities of modern medicine. This field of philosophical thinking refers to one of the presumably most existential topics overall in that its core lies in the question of the end of life and therefore, the question of death, that is: When is a human being dead? When does a human life end? What do such findings mean with regards to handling dying and dead bodies?

For almost half a century now, the field of transplantation medicine has raised and revitalized these questions in a distinctive and irrefutable way. Technologies for implantation of vital organs from dead donors demand a definitive answer to the question of how to draw the line between life and death. So we have to ask, what kind of signs and criteria could and should indicate that existential transition in a scientifically reliable and ethically responsible way, but also in a way that fits in – or challenges – our grown sociocultural understanding and phenomenological experience with dying and dead bodies? Lastly, it is the question of how to comprehend and how to conceptualize human life and death.

T. Eichinger (✉)
Institute for Biomedical Ethics and History of Medicine, University of Zurich, Zurich, Switzerland
e-mail: eichinger@ethik.uzh.ch

R. J. Jox et al. (eds.), *Organ Transplantation in Times of Donor Shortage*,
International Library of Ethics, Law, and the New Medicine 59,
DOI 10.1007/978-3-319-16441-0_2

2.2 Brain Death: Paradigm and Problem

In 1968, the *Ad Hoc Committee of the Harvard School* established the *brain death syndrome* to define and determine the death of individuals who are in a state of an irreversible coma and who manifest "the characteristics of a permanently non-functioning brain" (Harvard-Committee 1968, p. 85). Thus, not only was a condition pronounced which can be tested and clearly detected on the basis of a set of medical-diagnostic parameters and data, but also death was no longer a phenomenon encompassing the whole body with all its functions and life signs, but rather being dead became a question of the functioning of the brain. According to the new paradigm of specifying death, waiting for final cardiac arrest and other signs of death (such as livor mortis, apnoea, or rigor mortis) is dispensable if the brain is extensively and irreversibly damaged.

This manner of identifying the life of a human with the life of its brain represents nothing less than a historical shift in conceptualizing life and death – a historical shift that challenges the comprehension and acceptance both of the public and of a circle of experts. Since its introduction, the brain death criterion has been the subject of controversial discussion not only among physicians, neuroscientists, and nursing staff, but also between social scientists, ethicists, philosophers, lawyers, and the public. A series of serious objections to this stipulative definition of death, which was invented under pressure of organ transplantation in times of donor shortage, has been propounded.

One of the earliest critics of the criterion was the philosopher Hans Jonas, who condemned the new definition only a few months after the report of the Ad Hoc Committee was released as being a purely, pragmatically motivated redefinition and "antedating of the accomplished fact of death [...] with certain extraneous interests in mind" (Jonas 1969/2009, p. 503 f.), namely transplant interests. Aside from the risk of the immoral exploitation of helpless humans, according to Jonas the brain death criterion transports a dubious "revenant of the old soul-body dualism" (Ibid., p. 504) in the contemporary form of a soul-brain dualism. According to that, establishing the brain death criterion represents another form of overestimating the importance of the brain for life, identity, and the self-concept of man, which goes along with a degradation of the meaning of non-cerebral and bodily conditions. Thus, he took a very firm stand in the debate early on. From a realistic and unemotional perspective, it is worth mentioning here that in his rather provocative essays Jonas uses drastic and partially inadequate wording to depict the worst possible outcome of an unscrupulous introduction of the brain death criterion in favor of the procurement of vital organs. He fears that dying patients could be used "as a bank for life-fresh organs" (Ibid., p. 503) or "as a mine" (Jonas 1969, p. 244), and transplant surgeons are described as "executioners" (Ibid., p. 245).[1] However, even now, if one considers this criticizable linguistic sharpness, over 40 years after he

[1] For a modest but clear critique of Jonas' vocabulary cf. Miller (2009).

wrote his essay, the essence of his concerns about a new way of defining death is still up-to-date.

As the German philosopher Petra Gehring recently pointed out in view of the historical, cultural, and political dimensions on the subject, the brain death criterion allowed some fundamental alterations in conceptualizing and dealing with death to take place. Mainly, she refers to the cerebralization, punctualization, and conventionalization of death (Gehring 2010). First, there is the fact that death is equated with – or reduced to – a state of the brain, and a cerebral condition (*cerebralization*). At the same time, death starts at a precise, determinable point in time, namely the moment the brain dead diagnosis is made (*punctualization*). Thus, the declaration of death no longer stands at the end of a more or less natural process – the process of dying – but it is a matter of reaching a decision, in which the criteria and preconditions are defined by a group of experts. So death has become a matter of specified tests and the adhering conclusion can only be arranged and performed by specialists (*conventionalization*). These points – cerebralization, punctualisation and conventionalisation, as features of the valid death criterion – are not *naturally given* and therefore indicate the arbitrariness of its stipulation.

The declarative moment of this new death designation is confirmed by difficulties within the everyday practice of handling brain dead individuals. We have to face the disturbing fact that massive conflicts exist in the perception of brain dead humans – or rather brain dead bodies. Such conflicts concern especially those people who work in hospitals and medical care units and have to deal with potential organ donors who are (brain) dead but, whose bodies are warm, who are still breathing, metabolizing, sweating and show nail and hair growth, not to mention that they could be pregnant and deliver a living child through a caesarean section. All of these are bodily functions, which are in some degree necessary to keep organs *alive* and transplantable.

This disturbing setting could get even more intense in the course of retrieval. To avoid bodily reactions by the donor, such as the remaining sensation of pain or indisposition, some argue for the anesthetization of brain dead patients. A concise statement is given by Philip Keep, an anesthetist at the Norfolk and Norwich Hospital (UK): “Nurses get really, really upset. You stick the knife in and the pulse and blood pressure shoot up. If you don’t give anything at all, the patient will start moving and wriggling around and it’s impossible to do the operation” (BBC News 2000). If you have to administer anesthesia to a dead body, it is not easy to understand and believe that the body is not alive, not even just a little bit. Linus Geisler, a German specialist in internal medicine and a critical voice, calls the medical-scientific fact that brain dead people “are only apparently alive but dead in fact (only feigned living)” a “massive violation of human intuition” (Geisler 2010, p. 2).

In addition to these aspects of handling people who are declared brain dead, in the more recent past strong doubts about the rightness of the brain death criterion came up in the light of new neuroscientific findings.[2] These doubts from the brain research camp arose mainly because the methods used to diagnose brain death are

[2] PCBE (2008); Müller (2010).

mostly clinical methods (this is the case in Germany), for example, determining apnoea and whether brain stem reflexes are still present. The diagnostic investigations do not require certain mechanical diagnostic procedures such as an Electroencephalogram (EEG) or angiography, which were apparently necessary to ensure that the patient is really brain dead. There have been reports of cases in which patients, who were clinically diagnosed with brain death exhibited persistent intracranial blood flow or electrical brain activity.[3]

On the one hand, serious concerns were raised about the difficulties of making a reliable brain death diagnosis, while on the other hand increasing doubts emerged about whether the connection between brain death and physical death is reasonable *per se* and empirically maintainable.[4] So far, it has been assumed that immediately after brain death, *actual, real* or *physical* death – in the sense of cardiac arrest – would also occur. Nowadays that notion of a tight and inevitable connection can no longer be maintained. One case is known in which 14 years have elapsed between brain death and death.[5] Furthermore, the proposition that the brain fulfills functions that maintain the integrity of the body as a living organism and the loss of which causes the body to disintegrate, leading to cardiac arrest over a period of days, has gone unchallenged for a long time and is one of the central arguments in defense of the brain death concept. However, this proposition is no longer maintainable. As the medical ethicists Franklin Miller and Robert Truog put it, "the human body does not need the brain to integrate homeostatic functions [...]. Patients who fulfill all of the diagnostic criteria for brain death remain alive in virtually every sense except for the fact that they have permanently lost the capacity for consciousness" (Miller and Truog 2008, p. 39).

Thus, the problems of the concept of brain death and its corresponding criticism, with or without neurological foundation, consists of two main questions. First, is the patient really brain dead? Second, is the brain dead patient really dead? Whereas the first question permits a more scientific-technical and neurological answer, the second one demands philosophical or anthropological, respectively ontological, considerations. Before turning to the latter aspects of the topic, the aspects of conceptualizing life and death, the ethical implications which both questions contain need to be given some thought.

2.3 Beyond Brain Death

In response to the diverse problems of the brain death criterion – the questionable diagnostic reliability, the equalization of death with the loss of certain brain functions, brain dead patients that are somehow still alive – some have asked: Why not abandon the cerebral criterion as a pre-condition for organ extraction and return

[3] See references in Müller (2010).

[4] Cf. PCBE (2008) and Müller (2010).

[5] Müller (2013).

to the traditional cardiopulmonary standard of death? These approaches propose the traditional concept of *Non-Heart-Beating-Donation*. This practice is already permitted and exercised in some countries such as Switzerland, Spain, the United States, and the Netherlands.[6] The retrieval of organs from Non-Heart-Beating-Donors requires the determination of death following cardiopulmonary criteria, i.e. the cessation of circulation and respiration, and therefore circulatory arrest. The delicate point of that kind of determination of death is the comprehension and the handling of irreversibility. In that context circulatory death results from the withdrawal of life-sustaining measures without attempts at resuscitation, the discussion here concerns the appropriate waiting time span after the withdrawal. Would it suffice to wait 5 min, 2 min, or even a mere 75 s after the onset of a systole to be certain that a heart rhythm and pulse will not resume spontaneously? Thus, it becomes obvious that proving lost reversibility is constituted by a decision the doctors make. To quote Truog and Miller again, "Whereas the common understanding of 'irreversible' is 'impossible to reverse', in this context irreversibility is interpreted as the result of a choice not to reverse" (Truog and Miller 2008, p. 674).

In the case of heart transplantations, that leads to a remarkable paradox, namely "the paradox that the hearts of patients who have been declared dead on the basis of the irreversible loss of cardiac function have in fact been transplanted and have successfully functioned in the chest of another" (Ibid.). In this case, the fundamental dilemma of the transplantation of vital organs is taken to the extreme: First, the transplantation dilemma consists of the ambition of getting functioning or living organs from dead donors. If the goal is to transplant a heart after cardiac arrest, the predicament occurs that the very organ whose failure – or death – is absolutely indispensable in order to start the whole procedure, in that it serves as the crucial condition for the explantation due to the pronouncement of the donor's death. This necessary non-functioning or dead organ is intended to save another man's life by functioning or living by itself.[7]

This paradoxical outcome makes some authors go one step further and consider slaughtering another sacred cow, namely abandoning the *Dead-Donor-Rule* for the removal of vital organs. This rule, which embodies perhaps the most fundamental ethical (and legal) principle of medical practice – and not only medical practice – stating that it is wrong to kill or cause the death of an innocent person even if that could save the life of another. In the domain of transplantation that means that patients must be dead (respectively declared dead) before the removal of any vital organ for transplantation.[8] As already discussed above, by permitting the *dead-donor-rule*, conceptual extensions and even revisions of the definition of death seem to be inevitable (concerning the concept of brain death as well as cardiac death).[9]

[6] Bos (2005).

[7] Cf. Veatch (2008).

[8] Robertson (1999).

[9] As Truog and Miller put it: "In sum, as an ethical requirement for organ donation, the dead donor rule has required unnecessary and unsupportable revisions of the definition of death" Troug and Miller (2008, p. 675).

Therefore, the determinability of death is not the main problem for transplantation medicine, but rather the *dead-donor-rule*. For Miller and Truog, who admit to the weakness of the brain death criterion for pronouncing death, the current practice of vital organ donation already violates the dead donor rule anyway, so for them it is an imperative of honesty to face that fact and to accommodate to the ethical norms: "[I]n order to sustain the lifesaving practice of organ transplantation without moral obfuscation, we must face the fact that this requires extracting vital organs from living donors" (Miller and Truog 2008, p. 44). So why not abandon the *dead-donor-rule*? This would dissolve the transplantation dilemma.

Unsurprisingly, the proposition, which seems no less radical or antiquated than the brain death criterion, does not only receive approval within the discussion. Among the resolute critics is Linus Geisler for whom the fall of the *dead-donor-rule* would stand for "a fundamental break of taboo" (Geisler 2010, p. 3). For him it would be a "monstrosity that, for the first time in the medical history of the civilized world, doctors would be allowed to cause the death of a patient in order to make use of him for the benefit of other patients. […] The license to kill would become a legal medical qualification" (Ibid.). These are sharp words, but one has to note that the vocabulary of *killing* is a result of the honesty that Miller and Truog have in mind. From their point of view, ending a patient's life by withdrawing life support in favor of getting usable organs should be seen as a form of *justified killing*. Even if they try to avoid the expression *justified killing*, due to its "emotionally charged and value-laden language" (Miller and Truog 2008, p. 42), as mentioned in the recent debate, Robert Truog introduced the phrase almost 20 years ago when he claimed that, "the process of organ procurement would have to be legitimated as a form of justified killing" and concluded "that killing may sometimes be a justifiable necessity for procuring transplantable organs" (Truog 1997, p. 34 ff.). The key concepts and guiding principles for this purpose are patient autonomy and informed consent. The patient has to have given his consent to becoming an organ donor by ending life-sustaining treatment if they are "catastrophically brain-injured" (Miller and Truog 2008, p. 39). As Miller and Truog stated, under certain conditions causing a patient's death could be part of the legitimate physician's responsibility: "[W]e endorse life-terminating acts of vital organ extraction prior to a declaration of death, provided that they are tied to valid decisions to withdraw life support and valid consent" (Miller and Truog 2008, p. 45).

2.4 Betwixt and Between

The above-mentioned proposals for dealing with the fundamental and persistent transplantation dilemma – abandoning the brain death criterion, establishing non-heart-beating donation, giving up the *dead-donor-rule* – *all* these approaches suggest that perhaps conceptual changes on a more fundamental level could be helpful, and it seems to be necessary to extend our thinking on life and death. This raises the question of whether an indication could be made to abandon the claim of a clear and unambiguous distinction – between being alive and being dead – if the matter in question requires it. Stephen Toulmin had a similar notion in mind when he emphasized the Aristotelean challenge and need for practical reasoning, which ethics and clinical medicine have in common: "Ethics and clinical medicine are both prime examples of the concrete fields of thought and reasoning [...] in which we should above all strive to be *reasonable* rather than insisting on a kind of *exactness* that 'the nature of the case' does not allow" (Toulmin 1982/1997, p. 104). Therefore, it seems to be an unavoidable demand of practical reasoning to transcend the concept of a strict dichotomy of *alive or dead*, if the nature of the case requires it. The case here is the question of the determinability of patients in an irreversible coma, patients whose hearts or brains have stopped functioning, but whose bodies are still living. This question is normally phrased as follows: are these individuals already dead (so that we can explant organs) *or* still alive (which would make it an illegitimate procedure)? Dead or alive – there seems to be no third option, *tertium non datur*.

Whereas Toulmin had the ethical conflicts of medicine in general in mind, his philosopher-colleague Hans Jonas voiced similar concerns about the inadequate exactness on the very occasion of the brain death criterion. According to this, he exclaimed the need for appropriateness when thinking about life and death: "Giving intrinsic vagueness its due is not being vague. [...] Reality of certain kinds – of which the life-death spectrum is perhaps one – may be imprecise in itself, or the knowledge obtainable of it may be. To acknowledge such a state of affairs is more adequate to it than a precise definition, which does violence to it. I am challenging the undue precision of a definition and of its practical application to an imprecise field" (Jonas 1969/2009, p. 500). So the fact that the transplantation-brain-death-problem is still a field of open and controversial questions, "an unsettled and unsettling situation" as Miller puts it (Miller 2009, p. 620), is the inevitable outcome of the intrinsic vagueness and imprecision of the life-death spectrum.

Now, in light of the transplantation dilemma and the problems of the approaches for a way out, it could be advisable to conceptualize a third category for the status of existence. A category, which puts humans in a new and ambiguous realm *between* life and death, as claimed by the requirements of the transplantation practice in compliance with fundamental moral commitments. Thus, brain dead patients whose bodies – respectively some relevant parts of their bodies – are in good, extractable shape but whose brains are irreversibly damaged, would be considered neither *still living* nor *already dead* or, what basically amounts to the same thing, they would be *both* already dead *and* still living at the same time. As the German philosopher Ralf Stoecker puts it, "these patients are in one respect still like living persons and in the other respect they are already like dead people" (Stoecker 2012, p. 5). The project of defining, introducing, and implementing this third category of living (or rather semi-living) in the complex medical practice of organ donation signifies a huge effort with no guarantee of success for many different reasons. One of the central obstacles here is the strangeness and anxiety of imagining the practice of explicit procedures dealing with human beings between life and death in a third state of existence.

2.5 The Zombification of Humans

Remarkably, the unease regarding living individuals who are brain dead found its own resolve in the consciousness – and rather unconsciousness – of the broad public right from the start of the medical discussion triggered by the report of the Ad Hoc Committee. It appeared on the silver screens of the western world where, since the late sixties, more and more protagonists appeared from an intermediate grey zone somewhere between the living and the dead. This zone is a sphere where a kind of no-more-living-but-not-yet-dead-state prevails, a territory where a special kind of creature walks around and causes trouble – creatures from the dark side of popular culture that are well-known, or rather notorious and dreaded: the undead or zombies. These figures from horror fiction, appearing mainly in comics and movies, are distinguished (in the classical model) by lacking any kind of consciousness and self-awareness, while being ambulant and able to respond to surrounding stimuli. Even if it is assumed that brain dead patients are not really or not completely dead, what they definitely do not possess any longer, is consciousness and self-awareness. With this in mind, the application of organ transplantation on the basis of the brain death criterion would, strictly speaking, amount to the *zombification of humans*.

That notion may lead to looking at both the case of transplantation (its philosophical or anthropological relevance) as well as at the meaning of the zombie narrative in a different light, especially the cinematic interpretations, and thus also the connection between these two fields. There is a significant amount of parallels between zombies and brain dead people; in fact there is a conspicuous and unlikely coincidental chronological link. In 1968, the B movie *Night of the Living Dead* directed by George Romero was produced and released, a movie that has not only revolutionized the horror film genre but also pushed the sub-genre of zombie movies in a unique way, which has remained unrivaled to this day. Movies with and about undead characters have existed since the nineteen-thirties, but with *Night of the Living Dead* the zombie genre got a huge boost and experienced a cinematic renaissance – the undead on screen were powerfully reanimated. It was in the same year, 1968, that the brain death criterion came into being and with it all the uneasiness, obscurities, and fears connected with the uncertainty of drawing the line between life and death in a new way. Now, given that film as an art form and mass medium always reflects on or even anticipates contemporary collective and societal issues and tensions, the metaphorical figure of the zombie could connect medicine with film in a way which could be enlightening for noting and comprising emotional abysses and personal fears, on a societal as well as on an individual level, which are evoked by dealing with this particular transplantation dilemma.

Acknowledgment I am grateful to Dr. Sohaila Bastami for her numerous helpful remarks and inspiring comments.

References

BBC News. 2000. Braindead pain fears 'upset families'. BBC News, Health v. 19.08.2000. http://news.bbc.co.uk/2/hi/health/886947.stm. Accessed 24 Feb 2013.

Bos, M. A. 2005. Ethical and legal issues in non-heart-beating organ donation. *Transplantation Proceedings* 37 (2): 574–576.

Gehring, P. 2010. *Theorien des Todes zur Einführung*. Hamburg: Junius.

Geisler, L. S. 2010. The living and the dead. Translation from: Die Lebenden und die Toten. *Universitas* 65 (763): 4–13.

Harvard-Committee. 1968. A definition of irreversible coma. Report of the ad hoc committee of the Harvard medical school to examine the definition of brain death. *Journal of the American Medical Association* 205 (6): 337–340.

Jonas, H. 1969. Philosophical reflections on experimenting with human subjects. *Daedalus* 98 (2): 219–247.

Jonas, H. 2009, orig. 1969. Against the stream. Comments on the definition and redefinition of death. In *Defining the beginning and end of life*, ed. John P. Lizza, 498–506. Baltimore: John Hopkins University Press.

Miller, F. G. 2009. Death and organ donation: Back to the future. *Journal of Medical Ethics* 35 (10): 616–620.

Miller, F. G., and Robert D. Truog, 2008. Rethinking the ethics of vital organ donations. *Hastings Center Report* 38 (6): 38–46.

Müller, S. 2010. Revival der Hirntod-Debatte: Funktionelle Bildgebung für die Hirntod-Diagnostik. *Ethik in der Medizin* 22 (1): 5–17.

Müller, S. 2013. Brain death and organ donation: "There is still a significant need for research". Interview in Medica Magazine (09/05/2011). http://www.medica-tradefair.com/cipp/md_medica/custom/pub/content,oid,33310/lang,2/ticket,g_u_e_s_t/~/%E2%80%9CThere_is_still_a_significant_need_for_research%E2%80%9C.html. Accessed 24 Feb 2013.

Night of the Living Dead. USA 1968. Dir.: G. A. Romero.

President's Council on Bioethics (PCBE). 2008. The controversies in the determination of death. A White Paper. Washington, DC.

Robertson, J. A. 1999. The dead donor rule. *Hastings Center Report* 29 (6): 6–14.

Stoecker, R. 2012. Der Hirntod aus ethischer Sicht. In *Forum Bioethik*, ed. Deutscher Ethikrat, 1–5. Berlin: Deutscher Ethikrat.

Toulmin, S. 1997, orig. 1982. How medicine saved the life of ethics. In *Bioethics. An Introduction to the History, Methods, and Practice*, eds. Nancy S. Jecker, Albert R. Jonsen, and Robert A. Pearlman, 101–109. Sudbury: Jones and Bartlett.

Truog, Robert D. 1997. Is it time to abandon brain death? *Hastings Center Report* 27 (1): 29–37.

Truog, R. D., and Franklin, G. Miller, 2008. The dead donor rule and organ transplantation. *New England Journal of Medicine* 359 (7): 674–675.

Veatch, R. M. 2008. Donating hearts after cardiac death—Reversing the irreversible. *New England Journal of Medicine* 359 (7): 672–673.

Tobias Eichinger is a senior research assistant at the Institute for Biomedical Ethics and History of Medicine, University of Zurich, Switzerland. He is also a research assistant at the Department of Medical Ethics and the History of Medicine, Freiburg University, Germany. Dr. Eichinger has degrees in philosophy and film studies from the University of Freiburg and Freie Universität Berlin. His research interests focus on philosophical and ethical questions of modern biomedicine and life sciences and on issues of the relationship of film and medicine.

Chapter 3
Bodily Integrity as a Barrier to Organ Donation

A. M. Viens

3.1 Introduction

Bodily integrity remains a central issue for organ transplantation. The process of removing an organ from one body and resettling it into another body necessarily requires transgressing the physical integrity of the human body. This process raises different psychological and moral issues with respect to ideas about how we should treat our bodies or the bodies of our loved ones. On the one hand, ideas about the physical integrity of the body play an important role in decision-making by individuals and their families as to their willingness to participate in organ donation programs. For this reason, it is an important consideration to take into account when understanding those factors that can limit the potential supply of available organs for transplantation. On the other hand, ideas of the physical integrity of the body also play an important role in setting constraints on what is viewed as permissible in relation to possible policies or intervention practices aimed at increasing the general availability of donor organs.

My aim in this chapter is to briefly explicate these two issues in relation to bodily integrity and organ donation, and explore some of the potential problems raised in relation to increasing the supply of high-quality organs for transplantation. In the first part of the chapter, I provide a pithy overview of the concept of bodily integrity itself and how ideas about the importance of the physical integrity of the body can come into play in the context of organ donation. In the second part of the chapter, I examine the extent to which the beliefs and attitudes of individuals and their families about bodily integrity act as an empirical barrier to their willingness to be involved with organ donation. In the third part of the chapter, I raise some

A. M. Viens (✉)
Ethics and Law (HEAL), Southampton Law School, University of Southampton, Southampton, UK
e-mail: adrian.viens@gmail.com

R. J. Jox et al. (eds.), *Organ Transplantation in Times of Donor Shortage*, International Library of Ethics, Law, and the New Medicine 59,
DOI 10.1007/978-3-319-16441-0_3

issues with respect to the extent to which bodily integrity should also be seen as a normative barrier for different practices and policies surrounding organ donation. I conclude by arguing that the idea of bodily integrity admits of different conceptions and interpretations. Not only is this true within philosophical and public policy discourse, but is also reflected in the beliefs and attitudes of lay people. There is a need for both further theoretical work to be done to develop a more nuanced conception of bodily integrity, as well as further practical work that seeks to modify beliefs and attitudes about bodily integrity in the context of organ donation in order to reduce its effect as a barrier towards increasing the supply of high-quality organs for transplantation.

3.2 Bodily Integrity

The physical integrity of the human body, and especially whether and in what way we could have a right to bodily integrity, is a topic that remains widely discussed and debated.[1] Given the processes involved with organ retrieval and transplantation, it is evident how ideas of bodily integrity are engaged. It is not so evident, however, how we should understand the nature of the body, its physical integrity, what kinds of interventions qualify as transgressing bodily integrity and whether all instances of transgression must be seen as harmful, wrongful or both.

As more scholarly and public policy attention is given to bodily integrity and its implications, it has become clear that there is a multitude of considerations and interpretations underlying how we understand the physical integrity of the body and what it will mean for policy and practice surrounding areas such as organ transplantation. So much so, it raises the question of whether bodily integrity is an essentially contested concept or whether, in many cases, scholars and practitioners are talking past each other when they believe they are talking about the same thing.[2] Bodily integrity has been claimed to be grounded in considerations such as ownership, sovereignty, dignity and privacy. The maintenance of the physical integrity of the body is said to be manifested in different ways, such as the preservation of the wholeness, functionality or inviolability of the body. Further, there are also various putative ways of transgressing the physical integrity of the body that are said to be constituted by particular modes of intervention, such as invasiveness, dismemberment, mutilation or destruction. More still, over and above the physical harm that can result from such transgressions of bodily integrity, it has also been claimed that distinctive moral harms, such as devaluation, defilement and deprivation, can also result.

[1] Much of this section is based on A. M. Viens, 'Introduction,' in: A. M. Viens (2014).

[2] We often find essentially contested concepts with respect to abstract ideas within normative domains such as moral and political philosophy concerning claims where there is general agreement on a concept, but not its realization—resulting in endless disputes and disagreements as to its proper use. For more on the notion of an essentially contested concept, see Gallie (1956).

For this reason, it is possible to get very different claims about the nature of physical integrity and just what would be permitted, prohibited or even required from the existence of a right to bodily integrity. This is not only theoretically significant in terms of clarifying and explaining the nature of bodily integrity, but it also has important implications for practice and policy. This is so because, depending on which claims about bodily integrity are being relied on, different answers to the questions of which interventions are acceptable to lay people or which interventions should be morally or legally permissible can be given. For instance, one might claim that bodily integrity is grounded in personal sovereignty in a way that makes the physical integrity of the body inviolable, thereby making any invasive intervention like organ removal after death impermissible without consent. Likewise, someone might claim something completely different. One might claim that a bodily integrity is grounded in human dignity in a way that requires us to maintain the wholeness of the body in a way that prohibits any defiling or destructive modification—even if one wants and would consent to such modification.[3] As such, how we conceive of bodily integrity will have important implications for organ transplantation with respect to how likely people will be to want to donate their own organs or the organs of their loved ones and the general acceptability of efforts to increase the supply of donor organs that may be enacted in an effort to save more lives.

3.3 Bodily Integrity as an Empirical Barrier to Donation

Bodily integrity can act as a barrier to organ donation in so far as people are psychologically disposed to reject interventions they view as transgressing the physical integrity of their body or the body of their loved ones. This is so even when they are thinking about their bodily integrity after death. For this reason, one's personal future intention to donate posthumously or one's actual family decisions in favor of posthumous donation are less likely to occur because of how transgressing the physical integrity of the body acts as a countervailing consideration.

The available empirical evidence shows that bodily integrity (i) is a strong and significant predictor of one's intent and actual decision to donate organs and (ii) has a direct and negative effect on signing donor cards and decisions to donate.[4]

---

[3] To be clear, this is a general conception of bodily integrity and not specific to organ donation per se. Virtually all theorists and practitioners view consent as necessary (and often sufficient) for permissibly taking organs posthumously—and most theorists and practitioners do in the case of live donation as well. Nevertheless, it has to be recognized that part of these conclusions are predicated on a particular conception of bodily integrity and the conditions under which it can be permissible transgressed.

[4] See, for instance, Stephenson et al. (2008), Newton (2011), Irving et al. (2012). To be sure, bodily integrity is only one of many potential barriers that might lead individuals or their families to decide not to donate organs for transplantation. Other barriers cited in the literature include low education levels, religious objections, irrationality and a lack of virtues and values such as generosity and solidarity.

According to Newton, "the two most commonly identified barriers [to organ donation are] the need to maintain bodily integrity to safeguard progression into the afterlife and the unethical recovery of organs by medical professionals" (2011, p. 1). This was found for both religious and non-religious individuals and families. For religious individuals who cite bodily integrity as a central motivating reason against choosing to donate themselves or the organs of their loved ones, they cite considerations such as the belief that one needs a whole body in order to be resurrected, that the human body is a gift from God and parts should not be removed and the belief that donating organs might interfere in some way with the ability to undertake certain burial rituals (e.g., open coffins). For non-religious individuals who cite bodily integrity as a central motivating reason against choosing to donate themselves or the organs of their loved ones, they cite negative emotive reactions associated with the idea of *cutting up the body*, such as fear, distress, disgust, repulsion, that removing organs amounts of mutilation, or that having someone else's organ put into your body would cause personality contamination. Indeed, the desire to maintain the physical integrity of the body is so strong in some cases that families have not provided consent for posthumous donation even when the prospective donor expressed a wish to be an organ donor.

In one sense, it is understandable why ideas of bodily integrity act as an empirical barrier to organ donation. It is much easier to rationalize not donating one's organs or the organs of loved ones when you are declining an intervention that one sees as being sinful or a mutilation. Of course, the legitimacy of such beliefs or attitudes depends on whether or not the transgression of the physical integrity of the body really is as impermissible or undesirable as one thinks it is. Interestingly, from the qualitative evidence on the topic that is available, it appears that concerns about bodily integrity only work in one direction. That is to say, a concern about bodily integrity does not seem to be a barrier to *receiving* an organ for transplantation.[5] When it comes to receiving donated organs, the possibility that some donor's bodily integrity will be transgressed to procure the organ—as well as the bodily integrity of the recipient to receive the organ—does not produce similar beliefs or attitudes of apprehension, revulsion or disapprobation. This asymmetry in beliefs and attitudes should indicate to us that the actual value we place on the physical integrity of the body and the extent to which we think its transgression is morally problematic is not as clear and stable as we might think. Indeed, this asymmetry reveals what amounts to a selfish hypocrisy that should be highlighted and criticized. If the transgression of the physical integrity of the human body for the purposes of organ transplantation

[5] Another relevant asymmetry is found in relation to how beliefs and attitudes change depending on whom the recipient will be and what organs are involved. While some individuals express a willingness to donate an organ to a family member, they would not donate to a stranger. As well, some individuals express a willingness to donate posthumously but only if they can select which organs are taken—for instance, many people often express a desire not to donate their eyes or the eyes of their loved ones. For more, see Irving et al. (2012).

is so morally problematic, one should be consistent in the rejection of both donating *and* receiving organs.[6]

Be that as it may, in an attempt to increase the possibility of more organs being donated for transplantation, efforts need to be taken to try to modify beliefs and attitudes concerning organ transplantation. Primarily, there is a need to address and augment how we conceptualize the body, its physical integrity and what it is permissible to do with the body in relation to organ donation. While much of this will need to take place at the level of scholarship and public policy development, which I will briefly touch on in the next section, there are also ways in which such ends can be furthered that involve public engagement and education. For example, public information campaigns need to focus on correcting and promoting a number of background beliefs related to bodily integrity that may foster a propensity within individuals or their families to think organ removal is an impermissible transgression of bodily integrity or involves treating a dead body in a disrespectful way. Such campaigns should focus on the widespread interfaith support for organ donation; most of the world's major religious at least permit and many advocate that its adherents participate in organ donation.[7] Religious leaders should take the time to clarify and educate followers about how participating in regulated organ donation programmes need not, for instance, violate religious requirements or prevent adherents from being able to take part in traditional burial rituals. The general public, religious and non-religious members of the community alike, also would benefit from being further educated on the professional and respectful process involved in procuring organs and preparation of the body afterwards.

3.4 Bodily Integrity as a Normative Barrier to Donation

In the previous section, I was concerned with providing an overview of a central psychological barrier that prevents many people from being willing to donate their organs or the organs of their loved ones. This barrier is empirical in the sense that, whether or not the beliefs and attitudes concerning bodily integrity are justifiable, these psychological states are sufficient to prevent the decision to donate. It is also possible for bodily integrity, however, to operate as a normative barrier to donation. This is so in terms of how it can operate at the level of philosophical thought or public policy as to which kinds of donation promotion and procurement strategies

[6] Christoph Schmidt-Petri has suggested to me that, even if my point holds, there is nevertheless a difference between the cases of donating and receiving organs: the body of the donor is incomplete at the end of the procedure, whereas the body of the recipient is not. If one's conception of bodily integrity is integrity *qua* wholeness, then I would agree that this might be what is underpinning the beliefs or attitudes of potential donors (or their families) in resisting requests to be a donor. Be that as it may, however, when it comes to whether or not such beliefs or attitudes are morally justified, I am still inclined to think that the problem remains. If leaving someone's body incomplete, in virtue of removing an organ after death, is morally problematic, then we would still need an account of why a recipient (or their family acting on their behalf) are not complicit in the putative immorality of benefiting from some other person's body not remaining whole.

[7] See, for instance, Cooper and Taylor (2000) and Ryckman et al. (2004).

will be justified and, hence, should be allowed as means of increasing the availability of donor organs.

While all reasonable people should agree that increasing the supply of high-quality organs that would allow more people to live longer and have a better quality of life should be pursued, there are certain constraints that are placed on the various strategies that would be permissible to achieve this objective. One such prominent normative constraint on which organ donation policies we should adopt include ensuring that methods for procuring more organs are not accomplished through means that would impermissibly transgress the bodily integrity of dead or live donors. According to some bodily integrity-based objections, independent of the resultant reduction in mortality and morbidity from an increase in organ transplants, there will be some transgressions of bodily integrity that should be avoided because they constitute a distinctive or significant form of wrongdoing. As such, any donation strategy that would result in transgressing bodily integrity in this way is morally impermissible and, as such, should not be seen as a viable public policy option.

So a key question remains—given our understanding of bodily integrity, when it is transgressed and when it is permissible to do so—are there any strategies for obtaining more organs that considerations of bodily integrity would prohibit? For example, one way to increase the availability of high-quality organs would be to adopt a policy in which organs were posthumously confiscated from every eligible candidate. This is, for instance, a view defended by Cecile Fabre.[8] She argues that just as we should seek to fairly allocate valuable resources to those who need them most, there are good reasons for viewing organs as valuable resources that should be allocated to those who are very ill and require an organ transplant. She argues that body parts, such as organs, can be viewed as a scarce resource that can substantially help the least advantaged and they should be taken posthumously even in cases where deceased persons have not expressed any wishes to donate. Fabre (2006, p. 73) maintains:

> … if one thinks that the poor's interest in leading a minimally flourishing life, and a fortiori in remaining alive, is important enough to confer on them a right to some of the material resources of the well off, by way of taxation and, in particular, by way of restrictions on bequests and inheritance, one must think that the very same interests is important enough to confer on the sick a right to the organs of the now-dead able-bodied.

On her view, considerations of bodily integrity should not be thought to be sufficient to justify such a strong sphere of protection that it would lead to so many people in need being denied a chance to live a longer life.[9]

Even if a clear argument can be made concerning why certain strategies for organ donation involving the transgression of bodily integrity can be seen as harmful and/or wrongful, it is often difficult to see why this putative harm or wrongness must always be, allthingsconsidered, impermissible. As such, the possibility of bodily integrity being transgressed should not be viewed as the conclusion of the debate, but the start of the debate as to which particular strategies in which particu-

[8] Fabre (2006).

[9] For an alternative account of how we should understand bodily integrity and its implications for organ transplantation, see Wilkinson (2011).

lar circumstances transgress bodily integrity to an unacceptable extent. It is only in cases where transgressing the physical integrity of the body would be all-things-considered impermissible that we should view it as a genuine normative barrier to organ donation.

3.5 Conclusion

While it is undeniable that bodily integrity currently acts as an empirical and normative barrier to organ donation in different ways and at different levels, it is also clear that the barriers it creates need not remain fixed. The extent to which it remains an empirical barrier can be reduced through improving knowledge and information of potential donors and their families. It is also possible to reduce the extent to which bodily integrity presents a normative barrier to pursuing certain policies through clarifying the concept of bodily integrity itself, what forms of intervention should be thought to impermissibly transgress bodily integrity and in what circumstances its transgression should be pursued in the context of organ transplantation. Efforts to reduce these barriers are not only philosophically important, but could also result in real change that can have practical significance for the lives of many individuals. It provides an instance whereby philosophy could be used in conjunction with other public health tools as part of an overall strategy to reduce the number of individuals who suffer with lower quality of life or die each year waiting to receive an organ transplant.

References

Cooper, M. L., and G. J. Taylor. 2000. *Organ and tissue donation: A reference guide for Clergy*. 4th ed. Richmond: SEOPF/UNOS.

Fabre, C. 2006. *Whose body is it anyway? Justice and the integrity of the person*. Oxford: Oxford University Press.

Gallie, W. B. 1956. Essentially contested concepts. *Proceedings of the Aristotelian Society* 56:167–198.

Irving, M. J., et al. 2012. Factors that influence the decision to be an organ donor: a systematic review of the qualitative literature. *Nephrology Dialysis Transplantation* 27 (6): 1–8.

Newton, J. D. 2011. How does the general public view posthumous organ donation? A meta-synthesis of the qualitative literature. *BMC Public Health* 11:791.

Ryckman, R., B. van den Borne, B. Thornton, and J. A. Gold. 2004. Intrinsic-extrinsic religiosity and university students' willingness to donate organs posthumously. *Journal of Applied Social Psychology* 34:196–205.

Stephenson, M. T., et al. 2008. The role of religiosity, religious norms, subjective norms, and bodily integrity in signing an organ donor card organ donation and religion. *Health Communication* 23:436–447.

Viens, A. M., ed. 2014. *The right to bodily integrity*. Farnham: Ashgate Publishing.

Wilkinson, T. M. 2011. *Ethics and the acquisition of organs*. Oxford: Oxford University Press.

A. M. Viens is Associate Professor in Law and Director of the Centre for Health, Ethics and Law (HEAL), Southampton Law School, University of Southampton. He is also an associate research fellow in the Institute for Medical Ethics & History of Medicine, Ruhr-University Bochum. Dr. Viens has degrees in philosophy and law from the Universities of Toronto, Oxford and London. His research interests lie at the intersection of moral, political and legal theory, with a particular interest in topics related to health, safety and well-being.

Chapter 4
The Role of Body Concepts for Donation Willingness. Insights from a Survey with German Medical and Economics Students

Sabine Wöhlke, Julia Inthorn and Silke Schicktanz

4.1 Introduction

The current debate on organ donation focuses mainly on the question of how to motivate more people to donate or to overcome the laziness of not filling out an organ donor card.[1] The German law (BZgA 2012), for example, follows the classical information deficit paradigm by assuming that more information about the possibility for organ donation (e.g., now issued regularly by the social health care insurance agencies) will lead to more organ donors as it conceptualizes public skepticism towards a particular technology to be based mainly on ignorance.

However, this paradigm can be put into question for several reasons. First of all, research in the last decades has identified other relevant factors for public support, skepticism, or even disapproval: Moral evaluations based on self-determination, human dignity, or risks are widespread among the public and the conception of consistently play a role in the assessment of a particular medical practice.[2] Second, anthropological positions, or more general, *Weltanschauung*, including the meaning of nature and its technological advancements, the body, or the belief in contingency or religious rules interfere with the public assessment of modern science and tech-

[1] Ahlert and Schwettmann (2012); Heuer et al. (2009).

[2] Lock (1993); Lundin (2002).

S. Wöhlke (✉) · J. Inthorn · S. Schicktanz
Department of Medical Ethics and History of Medicine,
University Medical Center Göttingen, Göttingen, Germany
e-mail: swoehlk@gwdg.de

J. Inthorn
e-mail: julia.inthorn@medizin.uni-goettingen.de

S. Schicktanz
e-mail: sschick@gwdg.de

R. J. Jox et al. (eds.), *Organ Transplantation in Times of Donor Shortage*,
International Library of Ethics, Law, and the New Medicine 59,
DOI 10.1007/978-3-319-16441-0_4

nology. Thirdly, public trust and mistrust in political or scientific structures, often related to historical events, are important factors that influence public behavior and attitudes.[3]

To gain a better understanding of what determines a layperson's skepticism or unwillingness to donate, it is important to understand the particular factors and possible sources of concern. With regard to organ donation, qualitative studies in ethnology and medical sociology have indicated the relevance of the body and its conceptualization in the context of organ donation. The medical possibility to transplant organs is based on particular anthropological and ontological assumptions that are still heavily influenced by Descartes: the body is seen as fragmented, replaceable, and separate from personality and identity.[4] Moreover, the corpse is detached from its social and religious meaning—and only seen as a *source* of organs and other valuable *materials*.[5] It is often implicitly assumed that this position is typical for any Western, secular tradition that is based on rationality and the Enlightenment, including laypersons' thinking. However, whether this Western medical paradigm has been adopted by everybody living in the Western, industrialized world must be critically questioned. The increasing understanding of modernity, its post and late versions in their complexities, provides a necessary framework to reject such a simplistic assumption of *Western* culture as something that is homogenous, solely scientific, secular, and rationality-based. Instead, moral and political pluralism based on self-determination, as well as a critical assessment of scientific pragmatism, are in themselves leading paradigms. Hence, cultural factors have diverse sources and various forms of expression must be expected when citizens hold a position towards complex social practices such as organ donation. In summary, culture comprises convictions, values, and codes of behavior as well as lifestyle practices, which have been acquired and are transmitted to future generations.

Armed with such theoretical background considerations, we can raise some general and more specific questions regarding public attitudes towards organ donation. For example, does people's willingness differ depending on which organ they want to donate or have transplanted? One can assume that a strict scientific attitude does not attach any meaning to organs. Hence, people do not differentiate between different organs. If they do, however, do they give organs an identity or associate personality-related characteristics to it? How often do people equate brain death with the death of a person and, as such, regard it as a morally acceptable condition for *post-mortem* donation. And is there a link between the underlying body concept—holistic or fragmented—and the acceptance of the brain death criterion to define death.

Various opinion polls suggest that a German majority responds in favor of organ transplantation, but the number of individuals holding an organ donor card has remained rather low for the past few years. One explanation for this gap in attitude change might be found in hidden cultural factors. Up until now, the impact of cultural factors such as body image, concepts of death, and identity on attitudes

[3] Wynne (2006); Bauer et al. (2007).

[4] Lock (2002); Hauser-Schäublin et al. (2001).

[5] Waldby and Mitchell (2006).

towards organ transplantation have not been well examined. Our study explores some of these cultural factors affecting organ donation willingness. Furthermore, we focus on the role of body concepts and the impact of attitudes towards brain death on the acceptance of organ donation. Furthermore, we were interested in the acceptance of incentives for increasing organ donation.[6] Young adults are an important group to elicit general active acceptance of organ donation with regards to the body and issues affecting identity formation. Among other reasons, this age group is important in that values and attitudes towards health are being shaped and acquired during this phase of life.[7] As a research sample, we chose medical and economics/business students. This combination allows us to test whether the responses from these two groups differ due to of prior knowledge that is based on their academic subjects.[8] In the following, we will present the most important results, which have been structured into three interdependent categories: (1) (Active and passive) willingness to donate and receive an organ, (2) Acceptance of different body concepts and their impact on attitudes towards donation and acceptance of an organ, (3) Acceptance of the concept of brain death to determine human death.

4.2 Methods

Public surveys are an important tool to assess both the acceptance and the (un)willingness to donate organs.[9] We conducted an extensive survey among students with the aim to assess young people's attitudes on deceased organ donation (DOD) and living organ donation (LOD). The survey was conducted with students from different courses enrolled in two different academic subjects at a university in a mid-sized town in central Germany, with a student population of about 23,000, during the winter term 2008–2009. Medical students were chosen as a sample group (490 asked to participate, 466 participants) and were compared to economics students (450 asked to participate, 289 participants) (total $n=755$, response rate: 80.3 %) (Table 4.1).

In total, the questionnaire consisted of 55 sets of closed questions addressing the following topics: prior knowledge about organ transplantation and allocation, attitudes towards LOD and DOD under different conditions, models of commercialization and incentives, concepts of death and bodily identity, consent models, pro-social behavior, and socio-demographic data. We used a 6-Likert-scale for attitude questions, and yes/no/don't know for knowledge and for simple questions on decisions or willingness. The questionnaire was pre-tested for comprehensibility and factor analysis was used to explore validity. The evaluation of the survey results took place from 2010 to 2012.

---

[6] Inthorn et al. (2014).

[7] Hoffmann and Mansel (2010).

[8] Gross et al. (2001).

[9] Strenge et al. (2000); Boulware et al. (2002); Schaeffner et al. (2004); Ahlert (2007).

Table 4.1 Profile of respondents, University of Göttingen 2008/2009

Respondents	Total	Total in %
Total	755	100
Medicine	466	61.7
Economics	289	38.3
Female	386	52.3
Male	352	47.7
Age: 0–19 years	101	13.5
Age: 20–24 years	473	63.3
Age: 25–29 years	149	19.9
Age: 30 years and above	24	3.2
Breakdown by years in each respective program	Medicine total and (%)	Economics total and (%)
1st–2nd year	228 (48.8)	250 (51.2)
3rd–6th year	238 (86.7)	35 (13.3)

Data processing software SPSS was used to analyze the survey.[10] The analysis is based on frequency analysis and the calculation of means for Likert-scales. Differences between groups (academic subject, gender) were analyzed by using a Chi-square test. *P*-values below 0.05 were defined as significant (*) and p-levels below 0.01 as highly significant (**). For questions where participants could choose between the options yes/no/don't know, the answers *no* and *don't know* were combined and Chi-square tests were conducted for 4-field matrixes. The main focus of analysis was placed on which groups agreed to certain positions. Subjects who would not or hesitated to agree were regarded as one group.

4.3 Results

4.3.1 Willingness for Organ Donation and Transplantation

Passive willingness means that a person is theoretically willing to donate an organ when asked during a survey. The passive willingness for DOD was 58.4% among all participating students, while 33.2% were undecided. If a person holds a donor card, indicating the holder's willingness to donate, we defined this as active willingness to donate. Significantly, more women (28.6%) than men (19.4%) were in possession of a donor card.

The willingness to agree to LOD was much higher among all students than DOD. In the case of a sick partner, 80.3% of men (men → women) and 85.6% of women

[10] Norris et al. (2012).

(women→men) were willing to help their partner with a LOD. The willingness to donate a living organ to one's own child was equally high in both groups (to daughter: women: 85.9 %, men: 85.1 %; to son: women 82.5 %, men: 78.4 %). The question on possible motivations for LOD showed a clear ranking of reasons (ranking each motivation from 1 = total approval—6 = total disapproval). The primary motivation was *love* (mean 1.32). The second most important motivation was *responsibility towards the family* (mean 2.24). *Moral duty* as a motivating factor was seen ambivalently (mean 3.24). Other motivations, such as to *meet expectation of the family, gaining social approval*, or *financial compensation*, gained low or no consent (mean ≥ 4.80). The most frequently cited reason against LOD was fear of medical complications (women: 74.9 %; men: 67.9 %) (sig. $p = 0.029$), followed by the statement that this constitutes an invasion of bodily integrity (women: 47.9 %; men: 42.9 %). 11.7 % of women and 15.6 % of men were of the opinion that this also invades one's *psychological integrity*. The majority of respondents believed that LOD would improve the relationship between donor and recipient (66.2 %).

Although anonymous LOD is prohibited in Germany, 44.3 % of all respondents were in favor of it (economics: 47.1 %; medical: 42.7 %) (sig. $p = 0.036$). Students agreed that LOD should also be allowed between individuals who are not relatives or friends, but are *on bowing terms*. (75.3 % economics; 63.9 % medical) ($p < 0.001$).

4.3.2 Images of the Body

To test if different images of the body have an influence on attitudes towards organ donation, attitudes towards different body concepts were the first to be assessed. A large majority of students (84.1 %) favored a holistic concept of the body in which the human body signifies more than just the sum of its parts (see Fig. 4.1).

Despite this rather clear result, there were significant gender differences: More women (87.6 %) than men (80.6 %) have a holistic conception of the body (sig. $p = 0.023$). When asked about their position towards a more technical concept of the body, only about 10.9 % of the respondents agreed to the idea that parts of the body can easily be exchanged like in a machine, with a much higher percentage amongst men rather than women. While only 6.3 % of women agreed with this statement, 15.9 % of men agreed (sig. $p < 0.001$, see Fig. 4.1). Medical students were also more in favor of this body concept (8.3 % economics, 12.5 % medical, sig. $p < 0.001$), while economics students showed a tendency of being unsure about their answers (15.1 %). Economics students also showed this uncertainty with regard to the idea that the heart is the location of the soul and should not be transplanted, 26.0 % were unsure about this. Uncertainty was also relatively high regarding the question of whether certain body parts are believed to be significant for identity. Thus, 25.3 % of respondents were uncertain whether specific organs determine a person's individuality. 41.1 % of respondents disagreed with this statement and 33.7 % agreed (see Fig. 4.1).

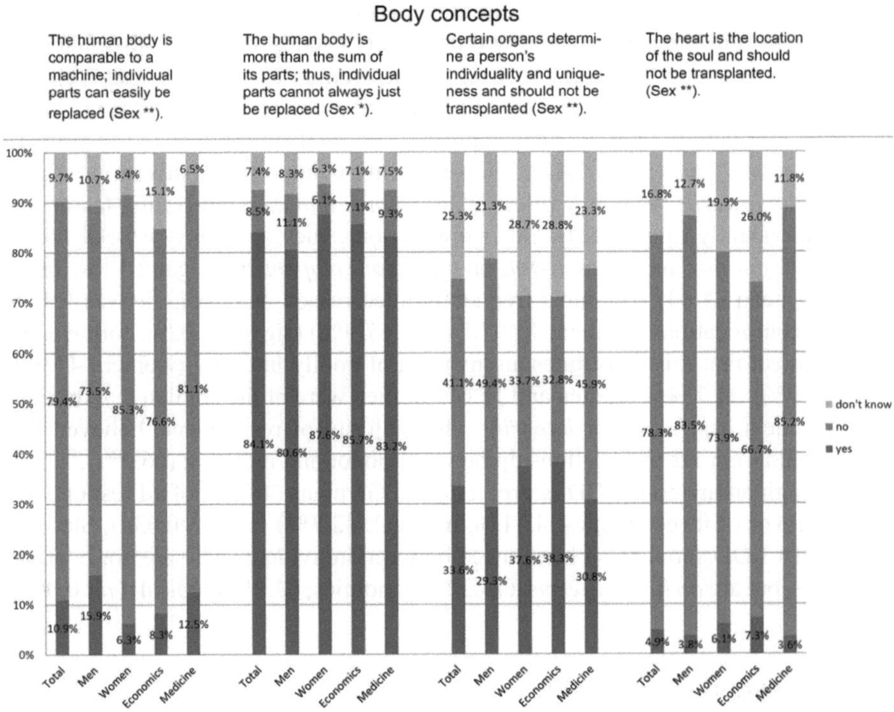

Fig. 4.1 Attitudes towards different body concepts showing differences between gender differences and differences between academic subjects

4.3.2.1 Preferences to Accept an Organ

Moreover, we asked what type of organ the respondents would accept in case of severe organ failure. There was a higher preference for human origin (postmortem or living, see Fig. 4.2) than for animal or artificial organs. Women opted for a living organ significantly more often (76.8 %) than men (71.9 %) ($p=0.014$). Respondents were more skeptical about other alternatives, e.g., animal organs, organs from stem cells, or a machine. Yet, more than half of the respondents stated that they would accept an organ grown from stem cells, but while 76.1 % of men would accept such an organ, only 58.9 % of women would agree to this option. Here, women were significantly more uncertain about it (32.3 %) than men (16.6 %) ($p<0.001$). The same level of uncertainty emerged on the question of whether an artificial machine would constitute an adequate surrogate organ (31.1 %) or about the option of an animal organ (36.1 %).

Apart from the origin of an organ, acceptance levels may also vary with respect to the type of the human organ. The answer options ranged from *fully acceptable* (1) to *do not accept at all* (6). The kidney showed the highest level of acceptance, scoring 1.3 (whole data set), as well as the liver with 1.4, followed by lung transplant and the heart (1.6). Transplantation of the cornea was also accepted, averaging 2.2. Transplanting single limbs was seen as *still acceptable* (3.2), as well as receiving a whole eye (3.2). Respondents were uncertain about the option of accepting face transplantation (3.8) and the transplantation of genitals, which showed a mean of 4.3.

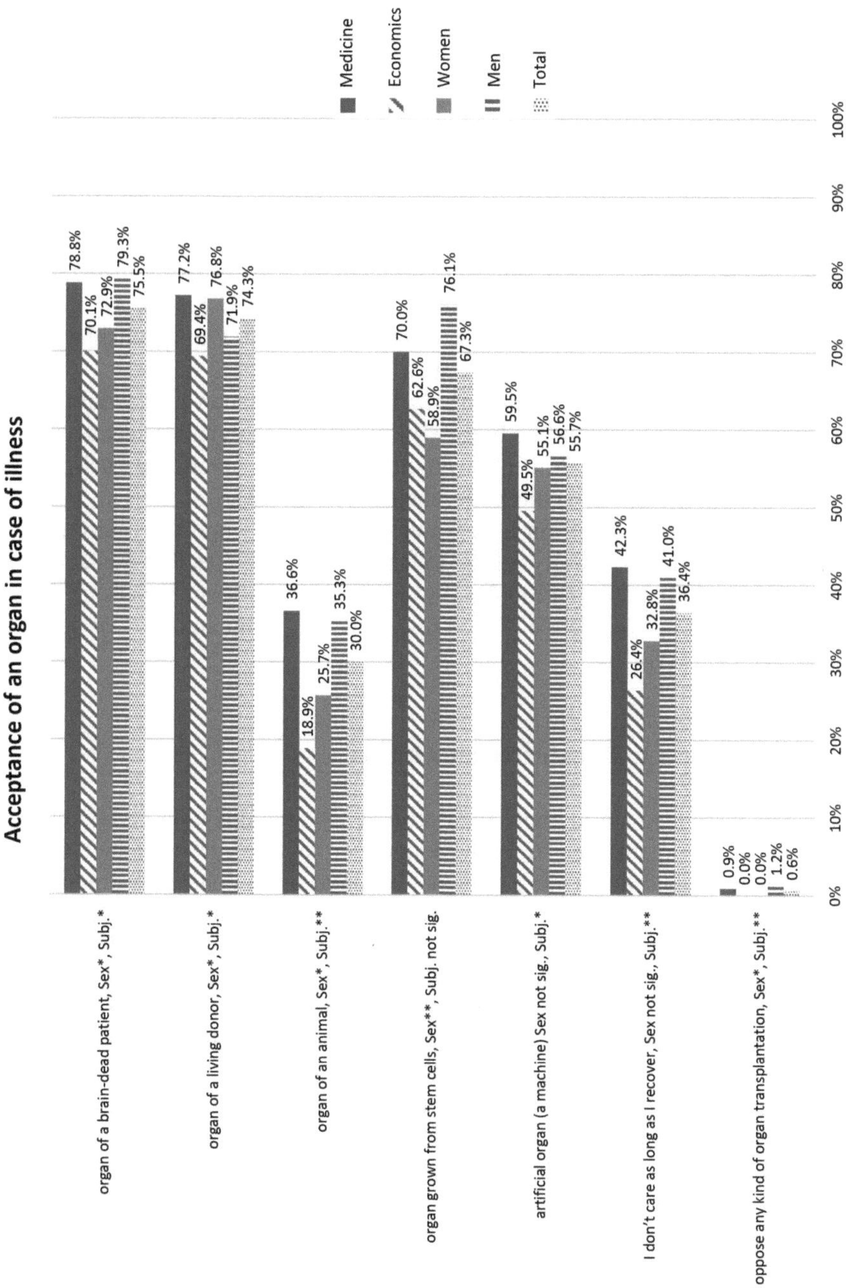

Fig. 4.2 Acceptance of an organ in case of illness. Positive answers in %, differences between gender differences and differences between academic subjects

Strikingly, the mean values of all options (except for the pancreas) showed that men were more willing to accept any kind of organ than women. While answers with regard to the kidney, liver, and lung only showed a slight tendency towards differing opinions, this difference became more pronounced in the option of accepting a heart transplant (1.5 for men, 1.8 women, sig. $p=0.003$). When it comes to externally visible organs, differences between men and women were even more significant. Values on the acceptance of a cornea transplant ranged from 2.0 among men to 2.3 among women (sig. $p=0.003$). These differences increased even more in responses to the option on the acceptance of receiving a whole eye transplant (2.8 men; 3.6 women, sig. $p<0.001$), acceptance of single limbs (2.8 men; 3.5 women, sig. $p<0.001$), a full face (3.4 men, 4.1 women, sig. $p<0.001$), or a transplantation of genitals (3.9 men, 4.6 women, sig. $p=0.001$).

Overall, the acceptance of an organ was highest for human organs and those organs that are *invisible* within the body, with men showing greater acceptance of transplantation than women. Students were also asked how important background information about the donor would be for them (see Fig. 4.3).

Answers (options ranging from 1-very important to 6-not important) showed that mainly information that is closely related to health, like health itself (mean 2.17), or smoking and drinking habits (mean 2.45) were regarded as being important. Other characteristics of a person were of little importance (e.g. skin color 5.4 or occupation 4.82, see Fig. 4.3).

4.3.2.2 Preferences to Donate Certain Organs

Respondents were also asked about their attitude towards donating certain organs (DOD), especially organs that, so far, have not been routinely transplanted. On the one hand, when asked about their personal willingness to donate an organ postmortem, answers showed a high willingness among respondents to donate internal organs such as the liver (73.1 %), heart (57.6 %), or kidney (75.7 %, see Fig. 4.4).

On the other hand, the willingness to donate visible body parts was generally much lower (cornea/eye 36.6 %, hand/foot 28.9 %, skin 31.7 % see Fig. 4.4). There was an overall difference between men and women. While the overall high willingness to donate internal organs was even higher among women (e.g. liver: 68.9 % men, 78.2 % women, sig. $p=0.004$; kidney: 71.8 % men, 80.8 % women, sig. $p=0.004$), the picture changed with more visible, external body parts. Here, men showed a slightly (but not significantly) higher willingness to donate than women (cornea/eye: 39.3 % men, 35.0 % women; hand/foot: 32.5 % men, 26.4 % women). The willingness to donate was strongly linked to personal views on particular body concepts. Overall, the willingness to donate organs postmortem was higher among those who had a fragmented, machine-like, or a holistic body concept than those who connected ideas of identity to certain organs (see Fig. 4.5).

Among respondents who were in favor of the idea that the heart is the location of the soul, only 8.3 % were willing to donate their heart postmortem. When asked about extending recent regulations on transplantation of organs which currently are rarely transplanted rarely or not transplanted at all, body parts such as genitals, the brain, or the face elicited strong rejection or uncertainty. Only 20 % of respondents

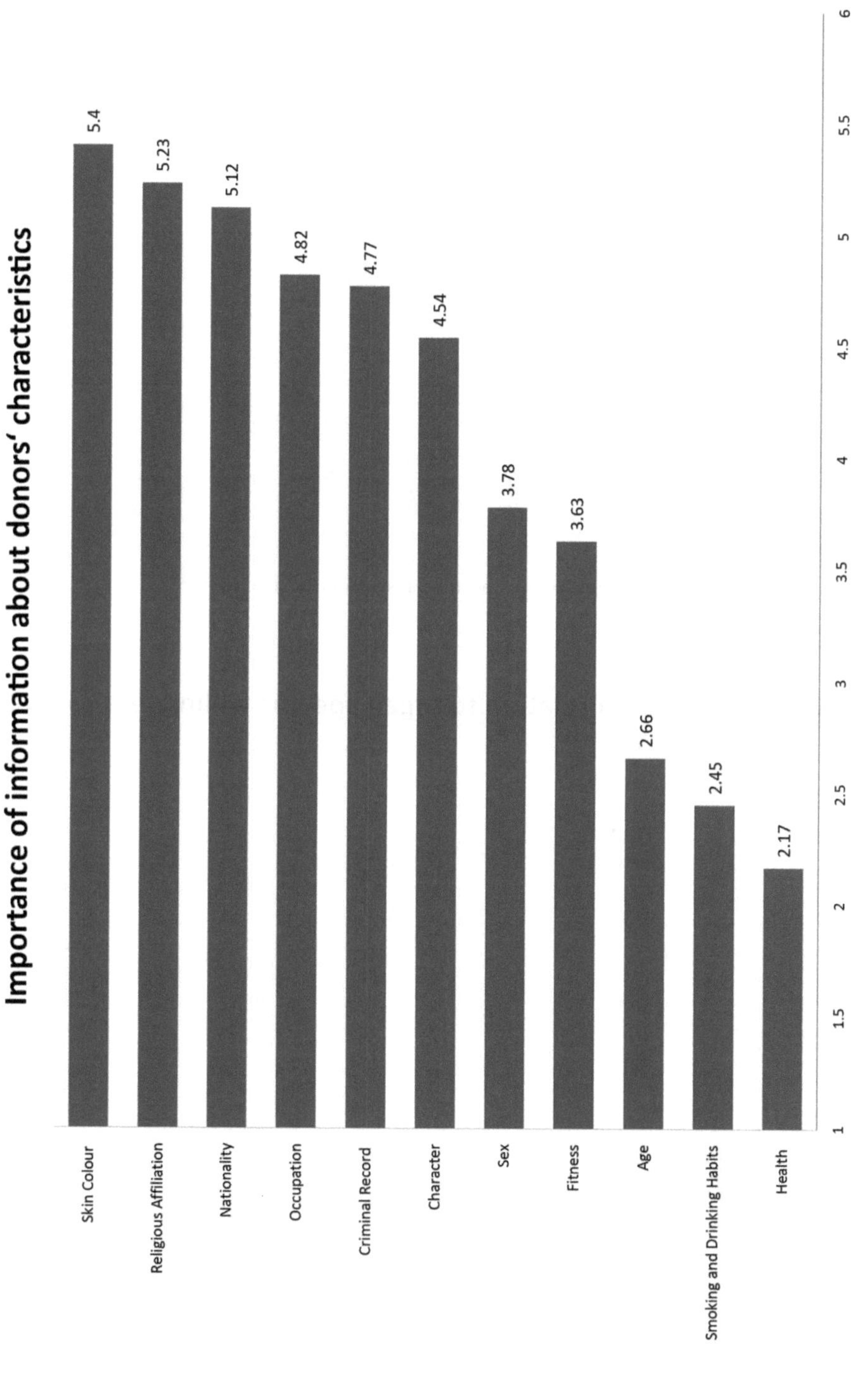

Fig. 4.3 Importance of information about donors' characteristics, total (n=755) (*1* = very important—*6* not important, means)

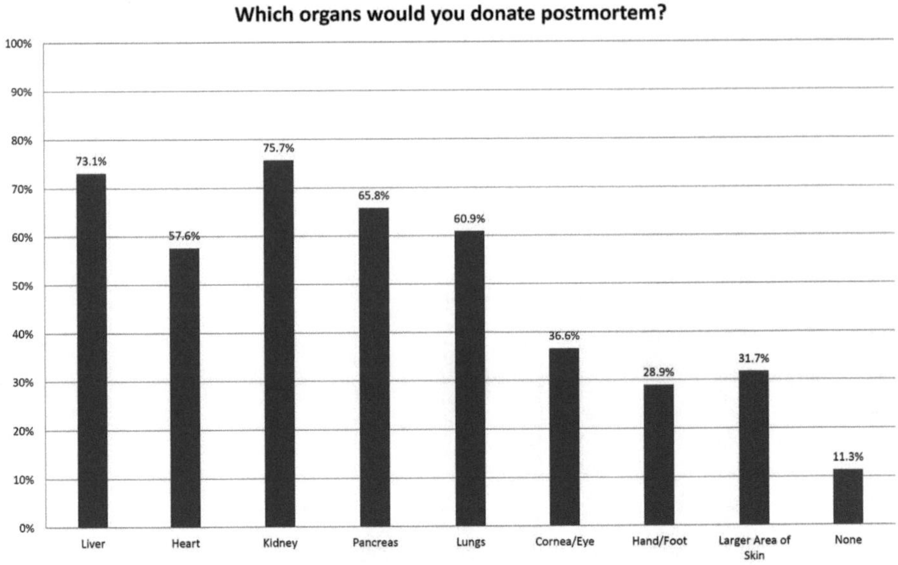

Fig. 4.4 Consent to DOD, organ specific, positive answers in %, total ($n=755$)

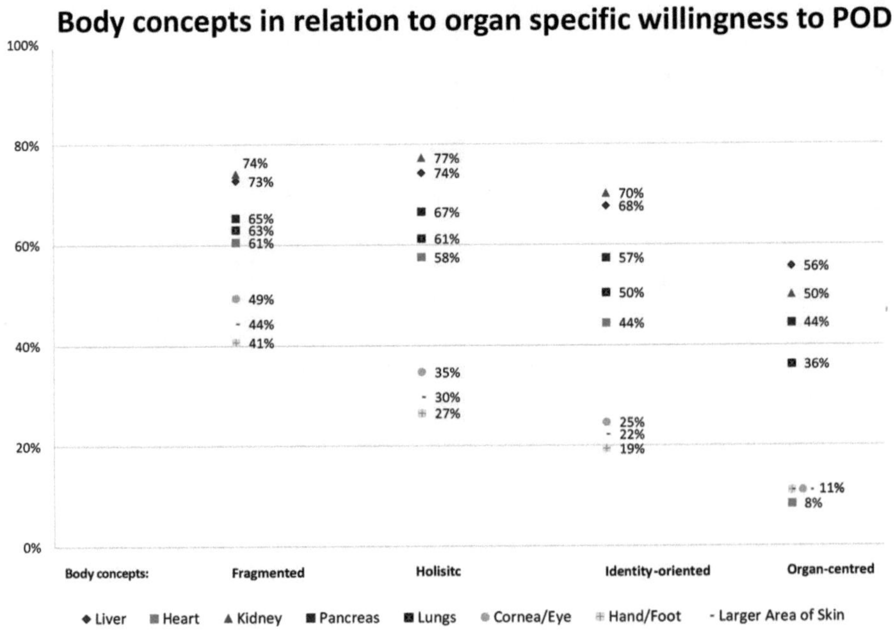

Fig. 4.5 Organ-specific willingness to DOD in relation to body concepts, positive answers in %, total ($n=755$)

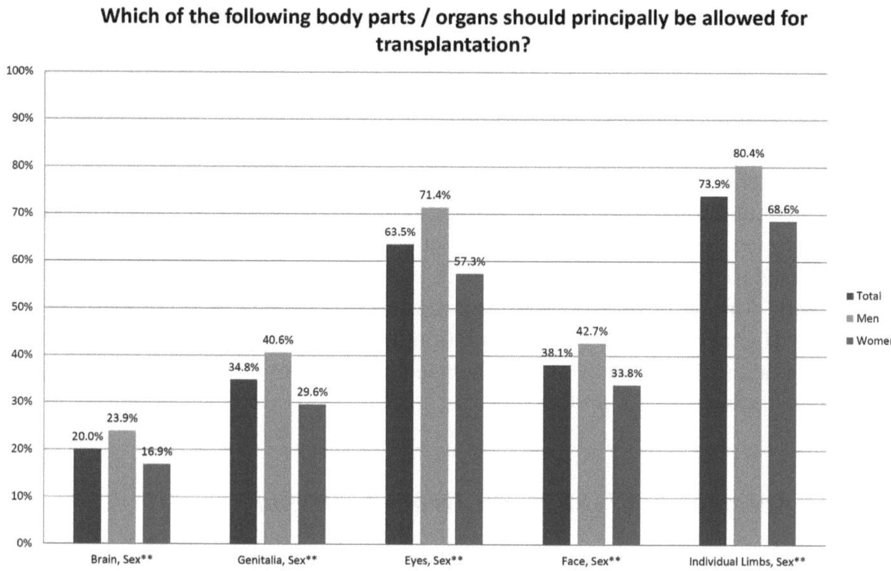

Fig. 4.6 Acceptance of transplantation of different body parts (in genereal), positive answers in %, total ($n=755$), gender differences

agreed to a brain transplant, one third remained undecided (27.7 %). Generally, there was a high uncertainty about extending possible options for donation. Thus, in every response option, one third of respondents stated that they could not answer the question. Responses here showed significant gender differences. Women tended to disagree more strongly than men concerning options to extend the scope of organs for transplantation (see Fig. 4.6).

On the other hand, they were less decisive in their responses to the questions. Thus, 23.9 % of men and 16.9 % of women answered positively about transplanting a brain, 21.9 % of men and 32.7 % of women were unsure (sig. $p=0.002$). 40.6 % of men and 29.6 % of women agreed with the transplantation of genital organs, while 32.2 % of men and 36.4 % of women were unsure (sig. $p=0.006$). In contrast, 71.4 % of men, but only 57.3 % of women answered positively to eye transplantation, 13 % of men and 14.5 % of women rejected this, and 15.6 % of men and 28.2 % of women were undecided (sig. $p<0.001$). 80.4 % of men and 68.6 % of women accepted the transplantation of single limbs, while 13.5 % of men and 21.8 % of women were undecided.

4.3.2.3 Comparing Willingness to Donate with the Acceptance of an Organ Donation

When we compared the question on the general willingness to donate organs post-mortem (passive willingness DOD) with the attitude towards generally extending the scope of organ transplantation to certain parts of the body, like the brain or a whole eye, which are currently not transplanted, results showed that those who themselves expressed a positive willingness to donate were generally also positive about expanding the spectrum of organ donation. For example, among those who would be willing to donate their cornea, 75.9 % approved of cornea donation in general, while among those who disapproved of cornea donation, only 56.1 % stated that they were principally positive about the possibility of eye transplantation (sig. $p<0.001$). Among the respondents willing to donate a hand or foot, 86.0 % principally approved of the possibility to transplant single limbs. In contrast, among those who rejected to donate a limb, 68.9 % still, in principle, consented to allowing limb transplants. Among those who were willing to donate larger areas of skin, 51.7 % approved of general full-face transplantation. In contrast, only 31.5 % of those who would not donate larger areas of skin themselves voted for the general possibility of a full-face transplant (sig. $p<0.001$).

4.3.3 Acceptance of the Brain Death Criterion

The willingness to donate organs postmortem seems to presuppose that people accept the definition of brain death in its current version. Thus, students were asked about their attitude towards different concepts of death (see Fig. 4.7; Table 4.2).

43.9 % of the respondents believed that a patient is dead when his or her brain is completely destroyed. Further, 20.9 % believed that a person is dead when those regions of the brain connected with personality stop functioning (brain stem death). 47.7 % of the medical students and only 37.6 % of the economics students agreed with the whole brain death criterion (sig. $p<0.001$). However, the survey also showed that 29.1 % of the medical students thought that brain death was not a safe criterion for death and agreed that a person is not dead as long as organs are still functioning. Questions concerning the criterion of brain death elicited significant gender

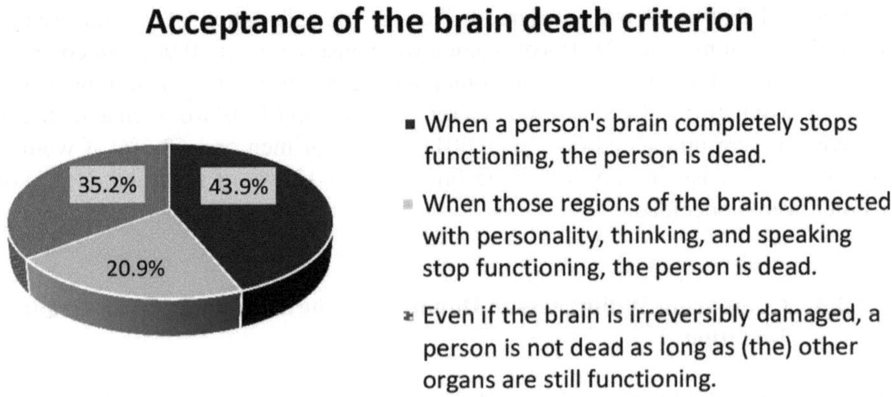

Fig. 4.7 Acceptance of different death concepts, positive answers in %, total ($n=755$)

Table 4.2 Acceptance of different death concepts, differences with regard to gender and academic subject

To remove organs after death, so-called brain death has to be determined. Which of these statements do you agree with?

in %	Total	Men	Women	Sig.	Medicine	Economics	Sig.
When a person's brain stops functioning completely, the person is dead	Yes	Yes	Yes		Yes	Yes	
	43.9	45.2	41.8		47.7	37.6	
When those regions of the brain connected with personality, thinking, and speaking stop functioning, the person is dead	Yes	Yes	Yes		Yes	Yes	
	20.9	24.6	18.2		17.2	23.2	
Even if the brain is irreversibly damaged, a person is not dead as long as other organs are still functioning	Yes	Yes	Yes		Yes	Yes	
	35.2	30.1	39.9	$P=0.012$	29.1	45.3	$P<0.001$

and differences between academic subjects. 39.9% of the female respondents and 30.1% of the male respondents doubted both brain death criteria ($p=0.012$). At this point, it is important to note that 6.9% of those who did not hold an organ donor card justified this with their doubts about the brain death criteria. Here, too, significant gender differences and differences between academic subjects can be observed. 9.1% of the female respondents held this opinion in contrast to only 4.5% of the male respondents ($p=0.016$). There also was a connection between body concepts and concepts of death. Those who think the body is similar to a machine accepted the idea of brain death more frequently (brain stem death plus entire brain death: 76.2%) than those who do not agree with this body concept (63.4%, $p=0.025$).

4.4 Discussion

In the following section, we will discuss our major findings in light of other studies' findings.

Willingness to Donate For DOD, we found that overall passive willingness to donate is much higher than active willingness. Passive willingness was expressed by a little under 2/3 of all respondents. This shows that willingness for DOD was not as high as has sometimes been assumed (e.g. the recent campaign of the German Federal Center for public health information states that four out of five German citizens would be willing to donate their organs[11]): only half of all economics and 63.5 % of medical students would donate organs after death. Notably, this ratio matches other German surveys.[12] Also, a more comprehensive representative study of 1000 German citizens[13] on attitudes towards presumed consent and market models for organ donation found that 59 % were passively willing to donate, but only 13 % held a donor card. This corresponds to practice: Usually, only 2/3 of family members agree to DOD (on behalf of the patient's anticipated wish), while 1/3 disagree with it.[14] Interestingly, the acceptance of an organ was higher (3/4 of students would accept an organ) than one's own willingness to donate. The willingness to agree to a LOD was much higher among all students than DOD.[15]

The German findings concerning the acceptance of LOD are remarkably higher than findings from other European studies (40 % in the Netherlands[16] and 80 % in the UK[17]). The high willingness contrasts with the current legal situation (LOD constitutes less than 1/3 of all donations[18]) and recent political activity in Germany, which intends to strengthen DOD but not LOD. German law continues to consider LOD as a second-rate option to DOD. The high potential for LOD, however, raises its own ethical and social concerns, perhaps because it has not been sufficiently discussed by the general public.[19]

Images of the Body Contrary to western medical constructions of the body and organ donation, medical laypersons' own concepts of the body are often shaped by culture. Our findings show that the majority of respondents (84.1 %) favor a holistic concept of the body. Only a clear minority of 11 % of respondents has internalized a fragmented concept of the body as an object.

Comparative studies of two groups—one consisting of people who hold a donor card, the other with people who do not—show that potential donors base their argument on a specific body concept and are less concerned with fears about their own death concerning their body.[20] There are still only few studies, which delineate potential donors' personal motivations and their culturally shaped body concepts. Thus, Sanner showed that one fourth of the students they interviewed rejected organ donation because of personal reasons, such as fear or respect for their own body.[21] Similarly, interviewees cited the fear of destroying their, albeit dead, body as an

[11] See campaign by the Bundeszentrale für Gesundheitliche Aufklärung, in Mobil Jun 2013, www.organspende-info.de.

[12] e.g. Rey et al. (2011); BZgA (2003, 2012); Ahlert and Schwettmann (2012).

[13] Decker et al. (2008).

[14] DSO (2012).

[15] See also: Ahlert (2007); Decker et al. (2008).

[16] Kranenburg et al. (2008).

[17] Mazaris et al. (2011).

[18] Mazaris et al. (2011).

[19] Wöhlke (2013).

[20] Kalitzkus (2003); Kaminer et al. (1978).

[21] Sanner (2001).

argument against organ donation. They felt that they were being robbed of their humanity. This also leads to questions on what happens to the body after death[22], considering a funeral or religious issues such as reincarnation. This can be linked to the belief in resurrection and the notion that the body has to be preserved as it was at the moment of death.[23] Furthermore, it is conspicuous that only qualitative studies actually link a certain body concept to a willingness to donate. Although these studies date back to more than a decade, our results endorse the continuing relevance of this question and underline the notion that there are many who feel uneasy about certain body concepts. This uncertainty is an important hint, which has to be taken seriously. It suggests that the respondents do not exactly know how to *frame* their *uncertainty* regarding the body.

Our findings on body concepts also highlight gender differences: more women preferred a holistic concept. This gender difference is interesting given that concerning LOD in Germany and other European countries, significantly more women donate their kidneys.[24] Furthermore, in Germany, more women hold a donor card than men. On the other hand, studies indicate that those who have internalized a concept of the body as an object are better at coping with organ transplantation and psycho-social organ integration.[25]

Preferences to Accept or to Donate Certain Organs According to our respondents, the donation of internal organs such as the heart, kidneys, and liver is seen as unproblematic. However, when it comes to visible body parts such as the cornea, a hand, foot, or the skin, the acceptance decreased, on average, to below one third. Women tended to give internal organs such as the heart, liver, and kidney. Interestingly, more men than women were willing to donate an external organ.

We can ask to what extent specific organs play a more significant role in establishing identity than others., considering the overall high passive willingness of DOD.

A qualitative study conducted in Sweden[26] showed that many respondents were afraid of having specific organs removed. This applied mainly to the heart or eyes, which can be felt or seen.[27] They were believed to have a symbolic meaning. Organs such as the liver or kidneys were seen as less personal. Skin was a special case in that it was hard to donate for some people because it is externally visible, while others found it easier to donate skin in that everyone has a lot of it and it regenerates.

Our results show a similar discrepancy in the high acceptance rate for donating internal organs, on the one hand, in contrast to a low acceptance of donating external organs, on the other hand. Our respondents have a high willingness to donate internal organs such as the liver (73.1 %), heart (57.6 %), or kidney, but are less willing to donate visible body parts such as cornea/eye (36.6 %), hand or foot (28.9 %), or skin (31.7 %). Interestingly, there was an overall difference between men and wom-

22 Sanner (1994); Siminoff et al. (2004).

23 Sanner (2001); Lock (1993).

24 See. Eurotransplant (2013); DSO (2012).

25 Decker et al. 2008

26 Sanner (1994).

27 Sanner (1994, p. 1145).

en. While the overall high willingness to donate internal organs was even higher among women, this changed with regard to more visible, external body parts. Here, men showed a slightly higher willingness to donate than women did. Künsebeck et al. (2000) conducted a survey among German medical and administrative staff in hospitals asking about their preferred organs for donation. In general, in comparison with our results there were no differences in the order of specific organs among the respondents. Kidneys gained the highest rate of acceptance with 61.7 % of laypersons, followed by the liver, pancreas, lung, and heart, for which 70 % of medical and 50 % of administrative staff signaled their willingness to donate these organs. The cornea was least accepted as a transplant with 61 % and 39.6 %, respectively.[28]

In correspondence to this study, our results show a high willingness to donate internal organs. These are organs such as the kidney or liver, whose transplantation is a well-established practice. On the other hand, our findings indicate a much lower acceptance of the donation of externally visible organs, such as the cornea, face, or limbs. Seeing as most of these transplants are still in their trial phase, we can assume that the higher disagreement for the donation of these organs may be due to insecurities about medical feasibility. However, in contrast to our data, Künsebeck et al. point out a significantly lower disagreement for organs such as the heart, cornea or, for example, organs that have not been transplanted before.

According to the respondents in the study by Künsebeck et al., organs which should not be donated at all include the heart (7.5 % medical; 12.7 % administrative staff), followed by the cornea (9.6 % medical; 6.8 % administrative staff). 4.1 % of medical and 2.1 % of administrative staff stated that the brain should never be allowed to be transplanted.[29]

Our results paint a similar picture when it comes to the willingness to accept an organ in the case of severe illness. Here, respondents clearly preferred human organs to artificially manufactured organs or animal organs. Moreover, the willingness to accept internal organs is significantly higher than the acceptance of externally visible body parts, such as skin or eyes. Other studies with patients show, that they believe it is important to receive information concerning the donor's health. Other traits, such as skin color, job, religion, or nationality, are deemed less important[30]. This contrasts with narratives by patients who, after transplantation, adopt formerly unfamiliar characteristics associated with the donor. While many surveys have focused on preferences in the donation of certain organs, only very few studies have explored the acceptance of specific organs.

A survey among German patients on the waiting list[31] showed that only 40 % of those interviewed expected that they would regard the transplant as being their *own* organ after transplantation. The high acceptance of kidney transplantations—among donors as well as recipients—might be due to the transparency and availability of organ transplantations and waiting lists to the public. On the other hand, our students' responses reflect cultural identity-establishing preferences. In west-

[28] Cf. Basu et al. (1989); Künsebeck et al. (2000); Lawlor and Kerridge (2011).

[29] Künsnbeck et al. (2000, p. 48); similar: Strenge et al. (2000).

[30] Sharp (1995, 2001).

[31] Schlitt et al. (1999a, b).

ern tradition, eyes are especially important; they are an integral part of social life. For many, the eyes are the windows of the soul, and perhaps more than any other body part, they embody the individual.[32] Additionally, the heart is highly charged with cultural symbolism,[33] which also explains why our respondents were reluctant when asked whether they would donate their heart. Although heart transplantation has been medically and technically established for many years, only about half of the respondents would make their heart available for donation. In our survey, students were also very undecided when confronted with the idea of donating their limbs or face. Up until now, there has not been a comparable survey, which specifically addresses the willingness to donate these body parts. This is surprising given that, in these fields, transplant technology advances rapidly. On the other hand, these body parts have a high cultural and symbolic value. Arms and legs figure into activity and mobility, and the face is one of the body parts that establishes identity.[34]

While theoretically reflecting on the fact that questions of organ donation and transplantation are always hypothetical, it seems important to understand the relevance of this question for the willingness to donate or the uncertainty of donation[35].

Acceptance of the Brain Death Criterion Regarding the ethical controversy about the validity of the criterion of brain death for determining human death[36] which arose after a decade of silence, it is important to realize that barely half of all respondents (45.2 % of the male respondents and 41.8 % of the female respondents) thought that a person is considered dead when his or her brain has been completely destroyed. More importantly, even 29.1 % of medical students thought that brain death is not a safe criterion to determine death. Also, among physicians, the current concept of brain death is not unanimously accepted.[37] Our results indicate that, for the public, even if they have medical background knowledge and are highly educated, brain death does not equal human death.

Some have suggested that the acceptance of brain death by defining death might be the central problem of postmortem donation.[38] From a philosophical and sociological point of view, death is neither a scientific nor a philosophical *truth* to be discovered or proven. Rather, it is a social construct whose cultural and normative aspects are as important as its biological and *rational* ones.[39] Similarly, a local survey indicates that younger people in particular were scared about not knowing what happens after death and thus avoided engaging in thoughts on their own death.[40]

Comparing several surveys, a consistent picture of public ambivalence towards medical definitions of death can be drawn. In a German survey by Fassbender in

[32] Lawlor and Kerridge (2011).

[33] Schipperges (1989).

[34] Sanner (1994, p. 1145).

[35] Schicktanz and Wöhlke 2015

[36] Stoecker (2010); Müller (2010).

[37] Muthny and Schweidtmann (2000).

[38] Müller (2010); Hübner and Six (2005); Ohwaki et al. (2006).

[39] Lock and Crowley-Makota (2008); Lock (2000); Ohnuki-Tierney (1994).

[40] GfK (2010).

2003, 62 % of respondents assumed that a person with complete irreversible brain failure is dead even if their circulation is artificially maintained. Cardiac arrest let 89 % regard the patient as dead. However, even after rigor mortis has set in, 11 % still doubted the onset of death.[41] The same study indicated that discussing death criteria with persons who had originally expressed a passive willingness to donate an organ let 18 % question their initial decision.[42] Overall, there are strong indicators that cultural attitudes on death are linked to attitudes on organ donation.

International surveys, also indicate that people are skeptical about brain death as the criterion that determines death. Although 98 % of respondents in a US survey stated that they had already heard of the brain death criterion, only one third (33.7 %) thought that a person who has been diagnosed as brain dead is really dead. 28.1 % of respondents assumed that the brain-dead person can still hear and 40.4 % thought that brain-dead patients are *really dead*, while 43.3 % thought that they are *as good as dead* and 16 % of respondents thought that those diagnosed with brain death are still alive.[43] According to Siminoff, the respondents held different personal opinions on when a patient is dead, and these differences cannot be simplistically reduced to ignorance or a confused definition.[44]

4.5 Conclusion and Outlook

In Germany, as in many other countries, there are two big discrepancies in the context of organ donation: first, between patients in need of an organ, on the one hand, and the number of those willing to donate, on the other hand, and second, between the high number of people stating that they want to donate an organ and the low number of donor card holders. The latter is often seen as a problem of ignorance or laziness.

However, the underlying problems might be much more complex and serious. First, it is very likely that the gap between general support for organ donation and personal commitment is also rooted in personal ambivalence, and moral and anthropological uncertainties concerning the status of the human body and death. Both topics, the concept of one's (and the other's) body and the understanding of death are deeply rooted in culture and can be understood as a part of implicit anthropological positions. These lay anthropologies—as we call them—can be summarized as *Weltanschauung*. They are sometimes more explicitly expressed, and more often they are implicitly acknowledged. The high levels of uncertainty and indecision in our survey with regard to these questions can also support this latter argument.

The ethical relevance of these lay anthropologies is obvious. They are an important key to understanding lay moralities and social attitudes. Philosophical or

[41] Faßbender (2003).

[42] Faßbender (2003).

[43] Siminoff et al. (2004).

[44] Siminoff et al. (2004).

cultural anthropological considerations are a necessary condition to develop consistent bioethical theories as bioethical positions consist not only of normative assumptions, but also of presumptions of what counts as a human being etc. However, the academic, legal, and ethical discourse, especially in the analytical and liberal tradition, has often neglected the relevance of such anthropological positions about the body by implicitly adopting a science-positivistic or (neo) Descartian stance.[45]

In contrast, on the basis of empirical evidence by qualitative,[46] as well as quantitative studies (as the one presented here), we assume that it is time for bioethicists to reconsider the importance of body and death concepts. Our survey study of highly educated students showed, in consistency with a few other surveys of the wider public asking similar questions, that images of the body and views about death are very likely to be a source of skepticism and behavioral inconsistencies. Moreover, in our study, we could show for the first time by means of a survey that body images, death acceptance, and the willingness to donate and to receive particular organs cannot be discussed separately.

Public bioethics and policies that aim at developing ethically justified models based on democratic norms should therefore not only consider consequentialist arguments to increase *social benefit* by increasing the number of available organs, but should also consider the citizens' right to have a particular stance on their bodies and death concepts. The existing pluralism in lay anthropologies might be an even bigger challenge for modern bio-politics. Whether the rational debate to determine the better argument (as we believe is an opportunity to deal with moral pluralism) will really lead to a broader social consensus on the understanding of bodies and death must be tested.

However, not all is lost for bioethics. Bioethics can work as a facilitator to allow more public debates on these underlying anthropological premises. Whether we thus gain a social consensus on some basic anthropological premises might be doubted. However, it might be worth a try. To our understanding, the recent problem is the one-sided presentation of anthropological premises or the total neglect of their relevance within the academic bioethics discourse. Second, it can encourage us to develop better ethical models of consent and donation by considering more concretely how to deal with plurality and moral uncertainty in such difficult issues as life and death.

Finally, it can result in the social acceptance that the need for organs can never be met—and thus, alternative paths in research, prevention and health care should be given priority in the next years to help those patients.

---

[45] Schicktanz (2007).

[46] E.g. Schweda and Schicktanz (2009).

References

Ahlert, M. 2007. Public and private choices in organ donation. *Homo Oeconomicus* 24 (2): 269–293.

Ahlert, M., and L. Schwettmann. 2012. Einstellung der Bevölkerung zur Organspende. In *Gesundheitsmonitor 2011. Bürgerorientierung im Gesundheitswesen*, eds. J. Böcken, B. Braun, and U. Repschläger. Gütersloh: Verlag Bertelsmann Stiftung.

Basu, P. K., K. M. Hazariwala, and M. L. Chipman. 1989. Public attitudes toward donation of body parts, particularly the eye. *Canadian Journal of Ophthalmology* 24 (5): 216–220.

Bauer, M. W., N. Allum, and S. Miller. 2007. What can we learn from 25 years of PUS survey research? Liberating and expanding the agenda. *Public Understanding of Science* 16 (1): 79–95. doi:10.1177/0963662506071287.

Boulware, L. E., L. E. Ratner, J. A. Sosa, L. A. Cooper, T. A. LaVeist, and N. R. Powe. 2002. Determinants of willingness to donate living related and cadaveric organs: Identifying opportunities for intervention. *Transplantation* 73 (10): 1683–1691.

BZgA. 2003. *Einstellungen Jugendlicher zum Thema Organspende*. Köln: Bundeszentrale für gesundheitliche Aufklärung.

BZgA. 2012. *Aufklärung zur Organ- und Gewebespende in Deutschland: Neue Wege in der Gesundheitskommunikation*. Köln: Bundeszentrale für gesundheitliche Aufklärung.

Decker, O., M. Winter, E. Brähler, and M. Beutel. 2008. Between commodification and altruism: gender imbalance and attitudes towards organ donation. A representative survey of the German community. *Journal of Gender Studies* 17 (3): 251–255. doi:10.1080/09589230802204290.

DSO. 2012. *Organ donation and transplantation in Germany*. Frankfurt a. M.: Deutsche Stiftung Organtransplantation.

Eurotransplant. 2013. Annual report. Den Haag.

Faßbender, J. 2003. Einstellung zur Organspende und Xenotransplantation in Deutschland. Dissertation, Universität Köln.

GfK Nürnberg für die Apotheken Umschau. 2010. *Repräsentativbefragung zum Thema "Sterben und Trauer"*. Baierbrunn: Wort & Bild Verlag.

Gross, T., S. Martinoli, G. Spagnoli, F. Badia, and R. Malacrida. 2001. Attitudes behavior of young European adults towards the donation of organs—a call for better information. *American Journal of Transplantation* 1:74–81. doi:10.1034/j.1600-6143.2001.010114.x.

Hauser-Schäublin, B., V. Kalitzkus, I. Petersen, and I. Schröder. 2001. *Der geteilte Leib. Die kulturelle Dimension von Organtransplantation und Reproduktionsmedizin in Deutschland*. Frankfurt a. M.: Campus.

Heuer, M., S. Hertel, N. Remmer, U. Wirges, T. Philipp, G. Gerken, A. Paul, and G. M. Kaiser. 2009. Organspendebereitschaft: Auswertung einer Umfrage zu Gesundheitsthemen. *Deutsche Medizinische Wochenschrift* 134:923–926. doi:10.1055/s-0029-1220249.

Hoffmann, D., and J. Mansel. 2010. Jugendsoziologie. In *Handbuch spezielle Soziologien*, eds. G. Kneer and M. Schroer, 163–178. Wiesbaden: VS Verlag für Sozialwissenschaften. doi:10.1007/978-3-531-92027-69.

Hübner, G., and B. Six. 2005. Einfluss ethischer Überzeugungen auf das Organspendeverhalten. Ein Erweitertes Modell der Organspende *Zeitschrift für Gesundheitspsychologie,* 13 (3): 118–125.

Inthorn, J., S. Wöhlke, F. Schmidt, and S. Schicktanz. 2014. Impact of gender and professional education on attitudes towards financial incentives for organ donation: Results of a survey among 755 students of medicine and economics in Germany. *BMC Medical Ethics* 15:56. doi:10.1186/1472-6939-15-56.

Kalitzkus, V. 2003. "Intime Fremde": "Organspende" und Organtransplantation im Spannungsfeld von Körper und Geist. In *Körperpolitik—Biopolitik*, eds. S. Beck and M. Knecht, 43–51. Münster: Lit Verlag.

Kaminer, I., H. Munitz, S. Tyano, and H. Wijsenbeek. 1978. The heart image as a model to internal-organ body image. *Psychotherapy and Psychosomatics* 30 (3–4): 187–192. doi:10.1159/000287298.

Kranenburg, L. W., A. Schram, W. Zuidema, W. Weimar, M. Hilhorst, E. Hessing, J. Passchier, and J. Busschbach. 2008. Public survey of financial incentives for kidney donation. *Nephrology, Dialysis, Transplantation* 23 (3): 1039–1042. doi:10.1093/ndt/gfm643.

Künsebeck, H.-W., U. Wilhelm, and S. Harborth. 2000. Psychosoziale Einflussfaktoren von Einstellungen zur Organspende bei Personen mit und ohne medizinische Ausbildung. In *Einstellungen zur Organspende und ihre klinische Relevanz*, eds. H.-W. Künsebeck and F. A. Muthny, 37–55. Lengerich: Pabst Science Publishers.

Lawlor, M., and I. Kerridge. 2011. Anything but the eyes: Culture, identity, and the selective refusal of corneal donation. *Transplantation* 92 (11): 1188–1190. doi:10.1097/TP.0b013e318235c817.

Lock, M. 2000. On dying twice: Culture, technology and the determination of death. In *Living and working with the new medical technologies. Intersections of inquiry*, eds. M. Lock, A. Young, and A. Cambrosio, 233–262. Montreal: Cambridge University Press.

Lock, M. 2002. *Twice dead: Organ transplants and the reinvention of death.* Berkeley: University of California Press.

Lock, M., and M. Crowley-Makota. 2008. Situating the practice of organ donation in familial, cultural, and political context. *Transplantation Reviews* 22 (3): 154–157. doi:10.1016/j.trre.2008.04.007.

Lundin, S. 2002. Creating identity with biotechnology: The xenotransplanted body as the norm. *Public Understanding of Science* 11:333–345. doi:10.1088/0963-6625/11/4/302.

Mazaris, E. M., J. S. Crane, A. N. Warrens, G. Smith, P. Tekkis, and V. E. Papalois 2011. Attitudes toward live donor kidney transplantation and its commercialization. *Clinical Transplantation* 25 (3): E312–E319. doi:10.1111/j.1399–0012.2011.01418.x.

Müller, S. 2010. Revival der Hirntod-Debatte: Funktionelle Bildgebung für die Hirntod-Diagnostik. *Ethik in der Medizin* 22 (1): 5–17. doi:10.1007/s00481-009-0044-5.

Muthny, F. A., and W. Schweidtmann. 2000. Einstellungen zu Hirntoddefinition, Organspende und Transplantation—Ergebnisse einer empirischen Untersuchung mit Ärzten. In *Einstellungen zur Organspende und ihre klinische Relevanz*, eds. H.-W. Künsebeck and F. A. Muthny, 55–68. Lengerich: Pabst Science Publishers.

Norris, G., F. Qureshi, D. Howitt, and D. Cramer. 2012. *Introduction to statistics with SPSS for social science*. Harlow: Pearson.

Ohnuki-Tierney, E. 1994. Brain death and organ transplantation. Cultural bases of medical technology. *Current Anthropology* 35 (3): 233–254. doi:10.1086/204269.

Ohwaki, K., E. Yano, M. Shirouzu, A. Kobayashi, T. Nakagomi, and A. Tamura. 2006. Factors associated with attitude and hypothetical behaviour regarding brain death and organ transplantation: Comparison between medical and other university students. *Clinical Transplantation* 20 (4): 416–422. doi:10.1111/j.1399–0012.2006.00494.x.

Rey, J. W., V. Grass, A. P. Barreisos, N. Haberstroh, C. Bahnemann, G. P. Hammer, U. Samuel, G. Otto, P. R. Galle, and C. Werner. 2011. Organspende in Deutschland. Eine regionale Umfrage unter Schülerinnen und Schülern. *Deutsche Medizinische Wochenschrift* 137 (3): 69–73. doi:10.1055/s-0031-1298796.

Sanner, M. A. 1994. Attitudes toward organ donation and transplantation. A model for understanding reactions to medical procedures after death. *Social Science and Medicine* 38 (8): 1141–1152. doi:10.1016/0277–9536(94)90229-1.

Sanner, M. A. 2001. Exchanging spare parts or becoming a new person? People's attitudes toward receiving and donating organs. *Social Science and Medicine* 52 (10): 1491–1499. doi:10.1016/S0277-9536(00)00258-6.

Schaeffner, E. S., W. Windisch, K. Freidel, K. Breitenfeldt, and W. Winkelmayer. 2004. Knowledge and attitude regarding organ donation among medical students and physicians. *Transplantation* 77 (11): 1714–1718. doi:10.1097/00007890-200406150-00015.

Schicktanz, S. 2007. Why the way we consider the body matters—Reflections on four bioethical perspectives on the human body. *Philosophy, Ethics, and Humanities in Medicine* 2 (30): 1–12. doi:10.1186/1747-5341-2-30.

Schicktanz S., Wöhlke, S. 2015. Leben im anderen: Übertragungsvorstellungen in der Organtransplantation zwischen kulturell Sagbarem und Unsagbarem. In: Kahl, A., Knoblauch, H., Weber, T. (Eds.) *Transmortalität und die Organspende*. Juventa [accepted]

Schipperges, H. 1989. *Die Welt des Herzens*. Frankfurt a. M.: Verlag Josef Knecht.
Schlitt, H. J., R. Brunkhorst, A. Haverich, and R. Raab. 1999a. Attitudes of patients towards transplantation of xenogenic organs. *Langenbeck's Archives of Surgery* 384 (4): 384–391. doi:10.1007/s004230050218.
Schlitt, H. J., R. Brunkhorst, H. H. J. Schmidt, B. Nashan, A. Havrich, and R. Raab. 1999b. Attitudes of patients before and after transplantation towards various allografts. Transplantation 68 (4): 510–514. doi:10.1097/00007890-199908270-00011.
Schweda, M., and S. Schicktanz. 2009. Public ideas and values concerning the commercialization of organ donation in four European countries. *Social Science and Medicine* 69 (6): 1129–1113. doi:10.1016/j.socscimed.2008.12.026.
Sharp, L. A. 1995. Organ transplantation as a transformative experience: Anthropological insights into the restructuring of the self. *Medical Anthropology Quarterly* 9 (3): 357–389. doi:10.1525/maq.1995.9.3.02a00050.
Sharp, L. A. 2001. Commodified kin: Death, mourning, and competing claims on the bodies of organ donors in the United States. *American Anthropologist* 103 (1): 112–133. doi:10.1525/aa.2001.103.1.112.
Siminoff, L. A., C. Burant, and S. J. Youngner. 2004. Death and organ procurement: Public beliefs and attitudes. *Social Science and Medicine* 59 (11): 2325–2334. doi:10.1016/j.socscimed.2004.03.029.
Stoecker, R. 2010. *Der Hirntod. Ein medizinethisches Problem und seine moralphilosophische Transformation*. Freiburg: Verlag Karl Alber.
Strenge, H., K. Laederach-Hofmann, B. Bunzel, and B. Schmeritschnig. 2000. Einstellungen zur Organtransplantation bei Medizinstudenten in Deutschland, Österreich und der Schweiz. In *Einstellungen zur Organspende und ihre klinische Relevanz*, eds. H. W. Künsebeck and F. A. Muthny, 22–37. Lengerich: Pabst Science Publishers.
Waldby, C., and R. Mitchell. 2006. *Tissue economies: Blood, organs, and cell lines in late capitalism. Science and cultural theory*. Durham: Duke University Press.
Wöhlke, S. 2013. The morality of giving and receiving living kidneys: Empirical findings on opinions of affected patients. In *Public engagement in organ donation and transplantation*, eds. G. Randhawa and S. Schicktanz, 144–153. Lengerich: Pabst Science Publishers.
Wynne, B. 2006. Public engagement as a means of restoring public trust in science—Hitting the notes, but missing the music? *Community Genetics* 9 (3): 211–220. doi:10.1159/000092659.

Sabine Wöhlke is a senior researcher at the Department of Medical Ethics and History of Medicine at the University Medical Center Göttingen. Dr. Wöhlke holds a degree in Cultural Anthropology and Gender Studies from the Georg-August-Universität Göttingen. In 2014 she finalized her PhD with the title: Medical anthropological and ethical perspectives towards decisions and motivations of living kidney donations, with a special focus on gender differences. Her main interests lie in ethical and medical anthropological research on organ transplantation, ethical aspects of genetic testing and predictive genetic testing and qualitative socio-empirical research.

Julia Inthorn is Senior Researcher at the Department for Medical Ethics and History of Medicine at University Medical Center Göttingen. Dr. Inthorn holds a degree in mathematics from the University of Munich as well as degrees in adult education and philosophy and received her PhD in philosophy from the Munich School of Philosophy in 2010. Her main areas of research in bioethics are ethical and philosophical questions of genetic risk, intercultural bioethics and empirical ethics.

Silke Schicktanz has been a full professor at the Department of Medical Ethics and History of Medicine at the University Medical Center Göttingen since 2010. Her research focuses on cultural and ethical studies of biomedicine. She studied biology and philosophy at the University of

Tübingen and finalized her bioethical PhD thesis on the ethics of xenotransplantation research in 2002. Her current research interests include cultural differences in bioethics (esp. organ donation, genetic testing, aging and dying, personalized medicine) and the normative structure of autonomy, trust, and responsibility.

Chapter 5
Foundations of a Duty to Donate Organs

Katherine Mendis

5.1 Introduction

Certain proposals designed to increase the supply of cadaveric organs suitable for donation, (e.g. confiscation of organs, an *opt-out* system, and various methods of compensation), are controversial in large part because many see cadaveric donation as a supererogatory act. The view that people are not obligated to make their organs available after death is based on Kantian respect for autonomy and a notion of rights derived from social contract theory. I look to both Kant and contractarian-informed views of free-riding to argue instead that making one's own organs available for donation after death is in fact a moral duty. According to a Kantian conception of a duty of mutual aid, we have a duty to respond to the true needs of rational beings when fulfilling such needs places little burden on us. And a refusal to donate organs entails the kind of indifference to interdependency that characterizes morally problematic free-riding. Accepting that cadaveric explantation is morally obligatory lends justificatory support to the proposals mentioned above, though I do not endorse any of them here.

5.2 Ethical Implications of the Organ Shortage

If the supply of suitable donated organs was sufficient to meet the need, arguing for a duty to make organs available would perhaps not be a wise allocation of philosophical capital. One might argue that although resolving the organ shortage would surely be a good thing, many other public health priorities are far more pressing. Still, the supply is woefully inadequate at present. This costly state of affairs has

K. Mendis (✉)
City University of New York, Graduate Center, New York, USA
e-mail: kmendis@gc.cuny.edu

R. J. Jox et al. (eds.), *Organ Transplantation in Times of Donor Shortage*,
International Library of Ethics, Law, and the New Medicine 59,
DOI 10.1007/978-3-319-16441-0_5

consequences that extend beyond aggregate suffering and loss of life, and raise concerns about justice and nonmaleficence.

According to the United Network for Organ Sharing (UNOS), as of January 8, 2010, there are 105,359 people registered on the waiting list for donated organs in the U.S. alone. More than 68 % of these candidates have been on the list for 1 year or more; more than 13 % have been waiting for more than 5 years. Yet each year for the last 10 years, the number of organ donors (both deceased and living) has hovered between 10,000 and 15,000, and decreased since 2006. The yearly number of transplants performed hovers between 21,000 and 28,000. Over 6000 patients die each year while awaiting transplants, an average of 18 patients each day.[1] The shortage of organs has additional costs: psychological harms to patients and loved ones, resources expended to provide continued care while patients wait, and resources expended on marketing campaigns to encourage more people to donate.

Recent years have seen an increase in the percentage of transplants performed with organs from living donors, due to both the shortage of cadaveric donations and advances in transplant medicine. In 1988, 14 % of transplanted organs came from living donors, while in 2008, 22 % came from living donors. Though exhaustive data on the outcomes is lacking, risks of morbidity and mortality are, of course, present for live donors. For example, a 2002 survey found that between January 1999 and July 2001, at least three kidney donors died and one was left in a persistent vegetative state as a direct result of their nephrectomies.[2]

The prospect of performing surgery on a healthy person, even in the most economically privileged of contexts, gives many of us pause for thought. But we cannot confine discussion of the organ shortage to its manifestations in the developed world. It is not surprising that some patients of means have not been content to languish on waiting lists, and have purchased organs on a burgeoning international black market, or through the ethically dubious Chinese system that harvests organs from executed prisoners.[3] These cases raise justice concerns insofar as they present an unfair advantage to the wealthy and exploit some of the world's most vulnerable citizens. They also raise nonmaleficence concerns, in that some of these donors are undoubtedly harmed (e.g. deceived, defrauded, coerced, or given inadequate follow-up care).[4] To perform transplants with the suspicion that the organs being transplanted may have been procured through shadowy networks that do not properly care for donors (who are also patients), or to provide follow-up care to patients who have procured their organs through these means, undermines the integrity of physicians, who, in addition to being charged with helping patients (under a duty of beneficence), are also to refrain from inflicting harm (a duty of nonmaleficence).[5]

[1] http://www.unos.org/data/.

[2] Leichtman et al., p. 138.

[3] Caplan (2012, p. 30).

[4] Rohter (2004).

[5] The idea of nonmaleficence dates back to the Hippocratic Corpus, and has been fleshed out more thoroughly in recent literature. Beauchamp and Childress (2008, pp. 113–119).

5.3 The Theoretical Foundation of a Duty to Donate Organs

My argument has some precedent in the literature on a duty to participate as a subject in biomedical research. Arthur Caplan draws on a Rawlsian view of *fair play*, in which "[t]he members of a cooperative group can legitimately expect each group member to accept the burdens and risks of participation" (Caplan 1984, p. 3). Rosamond Rhodes makes a more comprehensive argument with three parts. The first, the argument from justice, acknowledges that the medical innovations, from which we all might benefit, require sacrifice of "our flesh, our privacy, our safety, our comfort, and our time," as human subjects (Rhodes 2008, pp. 12–13). The argument from beneficence grounds our obligation in the Golden Rule and the interdependent reality of the human condition. Finally, the argument from self-development claims that it is essential to the exercise of our autonomy that we acknowledge our fragility, will that we be able to "fend off disease and disability," and will the necessary means to achieve it, i.e., a robust system of biomedical research (Rhodes 2008, pp. 12–13).

In ethical terms, organ transplantation differs from biomedical research in two important ways. First, principles of justice and self-development elegantly accommodate the case of biomedical research—from which we all benefit whenever we purchase over the counter painkillers. But it is less obvious that the system of organ donation and transplantation is a cooperative group that benefits all or even most of us. Second, the patient who languishes on a waiting list for an organ is a clear case of someone in need of direct assistance from another person; a general public group/class that hopes to benefit from biomedical research broadly is more difficult to cast in such a role. Still, there are similarities between the argument for a duty to participate in research and the argument I present in the following sections.

5.3.1 Mutual Aid

A Kantian approach helps us to account more fully for the unique moral facets of organ donation. The idea of respecting autonomy, on which some opposition to mandated organ donation is based, has deep roots in Kantian theory. It is important to keep in mind that autonomous agents are entitled to respect because they possess the capacities to formulate and abide by rational maxims. A Kantian examination of cadaveric organ donation shows that most maxims of non-donation are clearly irrational in a distinctly moral sense.

The CI-Test The First Formulation of the Categorical Imperative is well known: "Act only according to that maxim whereby you can at the same time will that it should become a universal law" (Ellington 1993, p. 421, cited as "*G*"). Evaluating a maxim according to this formulation is called the *CI-test*. There are two ways a maxim might fail:

> Some actions are so constituted that their maxims cannot without contradiction even be thought as a universal law of nature. In the case of others this internal impossibility is indeed not found, but there is still no possibility of willing that their maxim should be raised to the universality of a law of nature, because such a will would contradict itself (*G*: 424).

Kant provides four examples of duties that follow from application of the *CI-test*: duties to not commit suicide and refrain from false promises, and duties to cultivate one's talents and give to those in need. The first two duties hold because their contrary maxims (committing suicide out of self-love and making a false promise for personal gain) fail the *CI-test* due to a contradiction inherent in the maxims themselves, i.e. they contain what Christine Korsgaard calls a contradiction in conception.[6] We are subject to the second two duties because the contrary maxims (indolently failing to develop one's talents and indifferently failing to help the needy), while perhaps internally consistent, are examples of a simple contradiction in the will.[7]

Korsgaard considers how there can be "a *contradiction* in willing the universalization of an immoral maxim." She endorses a "Practical Contradiction Interpretation," in which the universalized maxim is seen as contradictory because it is self-defeating, "[…] your action would become ineffectual for the achievement of your purpose if everyone (tried to) use it for that purpose. Since you propose to use that action for that purpose at the same time as you propose to universalize the maxim, you in effect will the thwarting of your own purpose" (Korsgaard 1985, p. 25).

This interpretation gives a unified account of the kind of contradiction present in both the *contradiction in conception* and *contradiction in the will* cases. Both types of contradictory maxims are self-defeating when universalized. "The purpose thwarted in the case of a maxim that fails the contradiction in the conception test is the one in the maxim itself […]. The purpose thwarted in the case of the contradiction in the will test is not one that is in the maxim, but one that is essential to the will" (Korsgaard 1985, p. 40). The maxims that fail are "just those actions whose efficacy in achieving their purposes depends upon their being exceptional"; once they are subjected to the *CI-test* and their exceptionality is removed, they are seen to contradict the agent's purposes (Korsgaard 1985, p. 36).

A Duty of Mutual Aid Barbara Herman takes up the specific maxim of indifferent failure to help those in need (a maxim on nonbeneficence). Her analysis spells out in more detail how such a maxim is irrational, drawing on Kant's discussion of a case in which a man:

> […] finds things going well for himself but sees others (whom he could help) struggling with great hardships; and he thinks: what does it matter to me? Let everybody be as happy as Heaven wills or as he can make himself; I shall take nothing from him nor even envy him; but I have no desire to contribute anything to his well-being or to his assistance when in need […] even though it is possible that a universal law of nature could subsist in harmony with this maxim, still it is impossible to will that such a principle should hold everywhere as a law of nature. For a will which resolved in this way would contradict itself, insomuch

[6] Korsgaard (1985, p. 24).

[7] G: 422–424.

> as cases might often arise in which one would have need of the love and sympathy of others, and in which he would deprive himself, by such a law of nature springing from his own will, of all hope of the aid he wants for himself (*G*: 423).

Herman rejects the initially plausible interpretation that the duty to help those in need boils down to an insurance policy that any rational being ought to purchase, given the likelihood of needing assistance at some point in her life.[8] Instead, Herman claims that *in general*, if either "(1) there are ends that the agent wants to realize more than he could hope to benefit from nonbeneficence or (2) there are ends that it is not possible for any rational agent to forgo (ends that are in some sense necessary ends)," then the universalized maxim is irrational regardless of whether the agent has a prudential interest in insuring herself against genuine future needs (Herman 1984, p. 584).

Herman views the CI procedure as a mechanism to highlight the features of rational agents' condition as "members of a community of persons"—features that "serve as the condition of our willings." Thus in the case of a maxim of nonbeneficence, the test demonstrates that, "for any of us, the availability of the help of others is not something it can be rational to forgo." To support this thesis, she appeals to two hypothetical nonbeneficent agents: a stoic, committed to independence, and a wanton, who does not care whether any of her or his ends are realized. Even for the stoic, Herman claims, the maxim is irrational because her independence is itself an end to which the stoic is committed, and she may come to need the assistance of others in fulfilling that end (in, for example, distracting her from temptation to seek aid in times of difficulty).

The wanton is a slightly more complicated case. We are unlike him insofar as we may be unwilling to forgo certain ends, but we are like him in that some of these ends to which we are attached may conceivably be forgone. But, Herman argues, "[e]nds that are necessary to sustain oneself as a rational being cannot (on rational grounds) be given up," for the practice of having ends itself entails that "one has already willed the continued exercise of one's agency as a rational being" (Herman 1984, p. 586).

These ends—the fulfillment of which is required for a person's continuing function as a rational, end-setting agent—are called *true needs*. We cannot guarantee that we will achieve these ends, but neither can we rationally forgo them.[9] And the evidence for these true needs comes not from contingent features of our experience, but from "the natural limits of our powers as agents [...]. I may not be indifferent to others not because I would thereby risk the loss of needed help, but because I cannot escape our shared condition of dependency" (Herman 1984, pp. 587–592). Humans vary in their actual needs, but it is a fundamental truth that humans are the sorts of

---

[8] Herman (1984, pp. 579–582). The distinction between the irrationality of a maxim of universal indifference from a prudential irrationality is important for two reasons. First, Herman defends Kant from the charge that his project (of grounding a system of ethics on our rational nature rather than contingent features of our experience) is undermined by an empirical foundation. Second, in the case of organ donation, it is important to establish the irrationality of non-donation even if the willing agent is certain that he will never need a donated organ himself.

[9] Herman (1984, p. 586).

rational beings that depend on others. We are subject to the Categorical Imperative because we are rational beings, and subject to certain duties because of the type of rational beings that we are.

What Does Mutual Aid Require? Herman thus grounds a general duty of mutual aid, and turns to the task of articulating its contents. The moral character of the non-donating action is to be judged according to the character of its end, or the principle instantiated by the action.[10] The sorts of needs relevant to the duty of mutual aid are those *true needs* upon which our continued rational activity depends. The good that the duty looks to is "the preservation and support of persons in their activity as rational agents. The needs for which a person may make a claim under the duty of mutual aid are those which cannot be left unmet if he is to continue in his activity as a rational agent." Morally acceptable (rational) reasons for not helping those in need are those reasons that are weightier than the claim of need. And the only moral/rational justification for failing to act to meet the true needs of one's fellows is that so acting would place the agent's own rational activity in jeopardy. (Herman 1984, p. 597)

While there may exist an imperfect duty to share one's bounty with the less fortunate—imperfect in the sense that the agent has discretion about when and how to discharge the duty, mutual aid seems to be something different. If I encounter a situation in which I can ameliorate a threat to others' true needs without undermining my own, I am obligated to help, regardless of whether I helped yesterday and may have to help again tomorrow. Though I am free to determine the best strategy for administering aid, I am not permitted discretion in selecting among needy fellows so as to discharge a duty of mutual aid to humanity generally. I must respond to each individual case as it is presented to me, even if I am forced to provide more help than others must provide.[11]

Mutual Aid offers two prescriptions about organ donation. The first is that the plight of patients on waiting lists is to be regarded with the utmost seriousness. As the continuation of one's life is necessary for one's continued activity as a rational being, when confronted with the possibility that people will die if they are not provided with suitable donated organs, we must consider their plea as a claim falling under the duty of mutual aid.

The second point is that we are only permitted to deny this claim if meeting it would undermine our own true needs, so a negative response must be based on the potential cost to ourselves. Given the risks and burdens (scarring, lifestyle adjustments, etc.) of donating a kidney or a piece of one's liver and the fact that maintaining control over one's body is essential to continued existence as a rational being, the duty of mutual aid does not require living donation.

Cadaveric donation is another matter. We must be careful to consider the possibility that explantation of one's organs after death poses a threat to one's ability to continue as a rational agent. Pondering the specifics of one's mortality may cause some emotional distress, but it is difficult to see how such unpleasantness would un-

[10] Herman (1984, p. 595).

[11] Herman (1984, p. 596, 597).

dermine one's rational agency, burdensome though the distress may be. The possibility that a donor's life may be cut short prematurely (by a medical team's failure to take necessary life-saving measures out of a desire to explant organs expeditiously) looms in the imaginations of some, but this is generally not a realistic concern in the United States and Western Europe.[12]

It is conceivable that donors or families of donors might experience psychological trauma over imagining their body, or the body of a loved one, being altered by the harvesting procedures. While costs of this nature could be quite high for some, it is hard to imagine that they are ever high enough to undermine one's continued function as a rational being—to meet this standard, the trauma would need to produce a significant mental breakdown. Furthermore, many such costs are preventable; even a simple cultural shift toward recognizing cadaveric donation as a moral duty might mitigate some of the trauma.

We must also consider the potential cost of one's salvation that underlies some religious or otherwise conscientious objections to organ transplantation. We can deny or be neutral as to the metaphysical, or eschatological, claims of the conscientious objector and regard the cost as another form of emotional trauma. Or we can accept such metaphysical claims and acknowledge that being denied the opportunity to, for example, continue to exist as a rational being in the afterlife would certainly be a weighty cost. Some sincere religious believers will assess the costs according to the latter calculus and reasonably conclude that transplant candidates do not have a claim to their organs under the duty of mutual aid. The assumptions that underlie a society of reasonable pluralism (and the assumptions that underlie Kantian ethics!) suggest that we ought to evaluate religious cost according to the former calculus, but perhaps acknowledge that emotional trauma of this type is likely to persist even in the face of a cultural shift. Other (non-salvation-based) religious objections to organ donation could probably be categorized as persistent emotional cost as well.

Finally we must consider whether on principle, a legal requirement of cadaveric explantation itself undermines the rational activity of autonomous beings. Must we be permitted absolute control over the treatment of our remains in order to exist as rational beings while we are alive? While such a caveat, were it to be true, might render a policy of confiscation unjustifiable, it seems unlikely that the discretion to prohibit explantation after death is essential to rational activity, given restrictions on our bodies and our property that we readily accept, e.g. taxation and autopsy.

5.3.2 Rights and Free-Riding

We should bear in mind the tremendous waste involved in allowing usable organs to be interred with the corpses of their former bearers. We might consider in a similar

[12] Procedural requirements to prevent such a scenario might include strict criteria for defining death and strict separation of treatment teams and transplant teams. Furthermore, even if this concern were realistic, it is worth pointing out that such behavior would be motivated by a shortage of suitable donated organs. Measures to address the shortage would reduce pressure on transplant coordinators, and should thus diminish the specter of overzealous procurement.

light a wealthy person without heirs who makes no bequests. In such a case, the state would assume control over the deceased's assets. While we accept, either as a natural right or a social convention, her claim over her property and right to distribute it as she wishes, she does not have moral or legal license to simply throw it away, or render it unusable. Even during her lifetime, the woman's property rights would not allow her to literally burn her money; indeed taking currency out of circulation is a federal crime in the U.S (U.S.C. Title 18, Section 333).

We might be tempted to argue that unlike the use of currency, or even the dependence on medical services generally, organ transplantation is not an institution in which we all participate, so refusing cadaveric explantation would not run afoul of the demands of cooperative citizenship. But the above analysis of mutual aid also illuminates why the failure to make one's organs available upon one's death implicates the same moral concerns as free-riding.

The quintessential free-rider is the turnstile-jumper in the subway; she literally rides for free on a transit system funded by others. But what feature of this case is most salient to our moral condemnation of her actions? It is not simply that she benefits without paying. We are not likely to let her off the hook if she reaches the platform, learns that the train is out of order, and must walk to her destination instead. And if her fares were legitimately waived by a transit-voucher program for people with disabilities, she would still ride free, but her actions would be on different moral ground. The moral problem stems not from the benefit she receives, but the intention behind her refusal to give to a system that depends upon widespread cooperation. Similarly, those who use the term free-rider to critique social welfare programs use it most frequently to refer to those who could contribute more to society than they do. If both Mark and John decline to register for cadaveric organ donation out of general squeamishness and then Mark contracts hepatitis and receives a donated liver, we might be inclined to call him, and not John, a free rider, but it does not seem to make sense to say that Mark's prior refusal to release his organs differed morally from John's.

It seems that while the term free-riding implies receiving some benefit, the attitude of moral condemnation that underlies pejorative use of it turns on the content of our maxims, i.e., our grounds for action. In a sense, all maxims relating to conduct toward others that fail the *CI-test* are cases of free-riding; the false promisor free rides on promising, while the indifferent person free rides on the possibility of assistance. But simply calling all immorality *free-riding* threatens to strip the term of a meaning that seems to presuppose an institution or practice on which we *ride*. I suggest that acting on maxims that, if universalized, would eliminate institutions that are central to our human purposes is irrational in the same way that the turnstile jumper's behavior is irrational; they are attempts at free-riding even if they are ultimately unsuccessful.

If we were to will as universal laws maxims of non-donation (e.g., I will not agree to donate my organs because I do not want to incur the inconvenience of making my wishes known), the practice of organ donation would cease to exist. Insofar as we would like to receive organs if we need them, or we would like for our loved ones to receive organs if they need them, universalization of these maxims does not merely frustrate our general purpose in relying upon the help of others. It also specifically undermines a practice on which we would like to depend, one that serves our general purposes in continuing to exist as rational beings.

5.4 Conclusion

My argument undermines concerns that proposals such as confiscation, an opt-out system, or some sort of donor or family compensation system violate rights or fail to respect autonomy. It also undermines the claim that these more *aggressive* policies would unjustly affect disadvantaged or vulnerable populations. Should an unconscious patient present at an Emergency Room with acute appendicitis, consent for appendectomy is presumed, because it is a stretch of the imagination to conceive of rational reasons that a person might have for refusing the operation. We do not concern ourselves with the fact that a given patient may be relatively disadvantaged in his ability to make his preferences known to medical professionals—in this case, the extreme irrationality of refusal makes us comfortable with presumed consent. Re-orienting our thinking on organ donation could lead to a similar level of comfort with one of these proposals.[13]

References

Beauchamp, T, and J. Childress. 2008. *Principles of biomedical ethics*. New York: Oxford University Press.

Caplan, A. 1984. Is there a duty to serve as a subject in biomedical research? *IRB: A Review of Human Subjects Research* 6 (5): 1–5.

Caplan, A. 1992. *If I were a rich man could I buy myself a pancreas*? Bloomington: Indiana University Press.

Caplan, A. 2012. Polluted sources: Trafficking, selling and the use of executed prisoners to obtain organs for transplantation. In *State organs: Transplant abuse in China*, eds. D. Matas and T. Torsten, pp. 27–34. Woodstock: Seraphim Editions.

Ellington, J., (trans). 1993. *Kant's grounding for the metaphysics of morals*. Indianapolis: Hackett. (cited within as "G").

Etzioni, A. 2003. Organ donation: A communitarian approach. *Kennedy Institute of Ethics Journal* 13 (1): 1–18.

[13] A system of organ procurement that accepts the moral irrationality of unwillingness to make one's organs available could have the effect of transforming social mores and eliminating that very unwillingness. It often happens that when something achieves recognition as a moral or even merely a legal duty, popular sentiment swiftly rallies in support. There is some evidence that Kant would agree with this point, as he argues that if one exercises one's duty of beneficence "often and succeeds in realizing his beneficent intention, he eventually comes actually to love the person he has helped [...] do good to your fellow human beings, and your beneficence will produce love of them in you (as an aptitude) of the inclination to beneficence in general". Gregor (1996, p. 162). There is also evidence that Kant viewed the state's role in cultivating rationality and "removing potential barriers to morality" as an essential component in an individual's moral development. Surprenant (2006, pp. 90–111).

Giles, S. 2005. An antidote to the emerging two tier organ donation policy in Canada: The public cadaveric organ donation program. *Journal of Medical Ethics* 31:188–191.
Gregor, M., (trans). 1996. *Kant's metaphysics of morals*. Cambridge: Cambridge University Press.
Harter, T. D. 2008. Overcoming the organ shortage: Failing means and radical reform. *HEC Forum* 20 (2): 155–182.
Herman, B. 1984. Mutual aid and respect for persons. *Ethics* 94 (4): 577–602.
Hester, D (2006) Why we must leave our organs to others. *American Journal of Bioethics* 6 (4): W23–W28.
Howard, R. (2006) We have an obligation to provide organs for transplantation after we die. *American Journal of Transplantation* 6:1786–1789.
Korsgaard, C (1985) Kant's Formula of Universal Law. *Pacific Philosophical Quarterly* 66:24–47.
Matas, A., A. Leichtman, S. Bartlett, and F. Delmonico 2002. Kidney donor (LD) morbidity and mortality (M & M). *American Journal of Transplantation* 2 (Suppl. 3): 138.
Merle, J. 2000. A Kantian argument for a duty to donate one's own organs. A reply to Nicole Gerrand. *Journal of Applied Philosophy* 17 (1): 93–101.
Nelson, J. 2003. Harming the dead and saving the living. *American Journal of Bioethics* 3 (1): 13–15.
Nelson, J. 2005. Trust and transplants. *American Journal of Bioethics* 5 (4): 26–28.
Rhodes, R. 2008. Response to de Melo-Martin: 'On a putative duty to participate in biomedical research.' *Philosophy and Medicine, APA Newsletter* 7 (2): 12–13.
Rohter, L. May 23, 2004. The organ trade. New York Times.
Surprenant, C. 2006. Cultivating virtue. *Kantian Review* 12:90–111.

Katherine Mendis is a doctoral candidate in the Philosophy Program at the City University of New York Graduate Center. She is also an Ethics Fellow at the Icahn School of Medicine at Mount Sinai, and an Adjunct Lecturer at Hunter College. Ms. Mendis holds degrees in philosophy and history from George Mason University and The University of Chicago. She specializes in biomedical ethics and moral theory, with a current focus on property rights and feminist theory.

Chapter 6
Why Altruism is not a Convincing Argument for Promoting Post-mortem Organ Donation: Responsibility and Solidarity as Key Concepts

Diana Aurenque

6.1 Introduction: Altruism and Organ Transplantation

Altruism has played a central role in transplantation medicine throughout the history of the field. Even today, altruism is still considered to be an essential moral concept in the field of organ transplantation. A large number of medical associations and organ procurement institutions—such as the United Network for Organ Sharing (UNOS), the American Society of Transplantation (AST), The World Medical Association (WMA) and The German Organ Transplantation Foundation (DSO)—emphasize that altruism is morally appropriate, which constitutes the basis for the choice of donating organs. Also the Nuffield Council on Bioethics emphasized once again the special role of altruism for the donation of human parts in their report *Human bodies: donation for medicine and research* (2011), even when they outlined altruism in a particularly broad sense.[1]

The fact that altruism is one of the leading ethical principles in transplantation medicine goes along with at least two deep-seated moral intuitions: Firstly, the idea that the human body and its parts have a particular value, and secondly, that each and every individual has control over his or her own body. The latter refers to every human being's ability to decide how to lead his or her life and shape his or her

[1] "Altruism, long promulgated as the only ethical basis for donation of bodily material, should continue to play a central role in ethical thinking in this field. While some of the claims made for altruism may be overblown, the notion of altruism as underpinning important communal values expresses something very significant about the kind of society in which we wish to live. Understood in this way, altruism has much in common with solidarity: an altruistic basis for donation helps underpin a communal, and collective, approach to the provision of bodily material for others' needs, where generosity and compassion are valued". Nuffield Council on Bioethics (2011, p. 5).

D. Aurenque (✉)
Deparment for Philosopy, University of Santiago, Avenida Libertador Bernardo O"Higgins Nr. 3363, 9170022 Estación Central, Chile
e-mail: diana.aurenque@usach.cl

R. J. Jox et al. (eds.), *Organ Transplantation in Times of Donor Shortage*,
International Library of Ethics, Law, and the New Medicine 59,
DOI 10.1007/978-3-319-16441-0_6

own body, a fact that should apply even after one's own death. The idea that every human being has basic bodily rights that we ought to respect caters to this. The second intuition is related to the fact that organs do not constitute a product in the traditional sense of the word, in that they can neither be created nor produced. Thus, it is considered unacceptable that both the access and the distribution of organs are organized in the same sense as trading markets. Due to the special status of organs, one cannot manage their use in a market paradigm context in which conventional products are sold and purchased. In contrast to a market paradigm, the field of organ transplantation prefers a *system of giving*.[2] Thus, organ donation is seen as an act of giving, as long as it implies the *gift of life*. Such an act is voluntary and solely a result of good will and is considered to be altruistic due to the lack of personal gain. Despite the fact that organ donation seems to be regarded as an altruistic act, recently, a number of doubts and points of criticism about this assumption have been discussed.[3]

In this chapter, I will examine to what extent altruism arguments are likely to increase the willingness to donate organs. The working hypothesis is that altruism arguments are unsuitable for this purpose. In order to demonstrate this, I will first deal with the concept of *altruism*. In a second step, I will look into the motivational nature of altruistic actions and present this as a problem in the face of organ shortage. Due to the ethical and political challenge to tackle organ shortage—which means making the survival of seriously ill patients possible or to improve their quality of life—we urgently need binding measures. In a third step, I will suggest that not altruism but *solidarity* is the key word in promoting organ donation. For that purpose, I will argue that a model based on the value of solidarity is suitable to justify other policy interventions that might increase donation rates. Finally, I would like to draw attention to the meaning of justice (as fairness) for the success of these actions.

6.2 What are Altruistic Deeds?

Before searching for an acceptable definition of the concept, it may be wise to make an important distinction when speaking of altruism. This concept can be understood as a *motivation* to act in a certain (altruistic) way, but it may also refer to an (altruistic) *outcome* or result regardless of whether the motivation was also altruistic. In this chapter, I solely address the motivational understanding of altruism, inasmuch as that is the meaning that is considered to be essential in the field of organ transplantation.

Altruism is a term that goes all the way back to the early Stoics and is prevalent in Judeo-Christian tradition, as well.[4] However, it was August Comte who shaped

[2] Mahoney (2009); NHS Blood and Transplant (2012).

[3] Goodwin (2013); Saunders (2012); Moorlock et al. (2013).

[4] Maurer (1971).

the specific modern and secular notion of altruism[5] ("vivre pour autrui" [Schischkoff 1991, p.17]). In philosophy as well as in bioethics, different approaches have been proposed to outline whether altruism refers to a rational,[6] an emotional,[7] or an evolutionary[8] concept. Although one can find varying notions of altruism in literature, there is a general consensus on the fact that altruism is a motivated action that is performed for the benefit of somebody else's wellbeing. Altruism is therefore contrary to the term egoism, in that whereas selfish acts are an expression of exaggerated self-love, altruistic actions aim at benefiting the wellbeing of others: "altruism, in ethics, a theory of conduct that regards the good of others as the end of moral action" (Altruism *Encyclopædia Britannica* 2013). Altruistic actions are characterized by a genuine concern for others in an objective and impartial way[9] and their wellbeing. In addition to the central place of the other in altruistic actions, a *lack of self-interest* also seems to be an essential constituent of altruism. This lack of self-interest means that the altruistic agent does something for the benefit of another person without expecting any kind of reward; it is about an act of selflessness or even self-sacrifice. The altruist acts without expecting to benefit from the action in any way, whereas the egoist is not capable of such selflessness.

Regarding altruism as a motivation for altruistic actions generally entails the presumption that altruism is a genuine disposition. If deeds are done for the benefit of others, but are motivated by an external force that one does not regard as compulsory, then these are, strictly speaking, not altruistic actions. Altruistic acts that are not guided by an altruistic principle, such as norms expected by society or the denial thereof, do not arise from internalized values that have altruism as their basis. In order to call an act altruistic, it must have the ultimate goal of benefiting the wellbeing of others, but must also entail a certain amount of selflessness or at least a lack of concern for self-interests. This means that for the agent an altruistic act can have more risks and costs than benefits in pursuing the wellbeing of another person.

Seeing organ donation as an act of giving implies that this act cannot be coerced in order to be considered an altruistically motivated action. With regard to post-mortem organ donation, the existence of *informed consent* is the ethically legitimizing reason for the removal of organs. A person who gives informed consent to organ removal makes it possible for another person to potentially benefit from this decision. The individual's willingness to donate constitutes a good and selfless act.

[5] For Comte, moral obligations are not derived from theological precepts; instead, they are understood in the context of social relations. As a result of socialization, human beings are able to have inherently altruistic inclinations and prosper.

[6] Nagel (1979).

[7] Blum (2009).

[8] Batson (2011).

[9] Nagel (1979); De Wispelaere (2002).

6.3 The Problem with the Intentional Nature of Altruistic Actions

Regarding post-mortem organ donation as an altruistic act causes a problem for transplantation medicine. As long as there is an enormous gap between the supply of available organs and the demand for them, one may legitimately infer a moral obligation to solve the organ shortage crisis. This obligation concerns both the individuals' moral decisions on organ donation as well as the decisions on the matter in the form of public health policy.

The model of altruistic giving has not yet led to an increase in the willingness to donate. Since altruistic acts are always selfless or even acts of self-sacrifice, they cannot be brought about by force or coercion. The voluntary nature of organ donation should be put to the test using autonomous consent. Given the ethical and political challenges of solving the organ shortage crisis, which would mean improving or even saving the lives of many seriously ill patients, there is a need for regulatory measures that go beyond the model of altruistic giving. For this purpose, the altruism argument does not suffice; we must call for stronger and more convincing reasons to increase donation at both an individual and a general level.

6.4 Why Organ Donation is not an Altruistic Action

First, it should be stressed that a right to receive donor organs does not arise from the moral obligation to donate. It is important to remember that rights and obligations do not always go hand in hand.[10]

Second, recognizing post-mortem organ donation as a strong moral demand means not regarding it as an altruistic act, in that altruistic acts do not constitute moral duties due to their lack of self-interest; they are rather acts of supererogation[11]: "Supererogation is the technical term for the class of actions that go 'beyond the call of duty'". Roughly speaking, "supererogatory acts are morally good although not (strictly) required" (Heyd 2013). Therefore, supererogatory acts go beyond an obligation so that the abandonment thereof is morally justifiable from the very beginning. For example, it would be completely understandable if one starving person kept his or her last bit of food for him or herself without sharing with another starving individual. Consequently, it must be stated that altruistic acts should be carried out in moderation because otherwise they would be self-destructive. Motivational altruism calls for maximum ethical practice, an *opera supererogationis*, which, however, can be neglected due to the extremes of its nature. The most fa-

[10] Birnbacher (2008).

[11] Also McBride and Seglow understand altruism in relation to supererogation. McBride and Seglow (2003).

mous example of an altruist can be found in the Parable of the Good Samaritan (Luke 10, 25–37).

Post-mortem organ donation cannot be put on the same level as a supererogatory act, such as that of altruism. If a donor agrees to post-mortem organ donation during his lifetime, he is not in any way making a decision that would cause damage or pose a risk or cost to him or her for the benefit of somebody else, so there is no self-sacrifice involved.[12] This has to do with the idea that brain-dead individuals—despite the controversy surrounding brain death criteria—according to scientific knowledge can neither pursue verifiable interests nor suffer a loss as a result.[13] As Saunders claims, "since people's organs are of little use to them after they are dead, posthumous donors seem to sacrifice little or nothing" (Saunders 2012, p. 378). In contrast to the lack of harm for the donor agreeing to the donation, there are undisputable possible benefits to consider in relation to organ donation. As a result of the organ donation, the potential donor may even benefit from it in that he or she is deciding to make the best of his or her own death. The idea that death through organ donation becomes a more *meaningful death* makes it plausible why donation may also benefit the donor. In view of this case, the action by the donor cannot—strictly speaking—be regarded as altruistic because there is no lack of personal gain. However, shouldn't this lack of personal interest be expected if one considers the fact that organ donation does not inflict any harm upon brain-dead individuals?

6.5 Asymmetrical Structures and Responsibility

If post-mortem donors are brain-dead and they do not suffer any harm, according to the harm-benefit ratio, it becomes questionable as to why organ donation still has to be considered an altruistic act. Here it is important to point out structures of power and responsibility. Imagining a setting in which there are two equally needy people and only a single way in which help can be administered to them, a decision that only benefits the wellbeing of one of them cannot be conceived as an obligation to the other. But, if one assumes an asymmetrical structure in which one person could do *more* for the well-being of somebody else without suffering, then he or she has the *majority of the responsibility* and consequently, the majority of moral obligations[14]: "The fact that we can do more gives rise to the moral obligation to use this ability for the benefit of everybody" (Birnbacher 2008, p. 313).[15] If there is a clear asymmetrical power structure in a relationship, meaning that one individual can en-

[12] The largest religious communities consider organ donation as a good act for charity's sake, so even religious persons believe that post-mortem organ donation should not constitute harm.

[13] Wiesing (2012).

[14] This is the quintessence of the ethical philosophy from the French philosopher Emmanuel Levinas. Levinas (1984).

[15] Birnbacher says, „daß in puncto Organtransplantation die Sache einen vermehrten moralischen Druck rechtfertigt." Birnbacher (2008, p. 314).

sure that he or she will receive the other's organs after death, then he or she has an increased moral obligation towards the person in need. Provided that post-mortem organ donation does not constitute a self-sacrifice and greatly improves the quality of life or even saves the lives of seriously ill patients, there are good arguments in favour of speaking of a strictly moral and not just a supererogatory obligation.

6.6 Solidarity Instead of Altruism

Given the organ shortage, post-mortem organ donation should not be linked solely to the principle of altruism, but instead to a more suitable concept, namely to *solidarity*. In the Nuffield Council of Bioethics report from 2011, dedicated to the increasing importance of solidarity for bioethical issues, Prainsack and Buyx define solidarity as "shared practices reflecting a collective commitment to carry 'costs' (financial, social, emotional, or otherwise) to assist others" (Prainsack and Buyx 2011, p. 46).

Prainsack and Buyx emphasize the more practical orientation of solidarity in contrast to other more abstract values or sentiments, like altruism. However, in one matter this definition incorporates an important aspect of altruism in that Prainsack and Buyx consider solidarity to be a selfless act, which is disputable. Then solidarity also means a "feeling of belonging" and "pulling together for the sake of mutual interests and performing tasks" (Schischkoff 1991, p. 673.); and it goes along with the idea that cooperative actions entail both mutual benefits and obligations. Precisely this understanding of solidarity might serve as a more suitable moral reason to donate.

In the context of organ donation, this practice should be seen as a cooperative, solidary action that boosts both the wellbeing of others as well as that of the person performing the action. It is indisputable that actions benefitting both the self and others come about much more easily than purely altruistic actions. The reason lies in the fact that people performing the actions with a *mutual benefit* have more of an advantage than those not performing it. Thus, cooperative actions equilibrate an individual's concern for the self (*cura sui*) and the wellbeing of others.

Organ donation should therefore be regarded as a cooperative and solidary practice and not as a supererogatory action. The formula *helping others is also beneficial to me* could have a greater chance of solving the organ shortage crisis than the altruism argument. If we are willing to accept that altruism is not the only ethically acceptable justification for organ donation, as Saunders rightly proposes, we might be able to introduce other policy involvements that might help increase donations.[16] There is no doubt that cooperative models based on the value of solidarity, such as the model of reciprocity in organ donation, could obtain well-founded ethical legitimacy. Beyer defines the model of reciprocity as follows: "In the process of allocating scarce organs [for transplantation], people with documented willingness

[16] Saunders (2012).

to donate have priority" (Breyer 2008, p. 320). Another intervention can also be "allowing directed donation" (Saunders 2012, p. 1). Therefore, the willingness to donate can be considered a further criterion of allocation. Indeed, people without documentation will also get on the waiting list, but donors have priority.

The biggest problem with a cooperative model lies in the fact that popular opinion favours the model of giving, which leads to the assumption that policy-makers may be unwilling to change it.[17] Therefore, one should first highlight the compatibility of the cooperative model's value with existing and generally accepted values. Especially in welfare governments supporting fair and equal access to healthcare, in which the principle of solidarity is still going strong,[18] the implementation of the cooperative model would be easier than in other contexts. It is likely that an organized society based on the principles of solidarity is capable of valuing the benefits of cooperative actions in the field of organ transplantation.

Secondly, the potential conflict between the cooperative model and the respect for the individual's autonomy must be differentiated, in that autonomy is a principle that is highly regarded in pluralistic modern societies. Seeing organ donation as a cooperative act, as is the case in the model of reciprocity, results in the avoidance of the basic conflict of other models, such as in *opt-out* (presumed consent) and in *opt-in* systems (individuals are asked to register their willingness), in which two obligations collide: the obligation to help save a human life and the obligation to respect an individual's autonomy. As long as the model of reciprocity only forces one to think about one's own death and to state whether one is a donor or not, it does not touch on autonomy. The state does not presume, as the *opt-out* regulation does, that everyone is a potential organ donor. In the model of reciprocity, autonomy is merely somewhat restricted because one is asked to decide in favour of or against organ donation. Because of the moral duty to solve the organ shortage crisis, this minimal restriction of autonomy is justified. An incentive to donate, which would not only lead to a significant increase in organ donation but would also preserve autonomy, could be provided by supplying a donor with a donor organ more quickly in the event of organ failure. The third convincing reason to include organ donation in a model based on the value of solidarity relies on the fact that solidarity is a concept that works both as a moral guide for individual actions in a society as well as a "value capable of justifying the comparably stronger involvement of state authorities in public health" (Prainsack and Buyx 2011, p. 22). That is not the case for altruism.

6.7 Conclusion: The Success of Cooperative Actions

Altruistic actions are often referred to as an *act of love* or as an *act of giving*. Since altruistic actions are selfless, they cannot be forced upon an individual. Due to the ethical and political challenge to tackle organ shortage, I have argued that we ur-

[17] Steinmeier (2012).

[18] Prainsack and Buyx (2011).

gently need to adopt another way to understand organ donation, a way that goes beyond the classic altruism-based model. In this chapter, I have argued that organ donation should be understood as a form of social cooperation based on the value of solidarity, because with this rationale we might be able to increase donation.

However, in order to gain the support of the general public for post-mortem organ transplantation in the context of a solidarity-based model, it has to be reliable and trustworthy. For this purpose, it is essential that organs made available through acts of cooperation be fairly allocated so that the system of cooperation does not collapse. The negative effects of a loss of trust in transplantation medicine can be seen very clearly when looking at the transplantation controversy in Germany in 2012. In order to gain or regain the trust of the community, the allocation criteria and the concrete procedure of procuring organs have to be transparent and easy to understand. Furthermore, an increased amount of announced as well as unannounced inspections need to be carried out in the transplantation centres (by way of *redundant supervision*). Abolishing economic incentives for medical staff to avoid conflicting interests would also be advisable.

References

Altruism. 2013. In *Encyclopædia Britannica*. http://www.britannica.com/EBchecked/topic/17855/altruism. Accessed 20 March 2013.

Batson, C. D. 2011. *Altruism in humans*. New York: Oxford University Press.

Birnbacher, D. 2008. Organtransplantation - Stand der ethischen Debatte. In *Ethik in der Medizin. Ein Studienbuch,* ed. U. Wiesing. Stuttgart: Reclam.

Blum, L. A. 2009. *Friendship, Altruism and Morality*. Reissue edition (Routledge Revivals). New York: Routledge.

Breyer, F. 2008. Möglichkeiten und Grenzen des Marktes im Gesundheitswesen. In *Ethik in der Medizin. Ein Studienbuch,* ed. U. Wiesing. Stuttgart: Reclam.

De Wispelaere, J. 2002. Altruism, impartiality and moral demands. *Critical Review of International Social and Political Philosophy* 5 (4): 9–33.

Goodwin, M., ed. 2013. *The global body market: Altruism's limits*. Cambridge: Cambridge University Press.

Heyd, D. 2013. Supererogation. In *The stanford encyclopedia of philosophy* (Winter 2012 Edition), ed. E. N. Zalta. http://plato.stanford.edu/archives/win2012/entries/supererogation/. Accessed 20 March 2013.

Levinas, E. 1984. *Totalité et Infini*. 4. Aufl. Berlin: Springer.

Mahoney, J. D. 2009. Altruism, markets, and organ procurement. *Law and Contemporary Problems* 72:17–36.

Maurer, R. K. 1971. Altruismus. In *Historisches Wörterbuch der Philosophie,* eds. J. Ritter, K. Gründer, and G. Gabriel, vol. 1, 200–201. Basel: Schwabe

McBride, C., and J. Seglow. 2003. Introduction: Egoism, altruism and impartiality. *Res Publica* 9 (3): 213–222.

Moorlock, G., J. Ives, and H. Draper 2013. Altruism in organ donation: An unnecessary requirement? *Journal of Medical Ethics* 40: 134–138.

Nagel, T. 1979. *The Possibility of altruism. Reissue edition.* Princeton: Princeton University Press.

NHS Blood and Transplant. 2012. Organ donation. The gift of life. http://www.organdonation.nhs.uk/newsroom/fact_sheets/language_leaflets/organ. Accessed 20 March 2013.

Nuffield Council on Bioethics. 2011. *Human bodies: donation for medicine and research*. London: Nuffield Council on Bioethics.
Prainsack, B., and A. Buyx. 2011. *Solidarity: Reflections on an emerging concept in bioethics*. London: Nuffield Council on Bioethics.
Saunders, B. 2012. Altruism or solidarity? The motives for organ donation and two proposals. *Bioethics* 26 (7): 376–381.
Schischkoff, G. 1991. *Wörterbuch der Philosophie*. Stuttgart: Kröner.
Steinmeier, F.W. 2012. Organ donation is true solidarity. *European Journal of Cardio-Thoracic Surgery* 41 (2): 240–241.
Wiesing, U. 2012. Plädoyer zur Organspende: Mehr Mut für ein hilfreiches Geschenk. Spiegel Online. http://www.spiegel.de/gesundheit/diagnose/organspende-ethiker-plaediert-fuer-mehr-transplantationen-a-835319.html. Accessed 20 March 2013.

Diana Aurenque is professor at the department of philosophy at the University of Santiago of Chile (USACH). She has worked as researcher and lecturer in medical ethics at the Institute for Ethics and History of Medicine at the University of Tuebingen and also as an external lecturer for graduate and undergraduate programs at the University of Stuttgart and Freiburg, Germany. She studied philosophy in Santiago de Chile and completed her PhD at the University of Freiburg. Her research fields include the investigation of philosophy of medicine, German philosophy, philosophical anthropology, theoretical foundations of medical ethics, as well as the evaluation of problematic medical treatment on children (intersex-treatments, circumcision, etc.).

Chapter 7
Why Not Confiscate?

Christoph Schmidt-Petri

7.1 Introduction

There are two seemingly radical ways of resolving the problem of the shortage of organs available for transplantation. One is to create a (heavily regulated, to be sure) market for organs, in which people receive a financial or other incentive to increase the supply of organs, the hope being that given the right level of incentive, more organs will become available at a price worth paying, all things considered. Many object to this idea because they fear the commodification of the body,[1] the body being one of the last parts of our universe that the logic of markets has not yet managed to take over. The other way is to simply do away with any actual, presumed or hypothetical consent and to confiscate all suitable organs. In this chapter, I will discuss the ethical legitimacy of the latter option, also known as routine salvaging.

The most significant advantage of a policy of confiscation is not that the supply of organs becomes (pecuniarily) cheaper than it would be if there were a market for organs—it might not, as some compensation for the donor might still be deemed appropriate[2]—but that it becomes plentiful. Considering just Germany, a policy in which all people who have suffered brain death become organ suppliers (provided they are medically suitable) would allow all current demand for organs to be met.[3] So, at least at first sight, organ confiscation does solve the problem of organ shortage.

[1] Cf. e.g. Radin (1996); similarly Sandel (2012).

[2] Given that only brain-dead patients are suitable donors, which might raise a fairness issue as brain death is often caused by accidents.

[3] The data is presented in Sec. 3.3. However, as more organs become available, the structure of demand might also change, of course. Either way there will remain issues of justice in the distribution of organs—resulting in shortages of some sort—so a policy of confiscation does not provide a panacea.

C. Schmidt-Petri (✉)
Department of Philosophy, Karlsruhe Institute of Technoloy, Karlsruhe, Germany
e-mail: christoph.schmidt-petri@kit.edu

R. J. Jox et al. (eds.), *Organ Transplantation in Times of Donor Shortage*,
International Library of Ethics, Law, and the New Medicine 59,
DOI 10.1007/978-3-319-16441-0_7

This observation by itself would, it seems, only sound like a good reason to cold-blooded utilitarians for whom (according to the cliché) the ends justify the means, whatever they are. To most people, by contrast, the very idea of confiscating organs will sound utterly absurd. However, or so I will argue, reflecting on two practices currently considered ethically legitimate—at least in many countries—illustrates that it might not be. Additionally, the acceptability of these practices doesn't seem to depend on specific philosophical theories. They are, first, inheritance taxes, and, secondly, mandatory autopsies. Neither would provide sufficient legitimization for a policy of organ confiscation on its own. However, considered jointly, they seem to justify both a transfer of resources and the use of a dead person's body for the benefit of the living, to put it loosely.[4] Inheritance taxes show that it is considered legitimate for the state to take resources from a dead person in order to provide other people with certain benefits. In other words, they may constitute an *involuntary transfer of resources after death.* Inheritance taxes, however, do not concern the *body* of the dead person, but only his or her *external* resources, and that is clearly an important difference. However, *autopsies* do concern the body. The medical procedures performed during autopsies resemble that of an organ transplantation in that the body is opened and some (or all) organs are removed. In roughly half of all autopsies, consent by the patient or his/her relatives is not required by law. Thus, mandatory autopsies constitute an *involuntary opening of one's body involving the removal of organs after death.*

Thus, neither inheritance taxes nor mandatory autopsies require the consent of the dead, both are typically performed in order to benefit other people, and autopsies also involve opening the body of the deceased. In comparison, these practices are not that different from transferring body parts. So it seems there is a good argument starting with these widely accepted practices—widely accepted even by non-utilitarians, it seems—going to the widely rejected practice of organ confiscation. I briefly illustrate this further in sections two and three. In section four, I go on to discuss objections against this proposal based on concerns about the brain death criterion. In section five, I conclude that given the legitimacy of inheritance taxes and autopsies, routine salvaging is also legitimate; or, to put it more cautiously, if inheritance taxes and mandatory autopsies are (considered) legitimate, then so should routine salvaging.

7.2 Inheritance Taxes

7.2.1 Introduction

Whether inheritance taxes are just or not is a widely discussed issue on which there is neither consensus in theory nor in practice. Thinkers of a broadly egalitarian outlook will tend to believe that the wealth disparities the absence of inheritance taxes would make it easier to achieve are unjust, given that they are

[4] The analogy to inheritance taxes is discussed in Fabre (2006), the analogy to mandatory autopsies in Hershenov and Delaney (2009). My use of 'benefit' in this paper is intended to be theory-neutral.

highly unlikely to be consistent with equality (of opportunity, access to advantage, (of opportunity for) welfare/resources etc., as the case may be). Traditional right-libertarians such as Nozick tend to adopt a more individualistic perspective and given that compulsory taxation in general is, as Nozick carefully phrases, "on a par with forced labor" (1974, p. 169), inheritance taxes too are illegitimate. It is impossible to discuss this debate even in its rough outline here, so for the purpose of the argument I simply take the legitimacy of inheritance taxes, in one form or another, for granted.

In what sense are inheritance taxes analogous to organ transplantations? Three things seem clear: (i) they both occur after the death of the person (but see also section four below), (ii) they are not undertaken to benefit the deceased but in order to benefit somebody else, (iii), they involve the *transfer* of resources. The analogy seems quite strong. However, inheritance taxes do not involve the *body* of the deceased in any way. So we may assume that the legitimacy of inheritance taxes shows that there are legitimate involuntary transfers of resources after death, but not that they may involve the body of the deceased person. I will address this issue in section three after clarifying my analogy to inheritance taxes by discussing some possible objections to it.

7.2.2 Taxing and Confiscating are Two Different Things

The first objection questions whether levying a tax may really be equated with confiscation. A tax, so the objection goes, would only amount to a certain *percentage* of the bequest, and that doesn't amount to a confiscation. Besides, at least in many countries (such as Germany), inheritance taxes are only raised after certain tax-free allowances have been taken into account, and hence very few bequests are actually taxed.

This intuitively plausible set of objections is ultimately unconvincing. Taxing at a rate of, let's say, 20 % just means confiscating 20 %, while 80 % would indeed remain untouched. However, also in the case of organ confiscations, only a rather small 'percentage' of the body would be taken. Besides, given that brain death has to precede organ removal,[5] and the patient has to be in intensive care around the time of brain death, only about 0.5 % of deaths (again, in Germany) would be affected by routine salvaging.[6] Inheritance taxes, by contrast, have to be paid in about 13 % of cases.[7] Therefore, it is not true that inheritance taxes affect fewer people or are less onerous.

---

[5] I am ignoring donations after the circulatory determination of death as these are not legal in Germany at the moment. Including them wouldn't, it seems, substantially change the argument.

[6] The precise German figures for 2011 are: 852,328 deaths, of which about 400,000 occur in hospitals, about 1 % of which are brain deaths. See the records of the German statistical office (Statistisches Bundesamt 2012a, p. 1) and publications of the German Federal Centre for Health Education (BZgA), at http://www.organspende-info.de/organ (last access 15 July 2013).

[7] See Statistisches Bundesamt (2012b, p. 11).

7.2.3 What Would the Organs be Worth?

To the extent that organ confiscation is supposed to be similar to the taxation of bequests, it would seem natural to put (for instance) *one beating heart* in the list of objects the inheritance tax is to be calculated on. But how would that work? The only prices we have for organs are from the black market or are uninteresting for other reasons. Would we need a proper market for organs just to calculate the tax burden on organs?

This objection also helps to clarify the view I am discussing. A market in organs is not required for this proposal to work, nor does the analogy from inheritance taxes (or mandatory autopsies, for that matter) provide any justification for a market in organs.[8] The confiscation of organs would not *be* an inheritance tax. It would be *analogous to* an inheritance tax in that there is something the dead person may not authoritatively decide on after his or her death. It isn't actually a *tax* in the sense that an organ needs to be assigned a monetary value.[9]

7.2.4 But the Body is not a Resource!

The final objection to be discussed in this section is the most serious one. Even taking for granted, as I do in this chapter, that health is a matter of justice and that we are indeed morally required to support other people by providing them with health services, drugs, and maybe even with artificial limbs, if necessary and possible, the proposal under discussion seems to illegitimately treat parts of the human body just like any other object (like a crutch, for instance). But there is a long tradition, often and famously associated with Immanuel Kant's distinction between the *price* of objects and the *dignity* of all humans,[10] that asserts that a human being and his or her body requires fundamentally different treatment than objects in general.

It would be preposterous to deny that there is a very important difference between the human body and other objects—even if it is hard to pinpoint what exactly the difference is and what consequences it ought to have. Not just for reasons of space, I cannot offer a detailed view here. The most important reply is, I think, that whatever objections one could raise against organ confiscations on the basis of this difference would, at least *prima facie*, equally apply to mandatory autopsies (to be discussed in the next section), as during autopsies, the human body gets treated just like during an organ explantation. We cannot consistently claim that in one case, the autopsy, the dead body is treated with respect, or in accordance with its intrinsic

[8] Though this would have to be explored, it seems that organ confiscation would not, as a free market in organs might, contribute substantially to the commodification of the body. The reason seems to be that confiscation does not offer any additional incentives to the donor.

[9] If the confiscation of organs is not a tax, one might object, how are inheritance taxes supposed to provide evidence for their legitimacy? Yet, the argument is comparative—the confiscation of organs is supposed to be sufficiently similar to the taxation of bequests, even if it is not in itself a tax.

[10] See Kant's *Groundwork* (1785, p. 235f.) and Schmidt-Petri (forthcoming).

dignity or inherent worth (again, to put it loosely), but that in the other case, that of organ explantation, it would not be. Before discussing that reply, however, I would like to mention some less striking ones first.

First, we need to accept that not all material objects are *merely* material objects. Some material objects may have the same emotional value, make the same contribution to shaping one's personality or identity, or equally affect one's view of the world and emotional constitution as one's original body does. So if these personality-affecting features are what makes the body special, so are some material objects.

A very good example for this are musical instruments.[11] It is a common theme in classical as well as modern music that some instruments are not *just* objects to be treated like sound-producing tools, but are connected to the musician in a more fundamental way. They become important partners of the musicians and often even get given names.[12] However, if you were to own a Stradivarius at the moment of your death and nothing else, because nothing else mattered to you during your life other than your music, and that Stradivarius was *the* instrument you actually needed to play in order to make the music *your* music—that instrument was part of yourself, as some musicians put it—you nevertheless do not have the right to dispose of it the way you would like to at the time of your death. People realise very well that a Stradivarius is not to be treated like any other object, but its material worth will nevertheless figure in the inheritance tax calculation. If it is possible to treat such quite unique material objects with the appropriate understanding of their peculiarities, but still treat them like material objects nonetheless,—in fact, it is appropriate in this case to say the Stradivarius gets treated like a commodity—it should be possible to respect the dead body as something very special but nonetheless treat it like a material object in some sense—not by putting a price tag on it, but by accepting that removing some of the organs for transplantation will provide benefits to other people.

Secondly, we shouldn't deny the fact that many people do not consider their own body be that special after all, especially after death. If almost 75 % of people say they are in principle agreeing to donating their organs after death,[13] it would be quite strange to claim that, for these people, the body actually is not a fungible resource in the relevant sense, at least at that moment. Certainly current practice and its general endorsement *presuppose* that it is entirely normal to treat the organs of a brain-dead person as resources (or if it's not normal yet, then at least those organisations which are promoting transplantations think that it ought to be normal). Though it is true that, currently, donors have to consent to the donation, people don't conceive of that decision as something that somehow *turns* one's organs into a resource and that *that* decision ought to be up to the person whose body it is. Rather, it seems everybody

[11] An even more obvious (though in its details slightly different) example would be a material object that takes over a function normally performed by an organ—a cochlear implant (a bionic ear), for instance.

[12] For instance, Eric Clapton's *Blackie* Fender Stratocaster or Neil Young's *Old Black* Gibson Les Paul. These are not special in any obvious sense (e.g., made of some particular or precious materials), they just happen to be the right guitars for these artists.

[13] The data is from 2010, see BZgA (2010, p. 37).

agrees that the body of a brain-dead person *is* a resource, but that the person whose body it is should have the right to decide what happens with it after their death. On that view, we do not have to decide *whether* to treat the body as a resource—it clearly is. We do have to decide who will be entitled to decide what happens to it. In that sense, my suggestion is to treat (some of the relevant parts of) the body like an external material good of a dead person.

7.3 Mandatory Autopsies

7.3.1 Introduction

The practice of autopsies has a documented history of about 5000 years. Even though it hasn't always been popular or even legal throughout human history, it is clearly an extremely well established method of medicine and widely practiced today. Several tens of thousands of autopsies take place in the USA and Europe every year. In Germany, about 5 % of all deceased (that is, currently about 40,000 people) are autopsied every year, and the rates are a multiple of that in many other countries (they are six times as high in Finland, for instance). At least in Germany, every deceased person has to be autopsied if the cause of death is unclear, which is the case in about 2 % of all deaths (that is, in about 16,000 cases). For any organ transplantation (there are about 1200 in Germany a year), then, there are about 33 autopsies, of which thirteen are mandatory.[14]

Mandatory autopsies and organ transplantation also appear analogous: (i) both occur after the death of the person (but see section four below), (ii) they are not undertaken to benefit the deceased but in order to benefit somebody else[15] and (iii) they involve the opening of the dead body and the removal of some organs.

We have already seen that inheritance taxes and organ transplantations share the first two features. In the present section, the third feature is of paramount importance. During an autopsy, the body of the deceased is treated more or less like it would have to be treated during an organ explantation. That is, the torso is cut open from the shoulders down to the pubic bone, the ribs are sawn to get access to the heart and lungs, which are then removed together with the other organs, either *en bloc* or individually, to be examined further. The only essential difference to organ transplantations, it seems to me, is that the organs don't actually get transplanted to anybody else. Their subsequent examination, however, might go well beyond what would be taking place in an organ transplantation: for instance, the organs might

---

[14] Such mandatory autopsies, which do not require even hypothetical consent of the deceased or his or her relatives cannot be undertaken at the discretion of a medical doctor only, but have to be authorised by a state prosecutor (or a coroner).

[15] Whether by enhancing national security through improving crime detection or by enhancing national health by improved disease detection, in the case of mandatory autopsies, or the organ recipients in the case of organ transplantations.

be cut into slices for further examination. Furthermore, the skull is usually opened (with an oscillating battery saw) to examine the brain, which will be removed from the skull—a rather shocking procedure which is never performed for organ transplantations, of course.[16] After the autopsy and organ explantation have taken place, the bodies are treated similarly. In neither case will all organs be put back into the body in their entirety as they will either have been transplanted or damaged. So it is safe to say that as far as the invasiveness (or impact on bodily integrity) of these procedures is concerned, an autopsy is at least as invasive, if not more invasive, than an organ explantation. So if nobody objects to mandatory autopsies, why do many people object to organ confiscation? In what ways are the two practices different, or at least appear to be different?

7.3.2 Crime Prevention is more Important

One objection which seems to appear valid to many people is the following: isn't it more important for society that autopsies are undertaken in order to detect and hence prevent violent crimes than to keep some people alive for a little bit longer through an organ transplantation? This objection to the analogy has a certain *prima facie* plausibility. There does seem to be an important difference here. It seems as though murder, which is typically violent, sudden and can potentially occur at any age, is in some sense worse for the person affected than dying because of organ failure, typically a slow process and with enough time to prepare oneself for death, and typically occurring at old age. Hence, it seems as though less needs to be done to prevent the latter. So it might turn out that mandatory autopsies are legitimate but organ confiscations are not.

The role of autopsies in crime prevention should not be exaggerated, however. There are 'only' about 1000 cases of murder or manslaughter in Germany a year of which more than 95 % are solved[17]; even if we grant—very generously, it seems—for the sake of argument that in half of these cases the autopsy of the victim was necessary to detect the murderer, it still seems unlikely that the net benefit of this policy in terms of lives saved (by deterrence of further crimes) will amount to 1000 lives, which is roughly the number of people who could be saved a year if enough organs were available. Yet, unless mandatory autopsies save significantly more lives than could be saved through organ confiscation, it seems strange to claim that they are much more important.

However, let's grant the hypothesis that 1000 lives are saved a year through the practice of mandatory autopsies, and let's also assume that it is worse to die by getting murdered than it is to die from organ failure. Even so, the figures don't seem to add up. 16,000 mandatory autopsies are performed to save (according to

---

[16] The actual procedures during an autopsy also depend on the objective and condition of the corpse. My description is supposed to present a typical autopsy where the cause of death is unknown.

[17] Consistently since at least 1998. See Bundeskriminalamt (2013, p. 31).

the generous assumption) 1000 people, but given that each organ donor provides us with three organs on average, we would only need about 330 donors (of about 4000 brain deaths annually in Germany) to save the 1000 people in need of an organ.[18] It can't plausibly be claimed that it's worth 16,000 mandatory autopsies to save 1000 potential victims of crime but it is not worth 330 organ confiscations to save 1000 people in need of an organ.[19] Dying from violent crime, if worse at all, is not *that much* worse. Thus, the alleged superior importance of crime prevention through mandatory autopsies is not a good argument against organ confiscation.

7.3.3 Crime Prevention is Indeed more Important, but in a Different Sense

However, there is a better variant of the preceding objection. It might be claimed that I deliberately misrepresented the point of the objection. The objection was not meant to be that death through murder is worse *for the dying person* than death from organ failure. The objection was also not meant to be that mandatory autopsies were more (or at least equally as) efficient in saving lives than organconfiscations would be. The objection was that murder is *politically* more important than organ failure.

There does seem to be something to this objection too. Organ failure, one might say, is a *private* problem; murder is a *political* one (in some sense to be explored, and assuming that organ failure is not caused by state action). We welcome and encourage help from other people in our private lives and in extreme cases, such as road accidents, even use the criminal law (at least in some countries) to enforce our moral duties to provide help to our fellow citizens when there is nothing of obvious political importance at stake, provided the help can be given at a comparably low cost to the helping person. However, such an extreme invasion of privacy like opening someone's body without consent, even if it takes place after their death, may only be performed if something of political importance is at stake.

This could be spelled out as follows: the prohibition of physical violence (such as murder, manslaughter, grievous bodily harm, etc.) is a fundamental rule that, more than any other rule, actually contributes to the functioning of our community and thus also symbolises how our community is supposed to work, namely that (to put it loosely, once more) the peaceful coexistence of all citizens is a non-negotiable precondition. And to protect this fundamental value, we will go *very* far—so far as to do things which are normally unthinkable, namely opening each other's dead bodies in order to find out whether the deceased has been a victim of physical violence.

[18] Obviously, this is a rough and ready calculation and valid only on average, as the organs supplied might not match the organs required.

[19] To put the point differently: if mandatory autopsies ought to be as efficient in deterring murders as organ confiscation is in saving lives, then, given that one confiscation saves about three lives, the 16,000 mandatory autopsies ought to deter 48,000 murders. If at the moment only about 1000 murders occur in Germany per year, that seems highly unlikely.

This is a very complicated issue and I can only offer hints as to how some of the replies to it might sound. On one reading, this objection simply begs the question. *Why* is the state only concerned with the *politically* important murder but not the *private* organ failure? What exactly is political about murder, and on what theory? Does it really make much of a difference to the dying person whether it's her organs that fail by themselves or whether she gets shot in one of them? Or is the state saying that it should make a difference? If she can't help herself in either case and thus needs and may be presumed to be requesting help from her fellow citizens, why differentiate between these causes of death? Would it then appear more important to her fellow citizens to concentrate on the murder rather than on the organ failure? Far from being politically justifiable, doesn't this appear deeply *unfair* to the victim of organ failure?

It seems easy to agree that if murder was so prevalent that our states were at the verge of breaking down, priority should be given to the detection of murder. But, as discussed, that is not how our societies look like at the moment. Nor is it even clear that it's in the non-victims' selfish interest to fight murder harder than organ shortage, given that they themselves are far more likely to die of organ failure than of violent crime. It seems that without a complete theory of the political realm, this objection is hard to assess. Though it seems misguided to me (especially for societies which do accept compulsory health care), I accept that I haven't refuted it.

7.4 The Brain Death Criterion

A much more serious objection may be raised by doubting the legitimacy of the brain death criterion. Brain death is a medically necessary precondition for organ explantation.[20] But what if somebody believes that a brain-dead human being is not *truly* dead? This is one of the oldest objections to transplantations after postmortem donation: organ transplantations are illegitimate because brain-dead humans are not *truly dead* (though their brain might be), and hence they are killed in the process of explantation.

This is a rather weak argument if it is directed against organ transplantations in general. But for the same reason it is in fact a very good argument against organ confiscation. Let's take it for granted that there is persistent disagreement about when a human being is *truly dead* (or, to put it less metaphysically, under what circumstance he or she is in the suitable condition for an organ explantation to legitimately take place) that we shouldn't simply ignore. Still, this disagreement needn't by itself lead to problems in practice. If, say, I happen to believe that the cardiopulmonary definition of death is the adequate definition of death, so that brain-dead humans are not *dead enough*, while acknowledging that others disagree with me, for instance the legislator, I should simply refuse to have my organs explanted. There is no need

[20] Again, I am ignoring the issue of donations after the circulatory determination of death. My objection would not apply to them, but other, stronger objections would.

to worry or to find an agreement about the *one and only* definition of death if people are given a choice when their organs may be legitimately explanted.

Confiscating organs means I am not given that choice. Thus, under a policy of organ confiscation, I run the risk of being killed (according to my standards) in the process of explantation if I disagree with the brain death criterion. The risk of my being killed is a valid reason, it seems, to find organ confiscation objectionable as a general practice (even if humans with a dead brain will typically die soon anyway).

So this is where the analogy to mandatory autopsies breaks down. Autopsies, whether voluntary or mandatory, are always performed on humans who are dead on *any* (reasonable) standard. To put it differently, autopsies necessarily satisfy the dead donor rule. Yet, a policy of organ confiscation would not. It would only satisfy the dead donor rule on the brain death criterion, which many people disagree disagree with (also see Truog 1997).

This is not to say that organ confiscation is illegitimate. The argument simply shows that there is a tension. To the extent that the brain-death criterion is considered legitimate, the case for organ conscription goes through. The difference between autopsies and organ explantation then is not being denied, it is just not deemed relevant. But it is relevant to whoever disagrees with the brain death criterion—a policy of organ transplantation that requires consent allows for such disagreement. Essentially, it allows people to choose the criterion of death they want to subject themselves to.[21]

7.5 Conclusion

I have argued for the following claim: if inheritance taxes and mandatory autopsies are legitimate, then so is organ confiscation. Inheritance taxes by themselves legitimise the transfer of resources but not of body parts specifically; mandatory autopsies by themselves legitimise organ removal but not their transfer. And neither of the two require consent. Taken together, organ confiscation turns out to be justified—at least if the brain death criterion is accepted.

References

Bundeskriminalamt (BKA). 2013. *Polizeiliche Kriminalstatistik 2012*. Wiesbaden: BKA.

Bundeszentrale für gesundheitliche Aufklärung (BZgA). 2010. *Einstellung, Wissen und Verhalten der Allgemeinbevölkerung zur Organ- und Gewebespende*. Köln: BZgA.

Fabre, C. 2006. *Whose body is it anyway?* Oxford: Oxford University Press.

Hershenov, D. B., J. J. Delaney. 2009. Mandatory autopsies and organ conscriptions. *Kennedy Institute of Ethics Journal* 19:367–91.

Kant, I. 1785. *Groundwork for the metaphysics of morals,* Thomas E. Hill Jr. and Arnulf Zweig (eds.), Oxford: Oxford University Press 2002.

[21] I discuss some of these issues at greater length in Schmidt-Petri (2013).

Nozick, R. 1974. *Anarchy state and utopia*. Oxford: Basil Blackwell.
Radin, M. 1996. *Contested commodities*. Cambridge: Harvard University Press.
Sandel, M. 2012. *What money can't buy*. New York: Farrar, Straus and Giroux.
Schmidt-Petri, C. 2013. Erbschaftssteuern, Obduktionen und die Posthume Konfiszierung von Organen. *Was dürfen wir glauben? Was sollen wir tun?—Sektionsbeiträge des achten internationalen Kongresses der Gesellschaft für Analytische Philosophie e. V.* M. Hoeltje, T. Spitzley und W. Spohn (eds.). Online publication of the University of Duisburg-Essen (DuEPublico).
Schmidt-Petri, C. (forthcoming). Kant on Owning and Giving Away one's Body. *Kant-Studien Supplement* (Kant Congress Vienna) 2015.
Statistisches Bundesamt. 2012a. *Gesundheit. Todesursachen in Deutschland*. Wiesbaden: Statistisches Bundesamt.
Statistisches Bundesamt. 2012b. *Finanzen und Steuern. Erbschaft- und Schenkungssteuer*. Wiesbaden: Statistisches Bundesamt.
Truog, R. 1997. Is it time to abandon brain death? *Hastings Center Report* 27:29–37.

Christoph Schmidt-Petri is lecturer in Practical Philosophy at the Karlsruhe Institute of Technology. He received his doctorate in philosophy at the London School of Economics and Political Science with a thesis on John Stuart Mill's *Utilitarianism*. His research areas are moral and political philosophy, and he has published in journals such as The *Philosophical Quarterly, Philosophy of Science* and the *Journal of Value Inquiry*.

Chapter 8
The Theological-Ethical Dimension of Organ Transplantation in the Context of Contemporary Discussions

Konrad Hilpert

8.1 Introduction: The Ethical Dimension

Organ transplantations are not only a highly complex and challenging matter from a medical point of view; they also raise extensive ethical questions. This has to do with the fact that the procedure of transplanting organs between individuals requires two separate processes—donating and receiving –, which both have to be arranged by the institutions that are responsible for each respective process. In other words, curing or relieving *one* human being's suffering depends on *another* human being giving up a part of his body and donating it to the recipient (directly in the case of a living donation, and anonymously in the case of a post mortem donation). This raises such questions as to what extent the body is a part of our ego (self) or also then becomes the ego of the other person. In addition, the question is raised whom our body belongs to and what we can accept and also expect from others. In conclusion, how should we handle the transplanted part that belonged to a stranger so that it becomes a part of us and that we can then consider our own? These are all questions that mainly concern the *recipient.*

A second round of ethical discussion concerns the *donor*: In contrast to other medical interventions, the removal of an organ is not a curative procedure. Thus, removing an organ from a living person contradicts the principle that an intervention should only be permitted if it serves the benefit of those involved. In the case of a deceased individual, it contradicts the principle of deference. Under what circumstances can the benefit of the recipient, which is undoubtedly a given fact, outweigh the principles of these fundamental rules? What role does respecting the autonomy of the donor play or what role should it have to play? How can the risk and damage for the donor be reduced?

K. Hilpert (✉)
University of Munich, Munich, Germany
e-mail: hilpert@kaththeol.uni-muenchen.de

R. J. Jox et al. (eds.), *Organ Transplantation in Times of Donor Shortage,*
International Library of Ethics, Law, and the New Medicine 59,
DOI 10.1007/978-3-319-16441-0_8

In the end, there is a discrepancy between the demand and need for transplant *goods* and the available supply of donor organs. However, when a commodity is sacre the question is raised of whether this scarcity can be remedied by increasing the amount of supply. If this is not possible then the question of the *distributive equity* of the scarce good arises. This is the third ethical round of discussion: What criteria does the distribution of organs have to follow in order to comply with the fundamental principle of fairness?

These are the three ethical rounds of discussion that serve as the categories that questions from contemporary dialogs on organ transplantation can be placed in.

8.2 Current Issues

It is a known fact that the organ transplantation system in Germany has been subject to criticism for quite some time.

It started with a few federal German states that advanced a legal reform in May 2011 concerning organ donation. The aim behind this initiative was to increase the provision of donor organs. The facts that led to the launch of this reform were the statistics showing that Germany ranked quite poorly in the overall comparison of organ donors in European countries. Among the approximately 12,500 registered recipients who are waiting on a donor organ, one out of every three—which amounts to approximately 1000 people per year—die before they are able to receive the life-saving transplant. These are just numbers, but these numbers also signify the fate of individuals including young people and children, who have to live their lives under restricted conditions on a daily basis, which most of us cannot even begin to fathom. Part of the blame needs to be placed on the mandatory consent(opt-in) law, which has been in place in Germany since 1997 (Transplantationsgesetz) and relies solely on the moral plea to all German citizens to fill out and carry a donor card with them at all times. The indication that one of the reasons behind organ scarcity lies in the "non-exploitation of donor potential" was mentioned in a statement made by the National Ethics Council in 2007 (Nationaler Ethikrat 2007, p. 18). A political effort to increase the number of organ donations led to a cross-party decision in the German Federal Parliament in May 2012, amending the German transplant law in the sense that all German citizens over the age of 16 are prompted by their health insurance provider every two years to declare their willingness to be a registered organ donor (cf. Gesetz). To what extent this so-called "declaration law" serves as an adequate instrument in resolving the problem of organ donor scarcity or at least abating it is yet to be determined.

In the meantime, another debate has ensued, which has a long-standing history but was considered to be resolved for the last few years,[1] concerning the question

[1] Cf. Johannes Hoff & Jürgen in der Schmitten (ed.), Wann ist der Mensch tot? Organverpflanzung und Hirntodkriterium, Reinbek 1994; Ralf Stocker, Der Hirntod. Ein medizinethisches Problem und seine moralphilosophische Transformation, Freiburg i. Br./München 22010; Thomas Schlich

of whether the prerequisite stated in most transplant laws that the donor has to be declared brain dead prior to removing vital organs means that the donor is actually dead. This is by no means merely theoretical, but rather an important practical question in that if one is willing to donate his organs then he would like to be 100 % sure that he will be dead when his organs will be removed. There have always been doubts concerning whether or not brain death permits the general declaration of death (Jonas 1985, pp. 219–241), but these are individual voices that can be refuted by the extensiveness of mandatory diagnostics in Germany on the one hand, and the clarification of the difference between brain death and a persistent vegetative state on the other hand. A much greater amount of diesquiet emanated from movies and television, which made the public conscious of the discrepancy between the expectation of what a deceased individual usually looks like and the actual perception of someone who is brain dead, especially in some very rare cases in which pregnancies of women who were brain dead were pursued over the course of many weeks. A significant amount of attention has been allotted to the arguments presented by individual neurologists (Shewmon 2009, pp. 18–24) who challenged the central assertion that the death of the brain equals the death of the individual. This usually justifies the diagnosis of brain death as the prerequisite for organ extraction in that the death of the brain signifies the failure of the *control center* responsible for the integration of the various internal circuits into the organism as a whole. These doubts and concerns received more attention after being taken into serious consideration in a memorandum (*Controversies in the determination of death*) presented by the President's Council on Bioethics appointed in 2008 by the former President of the United States George Bush. Pro-life activists all over the world have adopted this memorandum, yet they have concealed the fact that the report does not directly oppose the practice of declaring brain death as such, but rather it addresses the need to substantiate each individual declaration more precisely, given the improved and advanced knowledge and research on the matter.

In my opinion, it is important to remember and be conscious of the following facts with regard to this discussion: It is not medically or scientifically possible to determine what death is and when exactly it occurs. Strictly speaking, the declaration of brain death is nothing more than a physiological indicator and an empirical criterion for the determination of the death of an individual. However, the same holds true for cardiovascular death, which for the last few centuries has been considered the ultimate end of life and the separation of body and soul.

Another question is how feasible the chosen indicator is and how sure one can be in determining whether or not it actually ocurred. The highest level of agreement, which has become a part of the official guidelines of the German Federal Medical Association, lies in the fact that the proof of the irreversible malfunction of the brain in all three areas (cerebrum, cerebellum, and the brain stem) counts as the defini-

& Claudia Wiesemann (ed.), Der Hirntod. Zur Kulturgeschichte der Todesfeststellung, Frankfurt a. M. 2001; Hans Münk, Das Gehirntodkriterium in der theologisch-ethischen Diskussion und die Transplantationsmedizin, in: ders. (ed.), Organtransplantation. Der Stand der Diskussion im interdisziplinären Kontext, Freiburg (CH) 2002, pp. 105–173.

tive sign of a person's death. Even if, given the most recent objections, one doubts that the brain's functionality is overestimated in the brain death concept and other organ's input in maintaining the entire organism is underestimated, it remains a fact that the malfunctioning of the brain in brain death is irreversible even when applying mechanical support, as is similarly the case with the body of a person who is brain dead and cannot use spontaneity and strength to keep vital functions going. In this respect, one can legitimately deny the brain death criterion in their individual case, but these doubts do not justify publicly discrediting this criterion as being *deceptive*.

At approximately the same time yet, without any apparent factual connection to the donor regulation and the brain death discussion, a third discourse was established concerning the appropriateness of established clinical transplant decision-making processes. Initially, this discourse was concerned with accusations against the board of directors of the German Organ Transplantation Foundation and whether the government should assume a stronger position of control within this sensitive field. Ultimately, the business of donating organs is nothing less than "the distribution of a chance at life" (Höfling 2012). The fact that the risks involved in this line of work are not fictitious by any means became evident in the irregularities that have occurred since July 2012 at the University Hospitals in Göttingen, Regensburg, Leipzig, and Munich, now known as the organ donor scandal. The ethical focus of these irregularities was that medical information was forged in order to grant certain patients (a few dozens in total) donor organs before it was their turn on the waitlist. This, in turn, means that those individuals who are next in line on the waitlist have to wait even longer and it could also lead to their death. This type of behavior is highly deceptive and makes people lose trust in the distribution system as a whole. It follows the aim to guarantee a fair distribution of the scarce amount of donor organs available, which in this case means that the person's standing and all types of financial motives are to be completely disregarded. Thus, it is vital to agree on both intensifying subpoena law and to observe false incentives within the system (cost pressure, premiums, number of cases, competition between hospitals, prestige, etc.) in order to improve the structure of making these decisions.

8.3 Theological Dimension

Ever since organ transplantation has become a realistic option, it has become the subject of intense theological reflection.[2] This reflection was mainly dedicated to the ethical evaluation of donating organs. After initial doubts and concerns, since

[2] Cf. Mark Achilles, Lebendspende—Nierentransplantation. Eine theologisch-ethische Beurteilung, Münster 2004, pp. 202–310; Walter Schaupp, Organtransplantation und Christliches Liebesgebot, in: Hans Köchler (ed.), Transplantationsmedizin und personale Identität. Ethische, medizinische, rechtliche und theologische Aspekte der Organverpflanzung, Frankfurt/M. 2001, pp. 103–114.

the late 1960s organ donation has become known and understood as a form of altruism and solidarity with critically ill patients.[3] Since then, not much has changed with regard to this concept and it has been affirmed and endorsed by high-ranking church documents.[4] There are three tasks that have become relevant in the recent past and that appear to be necessary according to contemporary discussions, which I will refer to here as key points. First, comprehending the fact that the donor is not just a vehicle for salvaging valuable human material, but also respecting the legacy of an individual whose dignity is to be appreciated after death and who should be handled deferentially (also with regards to language use). Second, remaining honest and humble, not only by contextualizing the success of the greater spectrum of possibilities and power within high-tech medicine, but also recognizing boundaries, fears, dependencies, and the possibility of failing. Third, providing spiritual guidance for the donor's relatives as well as the organ recipient, who will have numerous questions both *before* and *after* the transplant. These questions could include concerns about one's own finite nature, living with something foreign in oneself, and the question of the reason behind getting the opportunity to live because of a donation made by a complete stranger.

8.4 Conclusion

Transplantation medicine has enjoyed great popularity and admiration in the public. Only in recent years it has come under criticism due to new questions and emerging breaches of the rules. This criticism has been so powerful that the readiness of citizens to donate organs has significantly decreased. The German politics tries to counteract this development by increasing the information and improving the citizens' motivation to donate. To regain or strengthen trust in this area of modern medicine, there are also other indispensable preconditions: enhancing transparency in the allocation of scarce resources, more prudence, more accurate concepts of death and dying, and the social visibility of a respectful interaction with the donor that leaves room for sorrows and anxieties of relatives.

[3] Cf. Richard Egenter, Die Organtransplantation im Lichte der biblischen Ethik, in: Franz Böckle & Josef Fulko Groner (ed.), Moral zwischen Anspruch und Verantwortung, Düsseldorf 1964, pp. 142–153; Richard Egenter, Verfügung des Menschen über seinen Leib im Licht des Totalitätsprinzips, in: Münchner Theologische Zeitschrift 16 (1965), pp. 167–178; Antonellus Elsässer, Organspende—selbstverständliche Christenpflicht?, in: ThPQ 128 (1980), pp. 231–245; Anton Schuster, Organspende von Lebenden. Eine kritische Auseinandersetzung mit R. Egenters Auslegung des Totalitätsprinzips, in: Münchner Theologische Zeitschrift 49 (1998), pp. 225–239.

[4] Cf. Pope John Paul II., Special Message on organ donation: Address of the Holy Father tothe participants of the Society for Organ Sharing 1991, in: Transplantation Proceedings 23 (1991), XVII–XVIII; Kirchenamt der Evangelischen Kirche in Deutschland & Sekretariat der Deutschen Bischofskonferenz (ed.), Organstransplantation. Erklärung der Deutschen Bischofskonferenz und des Rates der EKD, Bonn/Hannover 1990; Katechismus der katholischen Kirche, Odenburg 2007, nr. 2296.

References

German Transplantation Law (last updated on 01.08.2012): http://www.gesetze-im-internet.de/tpg/. Accessed 1 Aug 2012.

Höfling, W. 2012. Interview with Joachim Müller-Jung. *Frankfurter Allgemeine Zeitung,* 31 July 2012.

Jonas, H. 1985. *Technik, Medizin und Ethik.* Frankfurt a. M.: Suhrkamp.

Nationaler Ethikrat. 2007. Die Zahl der Organspender erhöhen. Zu einem drängenden Problem der Transplantationsmedizinin Deutschland. Berlin.

Shewmon, A. 2009. Brain death: Can I be resuscitated? *The Hastings Center Report* 39 (2): 18–24.

Konrad Hilpert is a Professor emeritus for theological ethics at the Ludwig-Maximilians-University Munich (LMU) since 2001. He studied Catholic Theology, Philosophy and German language and literature studies in Munich and Freiburg, where he also received his doctoral degree in 1978 and his habilitation in 1984. His research interests are systematic ethics, bioethics, medical ethics, human rights, history of moral theology, social ethics as well as relational ethics.

Chapter 9
How to be a Virtuous Recipient of a Transplant Organ

Barbro Fröding and Martin Peterson

9.1 Introduction

This chapter investigates to what extent recipients of transplant organs ought to be held morally accountable for lifestyle choices that jeopardize the function of their new organ and, further, if recipients of transplant organs should in some cases be punished for not taking proper care of their bodies. Consider, for instance, a patient suffering from a life-threatening cardiovascular condition. The patient needs a new heart in order to survive. By prioritizing one patient in what is effectively a zero-sum game, the needs of others will be forgone. It therefore seems that it would be reasonable for the healthcare provider to have some say with regards to the lifestyle of the patient who receives transplanted biological material of which there is limited supply. How much of a say they get is, however, highly controversial.

One, arguably quite extreme, option would be to defend a strong paternalistic position. On such an account, the point of view of the healthcare provider would frequently override the preference and ideals of the patient and, consequently, give the healthcare provider the right to dictate a certain lifestyle for the person in question.

At the other end of the spectrum, we find people rejecting any type of interference in the private sphere. As soon as the patient has received the new organ, it is indeed *her* organ. The recipient is therefore free to choose any lifestyle she

B. Fröding (✉)
Division of Philosophy, Royal Institute of Technology (KTH), Stockholm, Sweden
e-mail: barbro.froding@abe.kth.se

Lincoln College Oxford, Oxford, UK

M. Peterson
Department of Philosophy, Texas A&M University, USA.
e-mail: martinpeterson@tamu.edu

R. J. Jox et al. (eds.), *Organ Transplantation in Times of Donor Shortage*,
International Library of Ethics, Law, and the New Medicine 59,
DOI 10.1007/978-3-319-16441-0_9

wishes—even if it is likely to have serious negative effects on her overall health and life expectancy. A more moderate, and in our opinion reasonable view, is that a certain set of moral obligations attach to the privilege that has been given to the patient. On our view, if taxpayers (in, say, Europe) invest in your health by paying for your treatment, then you are under at least *some* obligation to refrain from a lifestyle that is likely to jeopardize your new transplant organ.[1]

In this chapter, we shall ignore the two extreme views sketched above and focus exclusively on our preferred moderate position. We will discuss the case of biological organs rather than artificial ones in that we find such scenarios more relevant from a moral point of view. While strained resources can also generate demands on patients receiving artificial organs, it seems plausible to argue that the biological version has a set of additional strings attached to it. That being said, it would be a mistake to conclude that recipients of artificial organs are under *no* obligation to take good care of themselves. Few people would deny that they are.

Our main point can be summarized as follows. From a virtue-ethical point of view, the donation of a biological organ is a gift made for a good cause by the donor (or by the family of the deceased donor), and as a consequence, a set of special obligations arise. This includes the obligation to take good care of that gift.[2] Similar obligations do not attach to all gifts, including other forms of medical treatment. What makes organ donation so special is the extreme scarcity of this life-saving resource. Notably, our position, according to which the recipient is under an obligation to *refrain* from certain choices, should not be conflated with the more demanding obligation to *actively* make certain choices. The latter would be far more restrictive and to a greater extent infringe on the freedom of the individual.

It deserves to be mentioned that we will not argue that anyone should be punished for a situation that they find themselves in due to unfortunate circumstances. Rather, what will be discussed here is whether or not restrictions on lifestyle choices (which plausibly can be linked to a certain condition) might be imposed by the state post treatment. Note that this is very different from the more extreme position that society can justifiably condition care or medicine on choices that are made prior to the treatment. In other words, while we are committed to the idea that any patient should be eligible for a transplant simply by virtue of being human, we still find it reasonable to impose (certain) restrictions on her future lifestyle choices.[3]

---

[1] Here we mean lifestyle choices that have a proven link to a specific condition of the patient, such as smoking and lung cancer, or obesity and cardiovascular diseases. Indeed this is already a reality. Consider, for example the country of Bhutan where selling tobacco as well as smoking has been illegal since 2005. In a similar vein, the New Zealand government has decided to make the country smoke free by 2025 and the Finish government has decided to do the same by 2040.

[2] As pointed out by a helpful reviewer, there is a longstanding discussion on the concept of a gift and how that affects relationships in the field of moral anthropology, see e.g. Mauss and Titmuss. For space reasons, however, we cannot include this literature in this paper.

[3] It should be stressed that our claim is a moral one, not a legal or political one. We leave it open how this moral claim, if accepted, should be incorporated into existing policies. For a more detailed discussion on this please see Fröding and Peterson (2013), "Should we restrict the life-style of transplant and prosthesis patients?", forthcoming.

On a more general note, the best solution to the current shortage of biological transplant material is of course medical and technological developments, e.g. in the fields of stem cell therapy and nanotechnology. Breakthroughs in these areas are highly likely to both cut costs and enable completely novel treatments to improve the lives of many. This contribution, however, focuses exclusively on the current situation where resources are under extreme pressure and choices, affecting the well-being of many, need to be made on a daily basis.

The structure of this chapter is as follows. In Sect. 9.2, we will sketch some key elements of Aristotelian virtue ethics. We will focus in particular on the doctrine of the mean, which we argue, in Sect 9.3, is relevant to our moral attitude to transplant organs. We will try to show that, from a virtue-ethical point of view, we have good reason to accept what we call *enforced medium levellifestyle infringements*. By this we mean reasonable limitations on the range of lifestyle choices made available to recipients of transplant organs. Finally, in Sects. 9.4 and 9.5 we will address four objections to our analysis and briefly discuss some practical implications of our conclusion.

Before we begin, it should be noted that the underlying motivation for committing to the life of virtue comes from the agent herself and, consequently, that it is voluntary. The desire to lead such a life, which on occasion quite plausibly would require certain efforts, is based on the conviction that a life in accordance with moral and epistemic virtues is the best and happiest life. In this view, the agent ought to seek to look after herself in every respect and this includes physical as well as mental wellbeing.

9.2 Virtue Ethics

The idea that the healthcare provider has a moral right to restrict the choices of the individual and, in particular, that it is in the *individual's interest* to accept this arrangement, is best explained from a virtue-ethics perspective.[4] In order to sketch a plausible account of why some restrictions are attractive for both parties (i.e., both the individual and the healthcare provider) some theoretical elements of virtue ethics will have to be introduced.

Virtue ethics tells us that the best life for any human being is a life of virtue. Given the choice, this is the life that would enable the rational agent to fare better than she otherwise would. According to Aristotle, agents need to develop a set of moral virtues (e.g., generosity, courage, justice) as well as a set of intellectual virtues (e.g., practical wisdom, sound reasoning, technical skills). Once properly integrated, these character traits will be stable and will always apply in action, one implication of which is that the virtuous agent cannot be tactically vicious on occa-

[4] Many utilitarians (and other ethical theorists) would of course agree that the state has a right to restrict the choices of the individual, but note that they might not agree that it is in each individual's interest to do so.

sion. The virtues become second nature and making the right choices, for the right reason, will become the only option worth considering for the agent.

According to Aristotle, an action X has to meet three necessary and jointly sufficient conditions in order to count as being virtuous. The agent has to:

(i) Have practical knowledge about X,
(ii) Choose X and choose it for its own sake and
(iii) X must flow from her firm character.

Conditions (ii) and (iii) entail that in order to assess if an action is virtuous we need to know how the agent perceived what she was doing and why. In a recent discussion of the Nicomachean Ethics, Hughes stresses that,

> At a pinch a person can on occasion exercise self-control and do what needs to be done even when they cannot do it in the way that the good person does it. It is therefore not the case that on each occasion a correct moral assessment of what should be done requires moral virtue, though it is true that moral virtue is needed to get things right consistently, day in and day out. (Hughes 2001, p. 220)

To be excellent, i.e. virtuous, is to have an unconditional disposition to act, to feel and generally respond in ways typical of the good person. The non-virtuous expert, on the other hand, simply has the ability to act and respond (and perhaps in some cases feel) in the ways typical of the sort of expert in question.

A key element in virtue ethics is the doctrine of the mean. This is the idea that doing the right thing is about striking the right balance among a certain set of parameters. The doctrine of the mean is a contested feature of Aristotle's theory and we shall therefore take some time to clarify how we think it should be understood, before we explain (in the next section) its relevance to the debate on organ transplantation.

Very generally speaking, one could describe the doctrine of the mean as saying that an excellence is an intermediate in an ethical triad. Flanked by two vices, one dealing with excessive behaviour and one dealing with deficient behaviour, the excellence in the middle sets in during actions that neither go too far nor fall short of what morality requires from us. (In some cases, there are more than two vices but in what follows we can, without loss of generality, restrict the discussion to bipolar cases). Aristotle uses the metaphor of the skilled archer hitting the mark. Just like the archer, we must take a great many things into consideration when we aim to shoot, i.e. the moral equivalents of hurdles such as trembling hands, crosswinds, effects of gravity and so on and so forth.

To understand what Aristotle most probably wishes to say with this metaphorical picture of the right balance in life, it is not particularly conducive to think of the virtuous mean as a single, eternally fixed spot on a line. To the contrary, the balance is relative to a number of dynamic aspects. For example, was it done at the right time, to the right extent, by the right person, for the right reasons, in the right way?[5] In order to hit the mean on the *grand scale* one must hit the mean on all the individual sub-scales. This is presumably what Aristotle has in mind when

[5] See e.g. NE1106b21-22, NE1109a28, NE1111a3-5, NE1135a25, NE1135b33.

he somewhat depressingly informs the reader that we can err in countless ways, but only get it right in one way. Notably, the doctrine of the mean does not say that one and the same person cannot display both corresponding vices (on different occasions). In fact, that seems a quite plausible scenario in that a person who fails to grasp the essence of the specific virtue is likely to go wrong in all kinds of ways. Indeed, such an agent lacks understanding of both proportion and context. It seems plausible that Aristotle intends his doctrine both as a practical rule of thumb and as a principle for classification.[6] This is a disputed claim, but Aristotle can reasonably be read as both classifying the ethics of a practice and as telling the reader how to use these classifications.[7]

Admittedly, the virtuous life can on occasion be both hard and demanding. Instilling the virtues, something which is done by practicing and looking to the example of the good man on whom one is to model oneself, is no quick fix. Indeed, one of the more contested issues in *The Nicomachean Ethics* is whether or not the happy life is a possibility for many or just a few (or no one). The arguments here are based on what could be called a *threshold view* where the idea is that if an agent has instilled most virtues to a high level, lacks in none and is firmly committed to improving, she could reasonably be considered to be leading a happy life in spite of not being *fully virtuous*. Very briefly, this idea rests on the combination of statements such as (i) a lot of people can be happy,[8] (ii) Aristotle's dialectical method, and (iii) Aristotle's usage of paradigm cases, which are deliberately extreme in order to be as clear as possible. We take this to speak in favour of the idea that *eudaimonia* might not be conditional on complete virtue.

To establish good habits the training needs to start very early and continue throughout life. Indeed, just like with physical health, moral fitness needs to be exercised for the agent to remain *morallyfit*. The virtues can be thought of as habitual dispositions that give rise to more or less stable patterns of behaviour.[9] When exercising the virtues the agent has something, which can be called *equity*. This ability can be understood as an overall good judgment and it enables her to know how to interpret the spirit of the law and thus avoid both making mistakes and becoming overly rigid by following it to the letter. She can adapt to the circumstances without losing sight of what is truly just in a situation. Equipped with this capacity, or decency, she would be able to determine the just action and thus deal with situations for which no laws have (yet) been written. In summary then, being virtuous is having the ability to reason coupled with a deep understanding for what it really means to be just. Taken together those qualities enable her to get it right even in very complicated situations.

[6] Pakaluk (2005, p. 108).

[7] For a good account of this, see Crisp R., Aristotle on Greatness of Soul, in Kraut (2006).

[8] See Book 1.9 of the NE.

[9] For example, brittleness, which is a dispositional property of glass and this influences the behaviour of glass when dropped, i.e. it shatters.

9.3 Why We Should Accept Medium Level Infringements

As explained above, virtue ethicists maintain that a life of virtue is the best and happiest life for all human beings. Consequently, it comes as no surprise that advocates of this view, once committed, should be willing to accept at least some rules and laws that help to promote virtuous behaviour. On this virtue-ethics approach to bioethics, there are particularly strong reasons speaking in favour of what we shall call *enforced medium level lifestyle infringements* on recipients of transplant organs. By this we mean reasonable limitations on the range of lifestyle choices made available to recipients of transplant organs. What we have in mind are habits that threaten to directly deteriorate the function of the received organ. Prime examples are the well-documented connections between tobacco smoking and lung cancer; obesity and heart coronary disease; high alcohol consumption and the occurrence of liver cirrhosis. So, in essence, the claim defended here is that people are under a moral obligation to, for example, stop smoking if they receive a lung transplant, keep a normal BMI if they receive a heart transplant, limit their intake of alcohol if they receive a liver transplant and so on.

These moral obligations, or medium level infringements, can be justified within a virtue-ethical context.[10] Consider for instance the virtue of respect. Here we include both respect for others and respect for oneself. Admittedly, while respect is not to be found in the list of virtues originally provided by Aristotle, it is highly plausible that the three social excellences identified by Aristotle involve key elements of what we today call respect. The first two social excellences are nameless, but the first is often called *friendliness* in that it has to do with the pleasing and displeasing of others. The second is about how one presents oneself while interacting with others, and the third—wittiness—explains how to be playful in a fitting way.

In the present bioethical context, the virtue of respect for others can be broken down into the three following considerations:

(i) Respect for the donor and the donor's family
(ii) Respect for the other patients in the transplant queue
(iii) Respect for the people who contribute financially to the healthcare system

All these forms of respect are connected to the display of appropriate gratitude. As pointed out in Sect. 9.2, a central element in virtue ethics is the doctrine of the mean. Generally speaking, for an action to qualify as virtuous it needs to fall in the

[10] It has been pointed out to us that if the agent is infringed upon she is not virtuous in her actions. While it might be true that she is not excellent or complete in virtue we justify this by pointing to a combination of the threshold view and the fact that Aristotle wrote that rules and even punishments could be necessary parts of the process of instilling the virtues. E.g. Aristotle remarks somewhat grimly in Book 10.9/NE1179b11-13/. Those who have developed a sense of shame and "[…] been prepared by habits for enjoying and hating finely […]" /NE1179b26/, i.e. to associate the noble with pleasure they, on the other hand, can be successfully trained to acquire phronesis. Here Aristotle relies on Plato's account of the middle part of the soul, the so called spirited one. This part develops in young people before reason does and it seeks to do the just and noble (The Republic, 440 cd).

mean between two extremes on a number of spectra and the agent needs to compute parameters such as *when*, *why*, *how* and *to whom,* etc. before she acts. Striking the right balance is, on occasion, likely to be difficult and demand a lot of practice. Such systemic challenges, however, do not work as an excuse for not trying to do one's best. To purposely squander limited resources, which have been secured at the expense of another, presumably equally deserving patients, would be a flagrant violation of respectful behaviour and appropriate gratitude in almost any interpretation.

Let us now turn to the inward-facing dimension of respect, i.e. respect for oneself. On the virtue account, the good agent is required to be her own friend and to treat herself well. In fact, she is expected to love herself *the most*. To Aristotle, leading the virtuous life equals being rational in that it is the only life that enables humans to function at their top capacity. All things considered, the virtuous life is the best and indeed most pleasurable life imaginable. To lead this life, however, agents are required to look after themselves both physically as well as mentally and it follows that engaging in self-destructive behaviour would not only be potentially vicious, but indeed tantamount to irrational.

Therefore, the virtuous agent is in fact likely to make adjustments to her lifestyle, which she has good reason to believe will promote her own wellbeing. As briefly mentioned above, the virtuous agent has equity. In addition, she would also master the intellectual virtue of *phronesis* (practical wisdom) and this combination will guide her when facing difficult choices.

It might be helpful to think of *phronesis* as an ability that enables the agent to take in all the relevant aspects and make an all-things-considered decision on which she then proceeds. In other words, she has a heightened sensitivity to the morally relevant factors in a given scenario. Now, given that the agent knows that her physical and mental health is central to her chances of leading the good life, it is quite likely that when given health recommendations (which she has good reason to trust) she would conclude that in spite of certain initial inconvenience she ought to accept them and, if necessary, change her lifestyle accordingly. On the virtue account, her reasons for complying can best be accounted for in moral terms in that her duty to look after herself physically cannot be separated from morality. A positive side effect of this is, of course, that this is also the decision that will give the virtuous agent the most pleasure (at least after the initial adjustment phase).

9.4 Four Objections

We recognize that our proposal is far from uncontroversial. It is therefore appropriate to briefly respond to what we take to be four of the most important objections to our claim.

The first objection starts from the observation that once the transplantation has been performed, the transplant organ is inside the recipient's body. The organ should therefore count as being *part of* the recipient's body. In this view, it follows that it is up to the recipient to decide how to lead her life. To impose restrictions on the recipient's behaviour just because she has received a transplant organ would, consequently, be morally unacceptable.

While we recognize that this objection might have some relevance for artificial organs, we reject it in the case of biological ones. In our point of view, the biological organ is different in virtue of the relationship it creates between the donor and the recipient. The recipient ought to be morally moved by a sense of respect and gratitude, which, for the virtuous agent, should translate to a certain type of lifestyle. Moreover, an additional motivation to change a risky lifestyle should come from the agent herself, not the donor or healthcare provider. The virtuous agent ought to be moved by *her own* understanding of the good life. To take care of her new organ is part of what is required for leading a good life, and hence it is in the recipient's own interest to do so. Virtue ethicists have reason to conclude that this gives rise to a special self-regarding obligation towards oneself.

We now turn to the second objection. Here the concern is that the exact nature of the causal link between one's lifestyle and a particular disease is, in many cases, not clear. In today's society, we are bombarded with a mish-mash of conflicting advice on how to behave. Consider for example the case of diet recommendations, where we find advice ranging from Weight Watcher's, LCHF and Atkins. Experts and gurus are pitted against each other, and in many cases, it is far from clear who is right and who is wrong. Our strategy for taking care of this objection is to question the truth of the premise on which it is based. While it is true that it is not always clear which diet is best for your health, it does not follow that there is *no* evidence for concluding that, say, obesity is bad for one's overall health. Although there might be some disagreement about experts on certain factual issues, this does not give virtuous people reason to completely ignore all the nutritional and medical knowledge available in today's society.

The third objection is related to the second. In the last few decades, numerous experiments have shown that human beings are biologically hard-wired to make poor decisions, biased, and generally ill suited for processing large amounts of contradictory information.[11] From a moral perspective, this poses a big challenge: Can we reasonably hold people accountable for being, for example, overweight and thus endangering themselves if society cannot give any clear recommendations on how to best avoid such a situation from coming about? Our response to this challenge is two-fold. Firstly, we acknowledge that this is a great challenge to moral theory as a whole, not just to virtue ethics. Secondly, and more importantly, we believe that these experimental findings give us even stronger reasons to aim for the virtuous life. Since humans are, as the experiments show, so easily confused and often irrational, the best way forward seems to be to instil a set of virtues to ensure that we live as good a life as we possibly can.

We now turn to the fourth and final objection. Here the point is that even if it could be proven without a doubt that there is a tight causal connection between the recipient's lifestyle and some damage to her new transplant organ, the medium level

[11] See Fröding (2012).

infringements defended here have no place in a liberal democracy. Therefore, our analysis should be rejected.

While this liberal point might be convincing in a minimal, neo-liberal state, we believe that it is not applicable to the type of modern, western (welfare) states discussed here. If it is the case that (i) citizens are expected to accept at least *some* joint responsibility for sectors such as healthcare, and (ii) that no single person ought to be held accountable for finding herself in a situation which she could not reasonably have avoided, then it seems plausible to maintain that the healthcare provider should have a say on the distribution of healthcare resources. We also note that there is currently much support, both among lay people and doctors, for the view that people should be held responsible for certain choices that previously might have been taken to fall wholly within the private domain. Examples include the recently introduced Danish fat tax, the Norwegian sugar tax, and various regulations in several countries that make people ineligible for receiving an organ donation under certain circumstances.[12]

9.5 Some Practical Implications

In the view proposed here, virtuous recipients of transplant organs have one outward-facing obligation towards others, namely to display appropriate gratitude and respect for the donor and other people affected by their lifestyle choices. The virtuous recipient also has one inward-facing obligation, namely a moral duty to look after herself and her new organ.

This position, according to which individual recipients of transplant organs have strong moral reasons to adjust their lifestyle such that it conforms to relevant healthcare recommendations, is less extreme than one might think. In a society with limited means and very high demand for healthcare, resources have to be prioritized. Consequently, could it not then be the case that we are morally obliged to forfeit our rights to certain treatments by actively choosing a destructive lifestyle? Indeed, potential patients are required already today to adjust their lifestyle in order to be eligible for certain treatments. Examples include state funded IVF treatment in the UK, which requires patients to quit smoking and to have a normal BMI. Admittedly, these examples pertain to elective surgery and as made clear already in the introduction we do not argue that life-saving treatments should in any way be conditional on certain behaviour on the part of the patient. Also, it is often hard to scientifically prove the connection between isolated habits or behaviour and a certain condition. More often than not, it is about the grand total. To focus on *the last nail in the coffin* would not have the desired effect. Then again, there are scientifically and medically sound reasons to argue the connection between lung cancer and tobacco smoking, obesity and diabetes type II.

[12] The fat tax was introduced in Denmark on October 1, 2011. The Norwegian sugar tax was introduced in 1981. Similar taxes have been discussed in Sweden (Dagens Nyheter, 1 April 2010).

However, it can be argued that in the above cases that what the state dictates is based on the chance of success of the surgery rather than a pre-set moral agenda. Analysing it from virtue perspective shows that it is not the state but the *individual* that decides which moral rules she wants to live by, the fact that they are very likely to overlap with good physical health is hardly an argument against the idea defended here.

In a very broad sense, to be virtuous is to be sensitive to morally relevant factors and, based on them, to reach the right decision and then proceed to act accordingly. On the virtue account, any rational agent would be highly motivated to comply in that her idea of the good and happy life makes it impossible to intelligibly separate morality from her physical and mental wellbeing. Thus, in a scenario where she has good reasons to believe that embracing lifestyle changes would promote her chances to lead the good life, it would really be rather perplexing if she refrained. In doing so, it should be noted that she is not moved by paternalistic reasons, fear of punishment or any other external factor. In fact, the most compelling reason to comply comes from within herself—an explanatory model which presumably is more palatable to most people than the idea of the state dictating life conditions.

References

Fröding, B. 2012. *Virtue ethics and human enhancement*. Berlin: Springer.
Hughes, G. 2001. *Routledge philosophy guidebook to Aristotle on ethics*. New York: Routledge.
Kraut, R. 2006. *Blackwell companion to the Nicomachean Ethics*. Oxford: Blackwell.
Froding, B., and M. Peterson. 2013. Why computer games can be essential for human flourishing. *Journal of Information, Communication & Ethics in Society* 11 (2): 81–9.
Pakaluk, M. 2005. *Aristotle's Nicomachean Ethics*. Cambridge: Cambridge University Press.

Barbro Fröding is an associate professor at the Division of Philosophy, Royal Institute of Technology (KTH) in Stockholm. She is also senior research associate at the Oxford Uehiro Centre for Practical Ethics and a former fellow at Lincoln College Oxford. Dr. Fröding completed her PhD in 2008 and then worked as a Marie Curie post-doc fellow in Oxford before returning to KTH as a senior researcher in 2010. Her research interests include moral philosophy, applied ethics, virtue ethics (modern and Aristotelian), epistemic virtues, ownership of biological material and human cognitive enhancement.

Martin Peterson is professor of Philosophy at Eindhoven University of Technology. Prior to that, he was a research fellow in the Department of History and Philosophy of Science at Cambridge University. His areas of expertise include normative ethics (consequentialism), decision theory and ethics of technology, but also extends to metaethics, experimental philosophy and epistemology. Martin Peterson's most recent book is *The Dimensions of Consequentialism*, published by Cambridge University Press 2013.

Part II
The Law and Politics of Organ Donation: Problems and Solutions

Part I concentrated on the investigation of the current ethical and moral limits to organ transplantation. Based on these analyses it presented various innovative answers to the problem of organ shortage based on ethical reflection. *Part II* investigates the complex and intertwined problem areas surrounding organ transplantation by taking a closer analytic look at the current legal and political solutions being undertaken to alleviate the shortage. Following the aim of this volume, the critique of the status quo is supplemented by possible solutions that are capable of repositioning the societal debate.

In his contribution, *Nathan Emmerich* starts by contesting that there is an increasing degree of strain on the dead donor rule, explaining this by conceptual confusion about human death. Because brain activity can be present when individuals are dead by cardiac criteria and cardiac activity can be present in patients who are brain dead, it seems counterintuitive that there are two independent but necessary and sufficient criteria for the medical *diagnosis* of death. Emmerich examines this confusion and argues that it cannot be entirely avoided. This introduces a moral or ethical dimension to the way we choose to define and determine death. It seems that if post-mortem organ donation is to be ethical then, for the purpose of ensuring the informed consent of those registered to be donors, this aspect of death must be openly discussed. This means introducing a greater level of complexity to Organ Donor Registers (ODRs) and requires a biopolitical response to the bioethical concerns about the dead donor rule. In this view, it is not simply the case that the state shapes the biological bodies of its citizens through biopolitical laws and policies that are ethically underpinned. It is also the case that those who constitute the democratic body shape themselves through engaging with law, policy and bioethics.

Thomas Breidenbach's contribution displays the legal and administrative structure of organ donation in Germany. According to the revised German Transplant Act of 2012, organ donation is specified as a common task and the law assigns various responsibilities to several organizations. The removal and transplantation of tissues is regulated by the Tissue Law from 2007. Therefore, organ donation and tissue donation are legally separated in Germany. Hospitals with intensive care units are legally obligated to report potential organ donors to the central procurement organization, the German Organ Transplantation Foundation (Deutsche Stiftung Organtransplantation = DSO), which coordinates the entire organ donation process. The allocation is implemented by the Eurotransplant International Foundation (ET), which allocates organs in accordance with the guidelines of the Federal Medical Council. In order to give a detailed insight into the system of organ donation, Breidenbach elaborates on the processes, responsibilities and tasks of the involved parties.

In her article, *Alexandra Manzei,* critically investigates the seemingly self-evident relationship between the undersupply and a low willingness to donate organs. In contrast to this often undoubted and repeated idea, Manzei points out that the donation of organs in Germany is not just a question of willingness, but is also bound to the problem of brain death. She critically discusses this controversial concept of death and argues that, even if each and every German citizen were willing to donate his or her organs, there would still be a rather high number of patients waiting for organs. This situation has been completely ignored by politicians. While the new law exclusively aims to increase the citizens' willingness to donate organs, the structural problems of organ shortage remain unaffected. Furthermore, Manzei argues that the increasing demand of organs can be understood as a result of three different processes that are often disregarded in public discussions or official statements. First, organ transplantation is considered the most effective therapy for more and more diseases and replaces other, traditional therapies. Second, she calls to mind that many organs (from unrelated donors) are rejected at some point in time. The re-transplantation rate continues to increase. Third, the number of multiple organ transplantations is also rising. Manzei concludes by claiming that it would be much more important and necessary to reduce the demand for organs by promoting prevention and alternate forms of treatment.

Thomas Hayes explores some of the arguments surrounding systems of consent for cadaveric organ donation by examining the National Assembly for Wales' (NAW) law. This regulation departs from the current United Kingdom system of 'opt-in' donation and favors a system of 'opt-out' donation, under which consent is presumed as the default option if there is no explicit refusal. This law is designed to increase the supply of organs and thus reduce the organ shortage. Hayes raises concerns about the assumptions behind the projected increase in the rate of donation as well as the practicalities of implementing the proposed law within an EU member state. He concludes by stating that, however desirable the objective of saving and improving lives through alleviating the organ shortage may be, the particular means by which the NAW attempts to achieve this are flawed and unjustified. As there is no empirical evidence for a causal connection between opt-out systems and organ donation rates, there is no guarantee that the donation rate in Wales will increase with a change in law. There is even the possibility that the rate will decrease, particularly if the change leads to a loss of public confidence in the transplant system.

In their article, *Jurgen De Wispelaere and Lindsay Stirton* propose to tackle the current deficit in the supply of cadaveric organs by addressing the family veto in organ donation. They believe that the family veto matters – ethically as well as practically – and that policies which completely disregard the views of the family in this decision are likely to be counter-productive. Instead, they propose to engage directly with the most important reasons why families often object to the removal of the organs of a loved one who has signed up to the donor registry – notably, a failure to fully understand and deliberate about the information and a reluctance to deal with this sort of decision at an emotionally distressing time. To accommodate these concerns they suggest to radically separate the process of information, deliberation and agreement about organ explantation from the event of death and bereavement through a scheme of advance commitment. The authors briefly set out their proposal and discuss in detail its design as well as what they believe to be the main advantages compared to the leading alternatives.

Ulrich Schroth and Karin Bruckmüller expose the impact of legal preconditions for organ transplantation as well as the interpretation and implementation of these conditions. They argue that, in practice, legal preconditions significantly affect the willingness to donate an organ and subsequently the quantity of organs available. Therefore, an innovative political approach to solve the problem of organ shortage has to include a critical reflection and, if necessary, a change of the legal framework or its interpretation and practical implementation. Based on a comparison of the German, Austrian, Spanish and Belgian laws on organ transplantation, they favor an opt-in approach, giving full consideration to cultural and religious principles. Furthermore, they advocate a change of the organization of the German transplantation process, focusing on the improvement of brain death reporting, since the number of available post-mortem organs primarily depends on this information.

Responding to the legal and structural questions raised by the 2012 transplantation scandals in Germany, *Ruth Rissing-van Saan* develops a set of legal measures suitable to improve the current practice and to preclude abuse. First, she describes the current legal situation in Germany, emphasizing that the law does not determine the allocation of organs, because the German transplantation statute commissions the German Medical Association to develop evidence-based criteria for the allocation of organs. The German Medical Association makes its decisions according to a set of guidelines, which vary with the different phases of the organ transplantation process: rules that verify the donor's death, measures taken for organ retrieval, guidelines for the process of organ procurement, and rules assuring that the organ is of adequate quality. Focusing on the so-called MELD-Score (Model End-Stage Liver Disease) that combines three laboratory results (creatinine, bilirubin, and international normalized ratio, INR) to assess the severity of liver disease and the need for transplantation, Rissing-van Saan explores the legal consequences of possible malpractice. She then concludes by proposing a set of legal measures, including regular as well as sporadic inspections of the transplantation centers, the coordinating center and the procurement organization. Furthermore, the instrument of an independent Confidential Counseling Committee for Transplantation Medicine should be maintained, and this committee should give patients, their relatives as well as the general public the opportunity to file personal complaints or to ask questions and receive competent answers.

A different juridical answer to the questions raised by the German transplantation scandal is presented in the contribution by *Bijan Fateh-Moghadam*. Concentrating on the overall question of justice in organ allocation and representing a position of legal justice, he argues that from a legal point of view, justice has to be measured primarily by the standard of the rule of law and fundamental rights as defined by the German Basic Law (Grundgesetz). Against this background, Fateh-Moghadam claims that the statutory and sub-statutory legal framework for organ allocation provided by the German Transplantation Code and the Guidelines of the German Medical Association are not in accordance with the rule of law and are therefore unconstitutional. To strengthen his position, he brings forward the argument that the science of medicine is neither qualified nor legitimized to generate normative rules for prioritization in organ allocation. He concludes by pointing out that, in fact, this would be the responsibility of the public health administration, operating within the regulatory framework of the German Basic Law (Grundgesetz). The political failure to take on this responsibility is also one of the reasons why it is difficult to hold doctors accountable for arbitrarily intervening in an allocation system which fundamentally lacks legitimacy. As long as the normative nature of prioritization decisions is denied and standard criteria for organ allocation are persistently veiled as medical criteria, it will, according to him, remain illusory to speak of justice in organ allocation.

In her article, *Sibylle Storkebaum* undertakes an investigation of the German system of organ transplantation and focuses on the problematic aspects leading to a loss of confidence in the whole system. She poses a series of critical questions such as: What is the most recent development on replacing the brain death criterion with the even more questionable non-heart-beating donation? Why is there such a steep increase in the demand for organs? Is it the hospitals' greed that makes them aim to perform a large number of transplants or is it the pharmaceutical companies' quest for profit? Thereby, ex negativo, she sketches conditions needing to be fulfilled in order to ensure that trust can be restored in the system, e.g. transparency and a reduction and centralization of transplant centers.

Chapter 10
Challenges to the Dead Donor Rule: Configuring a Biopolitical Response

Nathan Emmerich

10.1 Introduction

Although the phrase *the dead donor rule* was not coined until 1988, Arnold and Youngner consider it to be "an unwritten, uncodified standard that has guided organ procurement in the United States since the late 1960s" (1993, p. 264). It represents two moral commitments that guide the retrieval of organs. The first is that healthcare professionals may not harm, kill, or hasten the death of a patient in the pursuit of organs. This is, of course, a basic moral commitment of medical practice—*first, do no harm*—that is being reiterated in the context of donation and transplantation. The second commitment is that the donor must be dead prior to retrieval and therefore beyond any possible harm that might result from doing so. Whilst this rule is obviously contravened in the cases of live donation of non-vital organs, it is maintained at the end of life. For example, the kidney of a dying patient would not be removed even if the patient wishes to be a (post-mortem) organ donor and doing so would not hasten their death.

The importance of the dead donor rule is not restricted to its role in the structural arrangements of healthcare practices, in conditioning the treatment of patients who are potential donors, or in constructing the ethics of donation. It is also an important part of what we might call the moral landscape of donation. For example, it plays a vital role in producing and maintaining the trust of the donating public. However, the existence of the rule and its role in the maintenance of trust should not blind us to the fact that our concept of death has not developed in a manner

N. Emmerich (✉)
School of Politics, International Studies and Philosophy,
Queen's University Belfast, Belfast, Ireland
e-mail: n.emmerich@qub.ac.uk

R. J. Jox et al. (eds.), *Organ Transplantation in Times of Donor Shortage*,
International Library of Ethics, Law, and the New Medicine 59,
DOI 10.1007/978-3-319-16441-0_10

fully independent of organ transplantation. It is well known that *whole brain death* and the accompanying criteria for its assessment were conceived, at least in part, for the purposes of facilitating the *post-mortem* donation of organs.[1] Whilst there was rapid cultural acceptance of this definition of and approach to death by the medical profession and *Western* societies more generally, it did not receive a universal welcome.[2] Furthermore, since its introduction there have been on-going concerns about the validity of brain death[3] and the dead donor rule,[4] concerns that have increased following the introduction of protocols for Non-Heart Beating Donation (NHBD), also known as Donation after Cardiac/Circulatory Death (DCD).[5] Whilst one can read the cessation of respiration as a *proxy measure* for brain death it requires a certain degree of contortion to think that the latter occurs within the time surgeons must allow to elapse following the final heart beat before commencing the retrieval of organs.[6] Consequently, whilst in the normal course of events we may be pronounced dead following brain death determination or due to cessation of cardiac function, we can be sure that one rapidly follows the other and that very little will happen to us in the intervening time. However, in the event of post-mortem donation, rapid retrieval of organs will take place following the pronouncement of death.

It is clear that there is an increasing degree of strain on the dead donor rule.[7] Brain activity can be present when individuals are dead by cardiac criteria and cardiac activity can be present in patients who are brain dead. Given our normal assumptions about death then, in the first instance, it seems counter intuitive that there are two independent but, nonetheless, necessary and sufficient criteria for the medical *diagnosis* of death. Furthermore, it is legal to treat the body of the post-mortem organ donor in ways that one is not allowed to treat the living—e.g. the harvesting of organs—but often under conditions that do not seem necessary if the body is *truly* dead—NHBD protocols often require the use of a shunt to cut off the blood supply to the brain. The strain on the dead donor rule is the result of conceptual confusion about human death. In this chapter, I will examine this confusion and argue that it cannot be entirely avoided. This introduces a moral or ethical dimension to the way we choose to define and determine *death*. It would seem that if post-mortem organ donation is to be ethical then, for the purposes of ensuring the informed consent of those registering to be donors, this aspect of death must be openly discussed. This means introducing a greater level of complexity to Organ Donor Registers (ODRs) and requires what we might call a *biopolitical* response to the bioethical concerns about the dead donor rule.

---

[1] Giacomini (1997) although see Belkin (2014).

[2] Lock (1998).

[3] Korein (1978); Veatch (1993).

[4] Arnold and Youngner (1993).

[5] Bernat (2006); Lynn (1993).

[6] The required waiting time varies between three and ten minutes Stiegler et al. (2012, p. 482).

[7] Gardiner and Sparrow (2010); Veatch (2004).

10.2 Death: Epistemic and Metaphysical

Death, one might say, is as much of a concern for philosophy as it is for medicine. However, whilst the latter is primarily concerned with how to tell if someone is dead, the epistemology of death, the former is focused on the metaphysics of death, with what it *really* is. Beyond determining what death might *mean*—whether or not death is *nothing to us* or *a great evil,*[8] the concerns of philosophy are usually *ontological* and directed towards the nature of human being (soul, person or organism) and, therefore, whether or not death should be considered: the severing of the soul from the body;[9] the end of personhood or *personal identity;*[10] or the dissolution of the human organism.[11]

In contrast, the primary concern of biology and, therefore, medicine is with the epistemology of death, with how to determine that death has in fact occurred in particular individuals or organisms. In the past, this has meant awaiting the first signs of biological decay. In 1833, Dungison advised "the only certain sign of real death is the commencement of putrefaction" (Cited in Ewin 2002, p. 109). However, at the present time death is determined in one of two ways: first, the irreversible cessation of respiration, most often determined by the irreversible cessation of cardiac function and, therefore, the circulation of the blood; second, via an assessment that the brain is no longer functional, so-called brain death or whole brain death. In such instances respiration is maintained, often mechanically, in order for a diagnosis. Given a diagnosis of brain death, ventilation is withdrawn and the remaining signs of life cease.

However, neither determination precisely reflects the ontological perspectives offered by philosophy. There is simply no empirical way to determine when the connection between a non-material object (the soul, the mind, or the essential component of personhood) has been severed from a material object (the body). Whilst we might connect personhood with brain function, the matter is not as simple as one might think. Some deny personhood to the fetus and even neonates, nevertheless their brains function in such a way as to not meet the criteria for brain death. We can think similarly for many other *higher* organisms. Furthermore, it is not clear that concepts of personhood can accommodate cases where there is a radical discontinuity in an individual's personal identity, cases of radical memory loss for example. Finally, it is likely that the cessation of personhood is primarily associated with neocortical function rather than with brain function *per se*. Although some might argue that they should be, patients who suffer an irreversible loss of neocortical function are not considered dead. Whilst the criterion for whole brain death seems to demand more than the loss of personhood those for respiratory death seem unconnected to anything of metaphysical significance.

---

[8] Warren (2006) for discussion.

[9] Kagan (2012).

[10] Schumacher (2010, Chap. 1).

[11] Becker (1975).

In fact, the metaphysics that underlies the biological perspective of modern medicine is likely Becker's (1975) understanding of the bodily integration/disintegration of human beings, or organisms than with the metaphysics of philosophical personhood. However, this biological ontology does not provide for a clear and bright line between *alive* and *dead*. Thus, it does not accord with our normal, everyday, or *ordinary*[12] intuitions (or 'folk philosophy') about death occurring at a precise point in time, albeit at the end of a process called dying. Nevertheless, we cannot simply abandon the determination made at specific points in time that death has occurred. First, there are strong cultural, epistemic and philosophical pressures to do so. This includes the need of medical professionals to decide when to stop medical treatment, particularly emergency treatment. Second, if we were to do so it may well rule out virtually all post-mortem organ donation. If organ retrieval teams were required to wait until all potential signs of life were absent the organs would no longer be in a condition suitable for transplantation. Consequentially, it is unavoidable that the epistemology used by biomedicine to pronounce that death has occurred conflates a variety of metaphysical views.[13]

Unfortunately, there is no obvious way for us to clear up this confusion. As more than 2000 years of philosophy and medicine demonstrate, the ontological and epistemic puzzle presented by death is not amenable to an easy solution. Some have responded to these problems by suggesting that death is not simply an ontological or epistemic category but also a moral or ethical category.[14] Such approaches do not obviate or supersede the ontological or epistemic analysis of death but, rather, reveal that there is another layer to the debate. The question of when a human being, as opposed to any other biological organism, is dead is not simply a search for an objective answer but also a question concerning their treatment. If an individual is dead then medical treatment can be withdrawn. If the individual is a registered donor then their organs can be retrieved for the purposes of transplantation. Whether or not someone is considered dead is an ethical event with ethical consequences.

10.3 Death and the Practices of Organ Donation

It is widely acknowledged, although complex, truth that the arrival of brain death criteria was not unrelated to the arrival of transplantation technology Belkin (2014). The potential good that could be served by the technological achievement of transplanting organs from one individual to another required a supply of viable organs. For organs to be sufficiently viable they must be retrieved a short time following *death* or, more accurately, following the cessation of an oxygenated blood supply to the organs. The contemporary technological achievements of the Intensive Care Unit (ICU) and mechanical ventilation had produced patients whose respiratory and

---

[12] Holland (2010).

[13] See Belkin (2014) for a more comprehensive account - and defense - of this practical reality.

[14] Gervais (1987, Chap. 4).

circulatory function could be maintained but, due to traumatic brain injury, were understood to have no prospect of recovery. Thus, the concept of brain death emerged from the moral challenge produced by this technology. However, further motivation to define criteria for its assessment was produced by a realization that *brain dead* patients could provide a source of transplant-viable organs. The respiratory and circulatory functions of brain-dead donors could be maintained until the last possible minute before organ retrieval, meaning that they would be in good condition for subsequent transplantation. For almost three decades, post-mortem organ donors were all patients who had been declared brain dead. However, in the mid-1990s protocols for NHBD began to be introduced.

Prior to the introduction of NHBD, the process of post-mortem donation involved a declaration that a patient was brain dead. Such patients are very likely to be undergoing mechanical ventilation and are in an ICU following some form of traumatic brain injury. The process of assessing a donor, consulting the family, allowing the family to say good-bye, making arrangements for a recipient, etc. could all be accomplished. Certainly it is not an easy time, but nevertheless there is time, and this is the process most people imagine when they register to be a post-mortem organ donor.

In cases of NHBD, this process can be quite different. There are two kinds of NHBD, controlled and uncontrolled. In the first, a patient is mechanically ventilated but is assessed as having no prospect of recovery. Although they may be dead neocortically they are not brain dead. In such instances there is enough time for the various processes that surround donation to be accomplished and the family can say good-bye to a patient who is still alive. In most cases, life support is withdrawn from the patient in the operating room where, according to the dictates of the local protocol, the surgical team will wait between 2 and 6 min following a final heartbeat before commencing retrieval. As a recent document concerning the legal issues surrounding NHBD acknowledged:

> [T]he care and treatment that a patient receives around the time of death may need to be adjusted if the patients' potential to donate is to be maintained or optimised. Such adjustments may include the timing and place of death (DHSSPSNI 2011: § 1.9).

Elsewhere I have argued that if it is to be reintroduced, the fact of elective ventilation ought to be brought to the attention of potential donors as part of the process of registration.[15] It seems important to do so if we are to secure the fully informed consent of donors. In light of such information, it may be that different individuals would make different choices and that they may do so for reasons they see as ethical. We can think similarly in cases where individuals donate following brain death or cessation of cardiac function. Potential donors should be made aware of the different protocols and given an opportunity to assent or dissent. Or, rather, to provide their active consent.

[15] Emmerich (2013).

10.4 A Biopolitical Response

The question of biopolitics is complex and there exists a diverse range of accounts, it is not a conceptually or theoretically unified field and thus resists easy definition.[16] That being said, the distinction between *bios* and *zoe,* terms which describe the ways human life is constructed by *sovereign power* particularly law, can be considered central. *Bios* should be considered qualified life, the life of one who is able to participate fully in the social and political dimensions of the state and is, in turn, legally recognized as a citizen. *Zoe* should be considered bare life, and is the life of the outcast, one who is not fully recognized by the state and who is unable to participate in society or politics. These terms are especially useful for thinking about the biopolitical dimensions of bioethics,[17] particularly the biopolitics of post-mortem organ donation. *Zoe*, or *bare life*, describes those who are on life support but who are not expected to make a recovery, particularly those who are brain dead but being kept *alive* on a ventilator. Thus, *zoe* describes the position of many of those who might potentially become post-mortem organ donors due to their medical status, Lock's living cadavers (2004) or those who are in a liminal state between being fully alive and fully dead. To be clear, it is not that the outcast has no legal status but, rather, that they have a particular legal status different to that of *qualified* life.

Beyond this basic distinction between *bios* and *zoe*, life and bare life, I am going to adopt a simple conception of biopolitics that involves the way in which the official policy and discourses of a state or society can shape the biology and biological self-understanding of its citizens. Such claims are usually made in relation to the psy-sciences,[18] genetics and genomics[19] and have, more recently, been reiterated in relation to the brain or neuro-sciences.[20] However, it is obvious that the discourses of philosophy, and therefore bioethics, are intimately linked to the social construction of the body. In this first instance, rightly or wrongly, we live within a culture of Cartesian dualism, which distinguishes between mind and body.

This dualism can be clearly seen in the ontological and epistemological aspects of death, discussed above. It is in play in the biopolitical construction of *bios* and *zoe*. It is in play in the idea of live and post-mortem organ donation. However, to suggest that individuals are, simply, Cartesian dualists would be misguided. Rather, they culturally instantiate and embody a variable form of dualism leading them to relate to themselves and their bodies as both subjectively or phenomenologically theirs, whilst also being objectively and biologically distinct from *themselves*. This idea is perhaps best captured by the phenomenological conception of *Leib* (self), *Körper* (body) and *Leib-Körper* (self-body or minded body), a view that can be considered as an attempt to understand the relationship of mind and body as one of

---

[16] Campbell and Sitze (2013, p. 2); Lemke (2011, p. 1).

[17] Bishop and Jotterand (2006).

[18] Rose (1998, 1999).

[19] Rose (2007).

[20] Abi-Rached and Rose (2013).

mutual constitution or embodiment. In this perspective the "body is not 'just another thing', nor is it pure feeling or pure subjectivity [rather w]e attend to the body as a feeling thing" (Ingerslev 2013, p. 165) and, we might add, as a meaningful thing.

As innumerable studies have shown, the body is inscribed with cultural meaning. The distinction between *zoe* and *bios* is one example of this. The difference between this aspect of biopolitics and (most) other forms of meaning inscribed in bodies is that it is rooted in sovereign power. In bioethics, philosophical debates about the ontological and epistemic nature of death are used as an attempt to rewrite sovereign power. It is a cultural discourse predicated on the generalized phenomenology of the human being as *Leib*, *Körper* and *Leib-Körper*. In the contemporary world of democratic (neo)liberalism[21] the individual is recognized as their own *sovereign power* and thus the *true* sovereign power of law requires, albeit minimally, the assent of the polity.[22] Thus, it is no surprise to find that whilst there are other ways in which *Leib*, *Körper* and *Leib-Körper* could be configured, the predominant configuration found in modernity is consistent with the contemporary interpretation of *bios* and *zoe* as life (subjectivity, personhood) and bare life (the absence of subjectivity, the irreversible cessation of personhood). The biocitizen is culturally enmeshed in the management of the self, where the primary resources for doing so are the discourses and constructions of not only biomedicine but of bioethics as well. What medical science and bioethics consider to be true and objective biological and moral facts are, in the wider cultural economy, resources with which biocitizens construct meaningful, which is to say *ethical*, relationships between their self (*Leib*) and body (*Körper*).

Such a perspective is in conflict with the dominant self-understanding of bioethics and the bioethical project. It is usual for (applied philosophical) bioethicists to claim that their debates are, or should be, understood as conceptually prior to any subsequent policy-formation discourses. Certainly this seems to be the implication of Radcliffe-Richards[23] recent methodological reflections, conducted in the context of presenting her views on the ethics of organ transplantations. However, if we accept that there is a moral dimension to any definition of death and that medicine and philosophy are unable to fully settle the question of what death is and how to determine it, then it would seem that the bioethical debates that surround the issue,

[21] In contexts such as these the term neo-liberalism usually carries critical, if not abusive, connotations. I am resisting such usage here.

[22] The implication of the biopolitical view taken here is that the sovereign power of the state historically precedes that of the individual. A view for which there is ample evidence when one considers that the idea of self-governance has its origin as an attribute of the state only later being applied to the individual (and thereby rendering the autonomous individual the sine qua non of morality and moral being). Schneewind (1998, p. 483). The more contentious corollary is that the state (or at least society or culture) constructs, and so brings into being, the individual who—morally speaking—is autonomous, self-governing, self-legislating and, therefore, their own sovereign power. Further argument and empirical support is needed but on this point one can, I think, consider the work of Reubi (2012, 2013) as providing at least some evidence for the existence of the relevant socio-cultural processes. However, these points must be put to one side for the time being.

[23] Radcliffe-Richards (2012, Chap. 3).

particularly in the context of organ donation, must carry over into debates about what policies we should adopt to govern donation. This is precisely because, as a matter of morality, the governmental context of (neo-) liberalism accords sovereign power to individuals. At least insofar as is possible whilst also maintaining the (bio-politically) necessary degree of true sovereign power required by (neo-) liberalism, both national and supra-national.[24]

The question at hand is not whether individuals *consent* to being pronounced dead according to specific criteria but, rather, whether all individuals are prepared to donate their organs in the various conditions under which death can be said to occur and donation takes place. At the present time potential organ donors are not told about the various ways in which donation takes place nor are they given any option to express their opinion or give their consent. Certainly, protocols have been developed through a consultative process involving doctors, bioethicists and, to a degree, patients and *lay* representatives. Nevertheless, no information regarding the various practices that constitute *post-mortem donation* is provided to those who register as donors. In the contemporary democratic milieu the individual, and not just the state, is the locus of sovereign power and therefore, although they can never do so in a fully *autonomous* manner—they are always subject to the discourses (biomedicine and bioethics), which contribute to the governmental dimensions of biopower—individuals have the moral right to govern themselves both as *bios* and *zoe*.

In this view, it is not simply that the state shapes the biological bodies of its citizens through biopolitical laws and policies that are underpinned by bioethical reasoning. It is also the case that those who constitute the democratic body politic shape themselves through engaging with law, policy and bioethics. In short, they are biocitizens accorded certain rights (and responsibilities) in the contemporary milieu of (neo-) liberalism. The government of the self, the construction of biocitizenship, occurs at the level of *true* sovereign power, through the formation or assembly of law and policy, and at the level of individual sovereign power, exercised subsequent to the formation of law and policy by individuals—biocitizens—engaging with these formations, structures or apparatus.

For example, at the present time, *bios* individual (bio) citizens can register as organ donors and thus shape the way in which they will be treated if they become *zoe*. In so doing, they are doing more than making bioethical decisions within a biopolitical apparatus. For the most part biocitizens do not make such decisions according

[24] It is on this ground that one can begin to articulate a biopolitical critique of the type I have put to one side (see: Fn. 21). The ground of such a critique is, as always, the degree of freedom individuals can be considered as actually having within (neo-)liberal systems of government and governance. Given the governmental power inherent in the true sovereign power of law, and the degree to which dominant discourses of biomedicine and bioethics are implicated in the formation, reformation and exercise of this power, to what degree might we consider the self-legislating individual as being able to legitimately exercise their own sovereign power? My argument here can be seen as suggesting that Organ Donor Registers ought to be expanded in such a way that such individuals—the neo-liberal subject—can exercise a greater degree of freedom, of sovereign power, and not have their choices closed off by the exercise of true sovereign power. Nevertheless the ODR remains, of course, a mode of biopolitical governance.

to methodologically rigorous criteria; they are not engaged in academic bioethical reflection and to think that they are (or, indeed, should be) is a form of intellectualism; it is to imagine that they adopt a scholastic point of view[25] rather than to make ethical decisions from within the horizons of their own lives.[26] For most people, registering as an organ donor is not the decision-making end point of a reasoned and theoretical analysis, but part of the process of reflecting on the issue, one aspect of their (ethical) engagement with organ donation. Potential organ donors (biocitizens) do not simply choose their preferred option amongst those presented to them by the ODR. Registering as an organ donor is one aspect of the biocitizens relationship to and conception of organ donation.

For post-mortem donation to be an option, biocitizens have to be in a position to make (ethical) sense of organ donation, and to understand themselves and others in relation to it. This reintroduces a philosophical aspect of death I alluded to, but did not expand on, in the introduction. Death is not merely an ontological, epistemic, or even moral, problem. It is also a problem of hermeneutics or meaning. This facet of death within human life is an expansion of the idea that death has a moral or ethical dimension and it finds its ground in the distinction between *Leib*, *Körper* and *Leib-Körper*. The problem of the hermeneutics—or everyday ethics—of death is a problem in the relation of the subjective self to the corporeal self, of the self to itself. It is not a problem of objectivist (bio)ethics nor of what Engelhardt calls a pluralist secular ethics,[27] i.e. an ethics that allows for cultural diversity and individual *choice* with regards to the moral concerns of contemporary society. The problem is biopolitical in the sense that it is a function of the biological self-understanding of its citizens and the way it is shaped by official discourses.

Thus, the biopolitical response to challenges to the dead donor rule is to see the value in, and necessity of, meaning in everyday life. The biopolitical response is one that acknowledges the ways in which the questions of bioethics are engaged and answered meaningfully, which is to say biopolitically, by the population at large, which should be considered as *ethically* legitimate perspectives. The correct *biopolitical* and *bioethical* response is to seek to engage with and facilitate this process. As a result, it is an argument for an expansion in the information given to individuals when registering as an organ donor and, therefore, the level of meaning such registers can capture. However, as mentioned, registering as an organ donor is one step in the relationship of biocitizens to organ donation. The biopolitical perspective I am articulating does not simply imply that the ODRs should be more comprehensive but that the infrastructure of organ donation should put into effect a greater level of engagement with the polity or *bios*. As phrases such as the *gift of life* imply, the post-mortem donation of organs is not merely an ethical choice but a meaningful one. At least at the time of writing, bioethics is in need of a greater sense of meaning as well as its meaning-making role in relation to the ethical dimensions of contemporary society, culture and biomedicine.

---

[25] Bourdieu (1990).

[26] Lambek (2010).

[27] Schumacher (2010, p. 45).

References

Abi-Rached, J. M., and N. Rose. 2013. *Neuro: The new brain sciences and the management of the mind*. New Jersey: Princeton University Press.

Arnold, R .M., and Youngner, S. J. 1993. The Dead Donor Rule: Should We Stretch It, Bend It, or Abandon It? *Kennedy Institute of Ethics Journal* 3 (2): 263–78.

Becker, L. C. 1975. Human being: The boundaries of the concept. *Philosophy and Public Affairs* 4 (4): 334–359.

Belkin, G. 2014. *Death before Dying: History, Medicine, and Brain Death*. New York, USA: Oxford University Press.

Bernat, J. L. 2006. Are organ donors after cardiac death really dead? *Journal of Clinical Ethics* 17 (2): 122.

Bishop, J. P., and F. Jotterand. 2006. Bioethics as biopolitics. *Journal of Medicine and Philosophy* 31 (3): 205–212.

Bourdieu, P. 1990. The scholastic point of view. *Cultural Anthropology* 5 (4): 380–391.

Campbell, T., and A. Sitze. 2013. *Biopolitics: A reader*. USA: Duke University Press.

DHSSPSNI (Department of Health, Social Services and Public Safety Northern Ireland). 2011, March. Legal issues relevant to donation after circulatory death (non-heart-beating organ donation) in Northern Ireland. Belfast.

Emmerich, N. 2013. Elective ventilation and the politics of death. *Journal of Medical Ethics* 39 (3): 153–157.

Ewin, R. E. 2002. *Reasons and the fear of death*. Oxford: Rowman & Littlefield.

Gardiner, D., and R. Sparrow. 2010. Not dead yet: Controlled non-heart-beating organ donation, consent, and the dead donor rule. *Cambridge Quarterly of Healthcare Ethics* 19 (1): 17–26.

Gervais, K. G. 1987. *Redefining death*. New Haven: Yale University Press.

Giacomini, M. 1997. A change of heart and a change of mind? Technology and the redefinition of death in 1968. *Social Science & Medicine* 44 (10): 1465–1482.

Holland, S. 2010. On the ordinary concept of death. *Journal of Applied Philosophy* 27 (2): 109–122.

Ingerslev, L. R. 2013. My body as an object: Self-distance and social experience. *Phenomenology and Cognitive Sciences* 12 (1): 163–178.

Kagan, S. 2012. *Death. Original*. New Haven: Yale University Press.

Korein, J. 1978. The problem of brain death: Development and history. *Annals of the New York Academy of Sciences* 315 (1): 19–38.

Lambek, M. 2010. Toward an ethics of the act. In *Ordinary ethics: Anthropology, language, and action,* ed. M. Lambek. New York: Fordham University Press.

Lemke, T. 2011. *Biopolitics: An advanced introduction*. USA: New York University Press.

Lock, M. 1998. Deadly disputes: Hybrid selves and the calculation of death in Japan and North America. *Osiris* 13:410–429. (2nd Series)

Lock, M. 2004. Living cadavers and the calculation of death. *Body & Society* 10 (2–3): 135–152.

Lynn, J. 1993. Are the patients who become organ donors under the pittsburgh protocol for 'non-heart-beating donors' really dead? *Kennedy Institute of Ethics Journal* 3 (2): 167–178.

Radcliffe-Richards, J. 2012. *The ethics of transplants: Why careless thought costs lives*. Oxford: Oxford University Press.

Reubi, D. 2012. The human capacity to reflect and decide: Bioethics and the reconfiguration of the research subject in the British biomedical sciences. *Social Studies of Science* 42 (3): 348–368.

Reubi, D. 2013. Re-moralising medicine: The bioethical thought collective and the regulation of the body in British medical research. *Social Theory & Health* 11 (2): 215–235.

Rose, N. 1998. *Inventing our selves: Psychology, power, and personhood. Reprint*. Cambridge: Cambridge University Press.

Rose, N. 1999. *Governing the soul: Shaping of the private self*. 2nd ed. London: Free Association Books.

Rose, N. 2007. *The politics of life itself: Biomedicine, power and subjectivity in the twenty first century*. New Jersey: Princeton University Press.

Schneewind, J. B. 1998. *The invention of autonomy: A history of modern moral philosophy*. Cambridge: Cambridge University Press.
Schumacher, B. N. 2010. *Death and mortality in contemporary philosophy*. Cambridge: Cambridge University Press.
Stiegler, P., M. Sereinigg, A. Puntschart, T. Seifert-Held, G. Zmugg, I. Wiederstein-Grasser, W. Marte, A. Meinitzer, T. Stojakovic, and M. Zink. 2012. A 10 Min 'no-touch' Time—is it enough in DCD? A DCD animal study. *Transplant International* 25 (4): 481–492.
Veatch, R. M. 1993. The impending collapse of the whole-brain definition of death. *The Hastings Center Report* 23 (4): 18–24.
Veatch, R. M. 2004. Abandon the dead donor rule or change the definition of death? *Kennedy Institute of Ethics Journal* 14 (3): 261–276.
Warren, J. 2006. *Facing death: Epicurus and his critics*. Oxford: Oxford University Press.

Nathan Emmerich is a visiting research fellow in the School of Politics, International Studies and Philosophy at Queen's University Belfast, where he is conducting research on the idea of Bioethical Expertise. His book 'Medical Ethics Education: An Interdisciplinary and Social Theoretical Perspective' was recently published by Springer.

Chapter 11
Organ Donation and Transplantation in Germany

Thomas Breidenbach

11.1 Introduction

Organ donation and transplantation are legally regulated by the German Transplant Act of 1997, which was revised in 2012 and 2013 (Transplantationsgesetz in der Fassung der Bekanntmachung vom 4. September 2007; letzte Änderung 15. Juli 2013). Organ donation is specified as a joint task and assigns various responsibilities to several organisations. The removal and transplantation of tissues is regulated by the Tissue Law from 2007 (Gewebegesetz vom 20. Juli 2007). Since then, organ donation and tissue donation have been legally separated. Hospitals with intensive care units are legally obligated to report potential organ donors to one central German procurement organization, the German Organ Transplantation Foundation (Deutsche Stiftung Organtransplantation = DSO), which coordinates the entire organ donation process. The allocation is subject to Eurotransplant International Foundation (ET), which allocates organs in accordance with the guidelines of the German Medical Association. The transplantation centres are responsible for waiting lists, organ transplantation and aftercare.

The general structure of the system (legal separation of organ donation, allocation and transplantation of organs) (Breidenbach and Banas 2011) was retained during the revision of the German Transplant Law (TPG) in 2012. However, critical discussions have increased due to the German transplantation scandals, where physicians in several hospitals were accused of systematically falsifying hospital data to speed up transplantation of their patients (Breidenbach and Banas 2011; Sigmund-Schultze 2012; Richter-Kuhlmann 2013). The discussion focused mainly on the lack of governmental supervision. In the meantime, some of the criticisms have been reconsidered because of an amendment of the law. For instance, the guidelines of the German Medical Association have to be approved by the Ministry of Health. Furthermore, physicians who manipulate the waiting list in order to give their patients

T. Breidenbach (✉)
German Organ Transplantation Foundation (DSO), Munich, Germany
e-mail: thomas.breidenbach@dso.de

R. J. Jox et al. (eds.), *Organ Transplantation in Times of Donor Shortage*,
International Library of Ethics, Law, and the New Medicine 59,
DOI 10.1007/978-3-319-16441-0_11

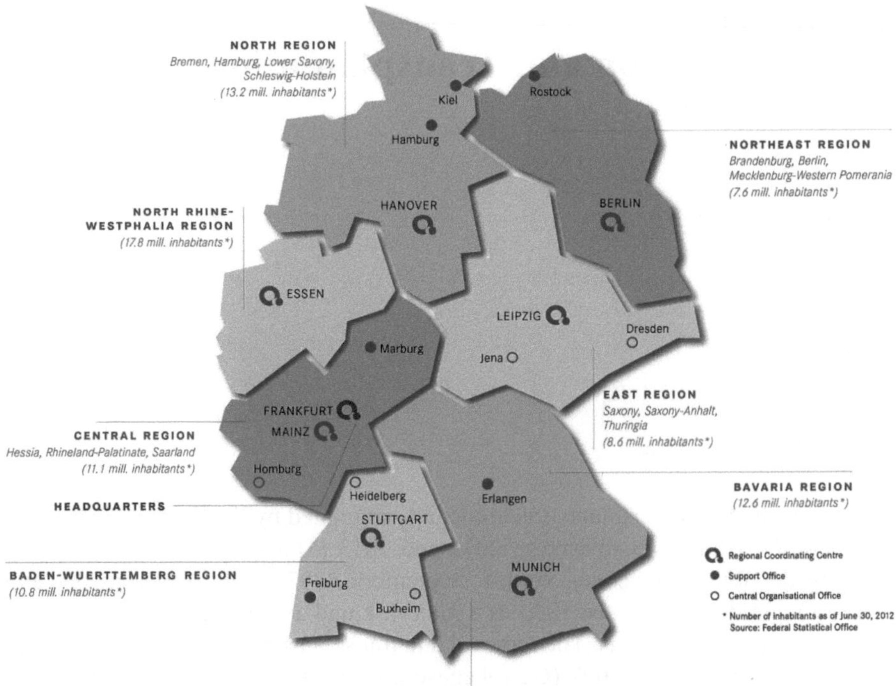

Fig. 11.1 Structure of the German Organ Transplantation Foundation (DSO)

preference can now be prosecuted by law. In the following chapter, processes, responsibilities and tasks of the involved parties will be presented in detail.

11.2 Division of Tasks According to the German Transplant Law (Fig. 11.2)

11.2.1 Hospitals

Hospitals are obligated to report every brain-dead patient as a potential organ donor to the German Foundation of Organ Transplantation (DSO) (Breidenbach and Banas 2011).

11.2.2 German Organ Transplantation Foundation (DSO)

The DSO is mandated by the Head Association of German Health Insurers (GKV-Spitzenverband), the German Medical Association (Bundesärztekammer) and the German Hospital Federation (Deutsche Krankenhausgesellschaft). The DSO is divided in seven geographical organ donor regions (Fig. 11.1). The DSO-coordinators

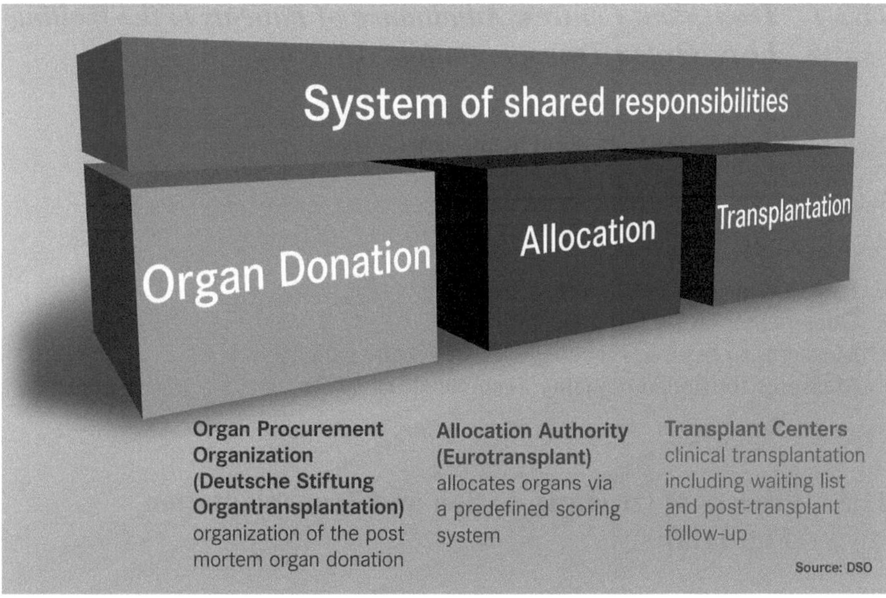

Fig. 11.2 Division of Tasks according to the German Transplant Law

are the main contact persons for the hospitals (Transplantationsgesetz in der Fassung der Bekanntmachung vom 4. September 2007; Breidenbach and Banas 2011; https://www.dso.de/.)

Tasks:

- Coordination of the donation process
- Measures to protect organ recipients
- Supporting transplant centres and hospitals in matters of quality assurance
- Collaboration with the allocating agency (ET)
- Publication of an annual report

11.2.3 Eurotransplant International Foundation (ET)

Tasks:

- Allocation of organs respecting state-of-the-art medical science
- Measures to protect organ recipients
- Collaboration with National Organ Procurement organizations, e.g DSO
- Regular reports to contracting partners

11.2.4 Transplant Centres: Admittance of Patients to the Waiting Lists, Organ Transplantation, Aftercare

Transplant centres are authorized by the federal states

Tasks:

- Patient registration on waiting lists
- Documentation for full traceability
- Measures to ensure psychological care for the patients
- Measures for standard quality assurance (Fig. 11.2)

11.3 Process of Organ Donation and Transplantation (Fig. 11.3)

11.3.1 Identification of a Potential Organ Donor

A potential donor has to be identified in the hospital at the first possible instance, and then be reported to the DSO (Transplantationsgesetz in der Fassung der Bekanntmachung vom 4. September 2007). Basically, every patient who suffered a massive primary or secondary brain injury resulting in death despite the maximum amount of medical care can be a potential donor. The circulatory functions need to be maintained artificially. Today, there are only a few absolute contraindications to organ donation (Breidenbach and Banas 2011; Dominguez-Gil et al. 2011; Guide to the safety and quality of organs for transplantation 2013) (see 3.4.).

Basic prerequisites for organ donation are:

1. Whole brain death
2. Consent to organ donation
3. Eligibility of the organs

Non-heart-beating-donation is not allowed in Germany (Bundesärztekammer 1998; Siegmund-Schultze and Zylka-Menhorn 2008).

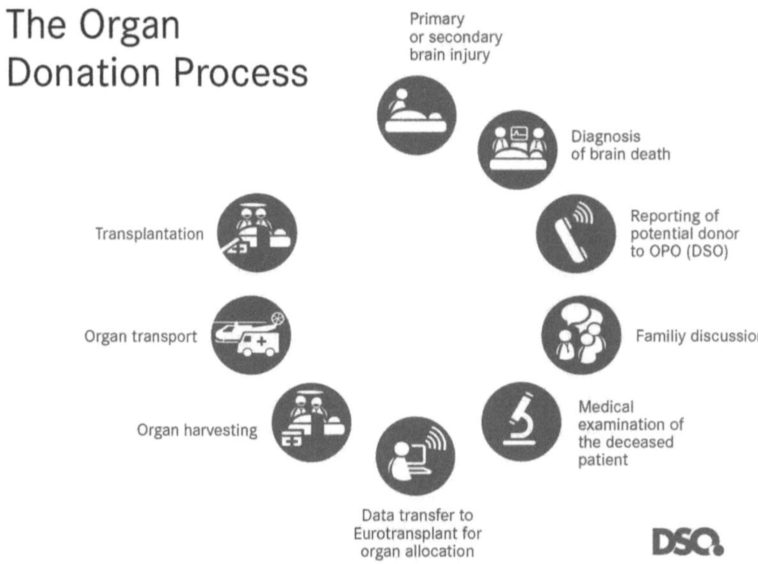

Fig. 11.3 The organ donation process

11.3.2 Brain Death

The German transplantation law determined that the declaration of whole brain death is a condition sine qua non for organ procurement (Transplantationsgesetz in der Fassung der Bekanntmachung vom 4. September 2007; Breidenbach and Banas 2011). It is defined as the irreversible end of all brain activity with maintained cardiovascular function and artificial ventilation. Brain death has to be examined in accordance with the guidelines of the German Medical Association (Siegmund-Schultze and Zylka-Menhorn 2008).

The guidelines require neurological examinations by two independently acting, qualified physicians, who have experience with patients who have suffered brain injuries. Furthermore, they cannot be actively involved in either organ removal or transplantation. The irreversible and unrecoverable end of all activity of the cerebrum, cerebellum and brain stem has to be attested. During the examination, the donor's dignity has to be respected at all times. Brain death is a medical-scientific as well as legal criterion for death (Richtlinien zur Feststellung des Hirntodes 1998; Magnus DJ et al. 2014).

11.3.3 Consent for Organ Donation

An essential, legal requirement is the information on the declared intention of the deceased person towards organ donation. If no written document, e.g. organ donor card, is available, the family will be asked for the patients' presumable will. But, in the majority of cases the patients' attitude towards organ donation is unknown. Merely 10% of potential donors have filled out a donor card. Hence, the dialogue with the next of kin and their consent are particularly important. In this respect, a certain statutory order of authorization has to be ensured: (1) marriage partners/registered partners, (2) children of full legal age, (3) parents, (4) siblings of full legal age, (5) grandparents. The respondents had to be in contact with the deceased for at least the past 2 years (Transplantationsgesetz in der Fassung der Bekanntmachung vom 4. September 2007).

During the dialogue the presumed will of the deceased has to be determined. In case there are no indications for the presumed will, the next of kin will be asked to decide according to their own discretion. A precondition for addressing the next of kin on the subject of organ donation is that they rationally understood the concept of brain death. Exception to this rule is when the next of kin addresses the subject before brain death was declared. Respectful and emphatic conversation skills are important when talking to the next of kin. Also, a separate and quiet room, the precise communication of the relatives' death, a clear explanation of brain death including checking whether it was understood, comprehensive information about organ donation and tissue donation with a clear priority on organ donation are all very important. The final decision of the next of kin needs to be respected. It is important to reach a stable decision in order to prevent a post-decision discordance (Breidenbach and Banas 2011; Breidenbach and Hesse 2011).

Knowing that their relatives' corpse is treated respectfully is very important for the next of kin. Also, the knowledge that there are no restrictions regarding the funeral is very important. As a matter of principle, next of kin should be given the opportunity to bid farewell to their loved ones in a dignified manner. This is recommended as it serves the interests of transparency and the prevention of misconceptions (e.g. disfigurement caused by organ removal). Hospitals might engage DSO coordinators to support the family approach. Moreover, the DSO provides family care by organising meetings. Experience has shown that sometimes questions arise weeks later. These questions can be answered at such meetings (Breidenbach and Banas 2011; Grammenos et al. 2012).

11.3.4 Donor Eligibility/Maintaining the Donor

In order to protect the organ recipient, the DSO initiates all necessary examinations to minimize the risk of transmitting infections or tumour diseases. The examinations include the check-up of organ functions, immunology, virology, bacteriology, blood typing and pathology. Due to the severe shortage of organs, the acceptance criteria have been expanded considerably over the last years. Accordingly, organ donation is possible up to a well-advanced age. The organ's functional state as well as its reserve is the deciding factor for donation. However, the medical history of the donor should be known. Organs with functional restrictions and/or patients with certain pre-existing illnesses are not automatically excluded from organ donation.

Many of such organs are well transplantable under favourable conditions such as short ischemia time (Breidenbach and Banas 2011; Dominguez-Gil et al. 2011).

Current medical contraindications for organ donation are untreatable systemic diseases or infections posing a vital threat for the recipient or functional restriction of the organs (Guide to the safety and quality of organs for transplantation 2013). In the case of impaired organ function, it has to be determined whether the impairment existed before the acute brain injury or occurred simultaneously. Additionally, the reversibility by an adequate intensive care therapy must be checked. If the reason for the limited function cannot be clarified, intraoperative biopsy may provide further insight.

An important factor for the success of the transplantation is an adequate organ protective intensive care treatment on the part of the donor. The goal is to prevent functional and structural damage and to maintain an optimal state of the organs. Cardiovascular function and thus the circulation of blood to and within organs must be maintained artificially (ventilation, hemodynamic therapy, and hormone substitution) (Breidenbach and Banas 2011; McKeown et al. 2012; Rey et al. 2012).

11.3.5 Allocation

The DSO coordinator submits all required donor information to the Allocation Agency (Eurotransplant) when brain death is declared, the donor's consent is available, and the eligibility of organs is tested positively. On the basis of a complex allocation system, Eurotransplant determines the potential recipient. The criteria for allocation are developed by the Standing Committee on Organ Transplantation of the German Medical Association (Richtlinien für die Wartelistenführung und die Organvermittlung). The allocation criteria incorporate medical as well as social values and universal ethical principles (fairness, transparency, validity, objectivity).

Eurotransplant is responsible for the allocation in Germany, as well as in Belgium, Croatia, Luxembourg, the Netherlands, Austria, Slovenia and Hungary. Depending on the organ, there are specific allocation criteria, which are highly complex and under continuous review. The current kidney allocation policy, for instance, considers the waiting time a main criterion in addition to the tissue match. There are special rules that apply to paediatric recipients, elderly donors and recipients, and highly immunized patients (Breidenbach and Banas 2011; https://www.eurotransplant.org/; Richtlinien für die Wartelistenführung und die Organvermittlung).

When allocating a liver, medical urgency matters the most. High urgency patients take priority. For patients undergoing an elective treatment, the allocation is based on the MELD-score (Model of End-Stage Liver Disease). The MELD scoring system is based on three objective parameters (Bilirubin, Creatinine, INR—International Normalized Ratio). It mirrors the 3-month probability of death on the waiting list. The patient with the highest score gets the organ. The allocation of the heart is subject to urgency followed by waiting time and the estimated ischemia time (time, an organ remains without the supply of blood). Lungs are allocated using a special score (Lung Allocation Score). The score incorporates urgency and prospects of success. The pancreas is allocated with regard to urgency followed by waiting time and estimated ischemia time. For the small bowel, the allocation is carried out in accordance with waiting time (Richtlinien für die Wartelistenführung und die Organvermittlung).

Within an allocation process, logistical and/or organizational delays are possible as well as a hemodynamic deterioration of the donor. The threat of losing an organ then requires an accelerated allocation procedure. The decision on the acceptance or refusal of an organ lies with the responsible physician at the transplantation centre. It is necessary to carefully balance the risk of a transmission of diseases against the probability of dying on the waiting list.

11.3.6 Organ Procurement/Transport

After the confirmation, that at least one organ was allocated, the DSO coordinator starts to organize the procurement procedure. The operation time has to be determined in consultation with the donor hospital, the procurement teams have to be informed and further steps planned. Thoracic organs are removed by the surgeons of the recipient centres, while abdominal organs are removed by regional procurement teams (Breidenbach and Banas 2011).

Organ procurement is possible in almost every hospital with an operating theatre. In rare cases, however, the donor can be transferred to a larger hospital. The procurement operation takes place under sterile conditions, similar to any kind of surgery. Great care is taken to ensure the reverential treatment of the body. Anaesthesia to eliminate consciousness and pain responses is redundant in brain-dead donors. Drugs administered only serve the dynamic stabilization of the donor as well as to facilitate the operation. After the procurement, organs are packed on ice and then transported as quickly as possible to the recipient centres. A fast transport to the transplant centres is essential for the success of the transplantation, due to the short period of time in which the explanted organ stays healthy (e.g. heart ~6 h, kidneys ~24–36 h). To ensure a smooth process, the DSO sets up all necessary logistics. The body is treated carefully and family members have the opportunity to bid farewell to their loved one. The possibility of a personal farewell after the removal operation must be provided to the families (Transplantationsgesetz in der Fassung der Bekanntmachung vom 4. September 2007; Breidenbach and Banas 2011).

11.3.7 Transplantation

After its arrival at the transplant centre, the organ is transplanted as quickly as possible. Thoracic transplant recipients are usually already in the operating room during the return transport. This facilitates the start of the transplantation right after the arrival of the organ. For visceral organs, an assessment and fine preparation of the organ is conducted before anesthesia is administered.

11.3.8 Aftercare/Family Care

Essential for the long-term success of the transplantation is an appropriate and qualified aftercare with organ function and medication being regularly viewed as well as a periodic check-up of the recipients' general health. The aftercare is usually done in the transplant centre, often in cooperation with resident physicians. If any question or problem should arise during a donation process, the DSO offers special debriefings and training programs to the donor hospitals. This appears to be appropriate, especially for those hospitals where organ donation is a rare event. Every employee involved in the donation process as well as the donors' relatives—if requested—receive a letter of thanks 4–6 weeks after the donation. The letter contains information on the whereabouts and the success of the transplantation but due to the german transplant law all data have to be anonymized. In case the relatives agreed to have their data saved, they will be invited to the beforementioned relatives' meetings after the donation. Experiences have shown that questions can arise after an initial period of grief. In the meetings, these questions can be discussed and processed with psychological support (Breidenbach and Banas 2011; https://www.dso.de/; Breidenbach and Hesse 2011; Grammenos et al. 2012).

11.4 Perspective

Transplantation medicine has been massively criticised within the last 2 years due to criminal manipulations of the liver waiting lists (Sigmund-Schultze 2012; Richter-Kuhlmann 2013). These manipulations have led to a loss of confidence within the general public and the medical personnel, which could be shown in a recently published study (Grammenos et al. 2014). Especially the severe uncertainty and loss of confidence within the medical personnel can explain the dramatic decrease of donation rates in Germany since they initiate the whole process.

But even before the scandals, German patients suffering from chronic or acute organ failure have been disadvantaged in comparison to their European neighbours (International registry in organ donation and transplantation 2013).

Unfortunately, the situation has tightened, leading to significant consequences for the suffering patients'—meaning many of them will have to die because they cannot receive a transplant in time. There is no doubt that everything has to be done to rebuild trust. This will only be achievable through maximum transparency and honesty by everyone involved. The processes of organ donation and transplantation itself are transparent and regulated in detail by the german transplantation law and the Standing Committee on Organ Transplantation of the German Medical Association (Transplantationsgesetz in der Fassung der Bekanntmachung vom 4. September 2007; Breidenbach and Banas 2011; Richtlinien für die Wartelistenführung und die Organvermittlung) as described earlier in this chapter.

References

Breidenbach, T., and B. Banas, eds. 2011. *Organspende und Transplantationsmedizin*. 1st ed. Grünwald: Börm Bruckmeier Verlag.

Breidenbach, T., and A. Hesse. 2011. Herausforderung und Chance. Das Angehörigengespräch Gespräch mit der Bitte um eine Organspende. *Bay Aerzteblatt* 9:2–4.

Bundesärztekammer. 1998. Organentnahme nach Herzstillstand. *Deutsches Ärzteblatt* 95 (50): A–3235

Dominguez-Gil, B., F. Delmonico, F. Shaheen, R. Matesanz, K. O'Connor, M. Minina, E. Muller, K. Young, M. Manyalich, J. Chapman, G. Kirste, M. Al-Mousawi, L. Coene, V. Duro Garcıa, S. Gautier, T. Hasegawa, V. Jha, T. Kiat Kwek, Z. Chen, B. Loty, A. Nanni Costa, H. Nathan, R. Ploeg, O. Reznik, J. D. Rosendale, A. Tibell, G. Tsoulfas, V. Anantharaman, and L. Noel. 2011. The critical pathway for deceased donation: Reportable uniformity in the approach to deceased donation. *Transplant International* 24:373–378.

Gewebegesetz vom 20. Juli 2007. (BGBl. I S. 1574), http://www.gesetze-im-internet.de/gewebeg/.

Grammenos, D., A. Greser, and T. Breidenbach. 2012. Informieren und begleiten. Angehörigenbetreuung in der DSO-Region Bayern. *Bay Aerzteblatt* 6:312–313.

Grammenos, D., T. Bein, J. Briegel, K.-U. Eckardt, G. Gerresheim, C. Lang, C. Nieß, F. Zeman, and T. Breidenbach. 2014. Attitudes of medical staff potentially participating in the organ donation process towards organ donation and transplantation in Bavaria. *Deutsche Medizinische Wochenschrift* 139:1289–94.

International registry in organ donation and transplantation. 2013. www.irodat.org. Accessed 20 April 2015.

Magnus, D. J., B. J. Wilfond, and A. L. Caplan. 2014. Accepting brain death. *New England Journal of Medicine* 370 (10): 891–894.

McKeown, D. W., R. S. Bonser, and J. A. Kellum. 2012. Management of the heartbeating brain-dead organ donor. *British Journal Anaesthesia* 108:96–107.

Rey J. W., T. Ott, T. Bösebeck, S. Welschehold, P. R. Galle, and C. Werner. 2012. Organprotektive Intensivtherapie und Simulatortraining. *Der Anaesthesist* 61:242–248.

Richter-Kuhlmann, E. 2013. Deutsche Stiftung Organtransplantation: Gefragt ist (neues) Vertrauen. *Deutsches Ärzteblatt* 110:18.

Siegmund-Schultze, N., and V. Zylka-Menhorn. 2008. Non-Heart-Beating-Donors: „Herztote" Organspender. *Deutsches Ärzteblatt* 105 (16): A–832.

Sigmund-Schultze, N. 2012. Transplantationsskandal an der Universität Göttingen: Erschütterndes Maß an Manipulationen. *Dtsch Arztebl* 109:31–32.

Transplantationsgesetz in der Fassung der Bekanntmachung vom 4. September 2007. (BGBl. I S. 2206), das zuletzt durch Artikel 5d des Gesetzes vom 15. Juli 2013 (BGBl. I S. 2423) geändert worden ist, http://www.gesetze-im-internet.de/tpg/.

Williams, M., and P. A. Lipsett. 2003. The physician's role in discussing organ donation with families. *Critical Care Medicine* 31:1568–1573.

2013. Guide to the safety and quality of organs for transplantation. European Committee on Organ Transplantation; (5th ed.).

Richtlinien zur Feststellung des Hirntodes. 1998. *Deutsches Ärzteblatt* 95 (53): 1861–1868.

Richtlinien für die Wartelistenführung und die Organvermittlung gem. § 16 Abs. 1 S. 1 Nrn. 2 u. 5 TPG. http://www.bundesaerztekammer.de/downloads/.

Thomas Breidenbach MD majored in biology in Hannover, Germany and Boston, USA, and went on to attend medical school in Hannover. He began his surgical career at the Department of General, Visceral, and Transplantation Surgery in Hannover under the direction of Prof. Rudolf Pichlmayr. He then continued as a surgeon at Augsburg Hospital, with Prof. Eckhard Nagel, where he lastly took on the position as the Assistant Medical Director at the transplant center. In addition, he was Lecturer at the Institute for Medical Management and Health Sciences at the University of Bayreuth. Thomas Breidenbach is currently the Regional Director of Bavaria for the German Organ Transplantation Foundation. He is also involved in different European projects regarding organ donation and transplantation medicine.

Chapter 12
Organ Shortage as a Structural Problem in Transplantation Medicine

Alexandra Manzei

12.1 Introduction

On November 1, 2012, legislative amendments to the German law governing organ transplantation came into force. From this date forward, the German transplantation law was no longer restricted to regulating the removal and donation of human organs and tissues. Instead, it is now declared purpose of the law "to promote the willingness to donate organs" (§ 1, (1) TGP). The amendments are intended to solve a problem which is typical not only for Germany: the problem of *supply shortage in transplantation medicine*, which is usually referred to as *organ shortage*. In the wake of this change in legislation, a lot of money is being spent on advertising to encourage people to sign a donor card—a measure which is considered as helpful for increasing the number of donor organs available for transplant. While many aspects of transplantation medicine are currently controversial in Germany, due to the scandals that occurred there in 2012,[1] this measure taken for itself is entirely beyond dispute: it seems to be unquestionable that the problem of organ shortage could be solved by increasing the number of donor card holders. The underlying idea is that if there were enough donor card holders—if, for example, every German citizen would sign a donor card—there would thus be enough organ donors to meet demands. However, what both political actors as well as the public do not realize is that not every donor card holder will become an actual donor. Unlike often suggested by the medical system, it is simply *not true* that everybody can donate organs after death. Actually, there is only a very small group of patients

[1] Due to a number of scandals in 2012 in which transplant clinics violated organ allocation guidelines.

A. Manzei (✉)
University of Augsburg, Augsburg, Germany
e-mail: alexandra.manzei@phil.uni-augsburg.de

R. J. Jox et al. (eds.), *Organ Transplantation in Times of Donor Shortage*,
International Library of Ethics, Law, and the New Medicine 59,
DOI 10.1007/978-3-319-16441-0_12

who is able to donate vital organs at all: until a few years ago, and in most countries worldwide, only patients who die after a complete brain failure—the so called *brain death*—are allowed to become donors for vital organs. But, only a very small number of patients meet this description. According to the German Foundation for Organ Transplantation there are approximately 2000 brain dead people in Germany per year, other studies speak of up to 3000–4000 brain dead patients. Yet, measured against the number of patients who are waiting for an organ (which is about 11,000 in Germany), and due to the fact that normally not every organ is transplantable, it is certain that there will never be enough organs to supply every needy patient.[2]

Most people are not aware of these facts, as I have come to learn from the many lectures I have held on this subject in the last years. Due to an inadequate information policy over the last 20 years, which equates brain death with the death of the human being, most people—and not only medical laypeople—believe that they could donate organs even after lying in the morgue for 1 or 2 days. Of course this is not possible. Organs of a corpse are not transplantable, as they would poison the recipient. The reason for this false assumption is not only a lack of information or ignorance. Moreover, it is the equation of brain failure with the death of a human being itself—the so called brain death concept—which causes this false assumption. However understandable the equation from an ethical point of view might be, as a consequence it leads to the wrong conclusion: that increasing the number of donor card holders would solve the problem of organ shortage.

In the following I will focus on this problematic assumption and its consequences. I will show that the exclusive orientation of health policy towards increasing the number of donor card holders does not solve the problem of organ shortage. Furthermore, it reinforces the problem by concealing the real reasons for supply shortage in transplantation medicine. These are, first of all, a rapidly growing demand for organs caused by the fact that for an increasing number of diseases, organ transplantation is seen as "the one best way" of therapy. The second reason is the lack of organs brought about by intrinsic problems of the transplantation system itself.

In a first subchapter, I will discuss the fact that not everybody is able to donate organs after death except the very small group of brain dead patients. In a second and third subchapter, I will recount the historical genesis of the brain death concept (which means the equation of the complete and irreversible functional failure of the brain and brainstem with the death of a human being) and outline new scientific doubts concerning this concept. Questioning the brain death concept is—then—a necessary prerequisite for realizing that organ shortage is a structural problem of transplantation medicine. In the fourth subchapter, I will show that the demand for organs is increasing for intrinsic reasons related to the transplantation system and not because of a lack of willingness to donate organs. As a consequence, the rising demand for organs results in morally questionable practices to obtain organs. I will outline a few of these practices in the fifth subchapter. After gaining an understanding of organ shortage in this way—as an unsolvable structural problem of transplantation medicine in its current shape—the article ends with a final plea

[2] See http://www.dso.de/nbsp/german-organ-transplantation-foundation-dso.html.

for the development of alternative forms of medical therapy. If we are to take the fact that there will never be enough organs for all needy patients anyway seriously, we must admit that we must substitute organ transplantation in the long run with medical procedures which do not require organs from living or dying human beings. If we do not do so, the moral pressure on living and dying human beings to serve as an organ and tissue reserve will increase, as well the negative consequences of organ shortage we have sadly become familiar with (e.g., organ trafficking).

12.2 Reasons Why *Not* Everybody Can Donate Organs After Death

It seems to be generally accepted that the problem of organ shortage could be solved by increasing the willingness to donate organs. This ostensibly proven knowledge remains largely unquestioned by politicians, the media, and the general public. Moreover, it seems to be unthinkable to doubt the relationship between the scarcity of organs and a low willingness to donate organs. Responsible for this taboo is the following argument, which—like some kind of ritual—is pointed out in the preface to almost any discussion on organ transplantation: "11,000 people are waiting for an organ. Each day, three of them die because there are not enough donor organs." Thus, everybody who dares to question this relationship, or worse, refuses to donate their organs, is deemed as being guilty for the so-called "deaths on the waiting list". For every person that thinks and acts morally, this is of course an intolerable notion—an accusation which nobody is willing to expose themselves to, not even on a theoretical level. At the same time, there seems to be broad skepticism about organ donation throughout society, which has not only become manifest since the number of organ donors has decreased during this past year. For years, there has been an enormous discrepancy between publicly stated acceptance of organ donation and a much lower percentage of donor card holders—and this is not only true of the general population, but also of medical experts. Insofar, there are good and objectively justified reasons to withstand the moral pressure for the time being and challenge the seemingly self-evident relationship between organ shortage and the lack of donor card holders.

The first fact that needs to be emphasized in this context is that people do not die because other people refuse to donate organs at the end of their lives (an accusation which is implied by the mentioned argument). People die because of diseases or old age, or both. People die because human beings are mortal—even the most advanced medicine has not changed this fact until today. However, what modern medicine does change profoundly is the question of *when and how* a human being dies—and this is where transplantation medicine plays a very special role. Unlike other medical therapies, organ transplantation requires *the availability of vital organs from other patients*. Therefore, ever since its development in the middle of the twentieth century, organ transplantation is characterized by a moral, legal, and medical dilemma: Human organs are not freely available spare parts, which can be manufactured and sold like an artificial knee joint or a hip endoprosthesis. Human organs are vital parts of the human body. Before they can be used to help a patient in need, they must be removed from another—living or dying—human being. This fact is the real reason of the so-called organ shortage: it is not true that vital organs can be obtained *after* death as suggested by the information policy of the medical system and by health policy. On the contrary, organs from a normal corpse—cold and stiff—can definitely not be used for transplantation.[3] An organ extracted from a dead body would indeed poison the recipient since the decomposition process of the corpse has already begun. Organs used for transplantation have to be vital and must not lack blood supply for a long time. With this in mind, the statements on the donation of "deceased donor organs" or "post mortem organs", which are propagated in information brochures, must be regarded as misleading. They conceal the fact that organs from a dead body cannot be transplanted.

Hence, it is a wrong conclusion to assume everybody could donate organs after death. Actually, no one can donate organs *after death.* There is only a very small group of people who are able to donate vital organs anyway: only those individuals who are dying but still have a well-functioning organism—as is the case with brain death—can donate vital organs at all. Thus, in Germany vital organs can and may only be obtained from persons who have officially been declared brain dead. Brain dead people are dying patients who are lying in an intensive care unit and do not exhibit brain activity any longer. For a very short time (only a few hours up to 1 day) the bodies of those patients can be kept alive by receiving artificial respiration. However, the number of patients that actually meet these requirements is rather small. The exact annual number of brain-dead patients in Germany can only be estimated; reliable data is not available. The few German studies on this subject assume that there are up to 3000 to 4000 brain dead patients per year at maximum.[4] However, even if all these people were suitable organ donors and all of their organs were transplantable (which usually is not the case), there still would not be enough organs to meet the demand. The *Eurotransplant Organisation* reported that there were 7919 patients waiting for a kidney in 2012, in Germany.[5] In other words, even if each and every German citizen would hold a donor card, there would still remain a rather high number of unprovided patients since—to repeat the argument—not everybody is able to donate vital organs but only very few terminal patients at the threshold between life and death. These structural reasons for supply shortage have been completely ignored by politicians. As long as legislation focuses exclusively on the increasing of the willingness to donate organs, the structural problems of organ shortage remain unnoticed.

---

[3] The only body parts which can be transplanted after being extracted from a real corps are ear ossicle, eye lenses and some other kind of graft but no whole organs.

[4] Föderreuther and Angstwurm (2003); Ohm et al. (2001); Wesslau et al. (2007).

[5] Active Eurotransplant waiting list, by organ, as per December 31, 2012, Table 4.5 (ii). See Eurotransplant Foundation (2014).

12.3 Dead or Dying? The Ambivalence of the Brain Death Concept

Another taboo in the political debate today is the essential ambivalence of the brain death concept as such, i.e., the question whether brain dead people are *dead* or *dying*.[6] The taboo surrounding this question is a phenomenon which emerged in Germany at the end of the 1990s. During the thirty years before, since the late 1960s, when the state of complete brain failure in intensive care patients was observed for the first time[7], the question of whether those patients should be considered as a dead or a dying human being has been the subject of highly controversial discussions—firstly in the medical system and later on in the public as well. Still in the early 1990s, during the preliminary stages of the ratification of the German transplantation law, the conflicts regarding the question when dead occurs culminated in bitter arguments between proponents and opponents of the concept of brain death.[8] Hence, there are good reasons why the transplantation law *does not answer the question* (whether brain dead people are dead or dying) until today. It does not offer a definition of death. Instead, the legislative body shifted the responsibility to defining death to the medical system.[9] Although there are statements in the law which *seem* to define brain death as the death of the human being a closer look shows the opposite.

There are three references in the law where the question of death is mentioned. In one article, the law dictates that prior to the harvesting of an organ, "the death of the organ or tissue donor must be ascertained in accordance with the current state of medical knowledge" (see § 3, [1] TPG). In the subsequent article it is stated that organs must not be obtained before the brain death of the donor is declared (which is described as "an unrecoverable failure of all brain functions in the cerebrum, the cerebellum, and the brain stem" (see § 3, [2] TPG). However, these two requirements are *not* discussed in relation to one another. It remains unclear whether brain death can be equated with the death of the human being, or not. Furthermore, § 16 TPG specifies that it is the duty of the *German Medical Association* (Bundesärztekammer) to provide a definition of brain death according to the current state of medical science in the form of guidelines. Correspondingly, the academic advisory council of the *German Medical Association* states in its *Guidelines for the diagnosis*

[6] To remember: Brain death concept means the equation of the complete and irreversible functional failure of the brain and brainstem with the death of a human being.

[7] See for example the famous critic from the ethicist Hans Jonas (1974).

[8] Manzei (2003).

[9] This is a completely different story than the development of the same discussion in the US. Here, the answer to the question when death occurs is provided in a special act, the "Uniform Determination of Death Act" (UDDA) from 1981: "§ 1. [Determination of Death]. An individual who has sustained either (1) irreversible cessation of circulatory and respiratory functions, or (2) irreversible cessation of all functions of the entire brain, including the brain stem, is dead. A determination of death must be made in accordance with accepted medical standards." See President's Commission (2008) 5.

of brain death: "In terms of natural and medical sciences a human being is considered dead when brain death has occured" (Deutsches Ärzteblatt 1998). But here, too, no explanation is given as to why the failure of the brain should be considered as equal to the death of a human being.

Whereas this absence of a definition of death—in the transplantation law as well as in the guidelines—at the first glance appears as a fundamental flaw, it is actually an adequate frame to implicitly reflect the ambivalence of the brain death concept. Fundamentally, medical science cannot provide a definition of death. What we understand as death (and as life) is a cultural, societal, or religious question. Medical science can *diagnose* death, but it cannot define it. In that sense it can be seen as a wise decision of the German legislator to *not* regulate organ donation strictly in form of the "opt-out-system" (as, for example, Austria or Spain do), meaning that anyone who has not refused would automatically be seen as an organ donor.[10] Moreover, the legislature implemented the "opt-in-solution" or, rather, the "expanded assessment solution" (Erweiterte Zustimmungslösung) which means that only those people can become organ donors who themselves (or whose relatives on their behalf) have given explicit consent. In this way, everybody should be given the opportunity to decide for themselves—freely and without pressure—if they can accept the concept of brain death and, under these circumstances, agree to consent to donate their organs at the end of life. This idea expresses the absolute and coercion-free acceptance of the individual right to self-determination. Even today, this still remains as the basis of the new legislation in Germany.

In this sense, the transplantation law was important not only in respect to medical and legal questions. It also served an important social function by enabling and creating a broad social consensus concerning organ transplantation. Since then, the ambivalence of the brain death concept has not been seriously discussed nor questioned by the public in Germany again. Only among German medical and ethical experts and in international debates beyond German public discussion the dispute has been carried forth. Since a few years now these discussions returned to Germany again, and today—accelerated by the scandals in the last years—the concept of brain death is being challenged once again. In particular, people in Catholic and Protestant communities are questioning the brain death concept again.[11] In the following chapter I will outline the—partly new and partly well known—arguments of this new debate.

[10] In any case, the opt-out-solution, too, would not solve the problem of organ shortage because it does not increase the number of brain dead people but only number of donor card holders. To be precise, it does increase the quantity of transplantable organs somewhat, as a comparison of several European countries shows, but the problem of organ shortage would remain—because the opt-out-solution does not increase the number of brain dead people.

[11] See Byrne (2009) and EFiD (2013).

12.4 New Medical Studies Prove the Problematic Nature of the Brain Death Concept

The "new" skepticism against the brain death concept is pushed by two main arguments. The first argument concerns the mentioned ambivalence of the brain death concept. Recent medical studies have demonstrated that brain death is not synonymous with the death of a human being, because death does *not* occur immediately after the failure of the brain functioning. At least 175 cases that have been documented up to the year 1998 provide scientifically evidence that brain dead patients may continue to live for up to 14 years if they are supported by adequate intensive care interventions.[12] Moreover, it is possible that the actual number of brain dead patients who are not really dead is much higher since, of course, only those cases can be reviewed in which no organs were removed after the diagnosis of brain death. Because, the removal of a vital organ foregoes the possibility of any result other than death. Therefore, in a white paper the American *President's Commission on Bioethics* (2008) accused the brain death concept of being a self-fulfilling prophecy.[13] Hence, the commission rejected the established justification which grounds the brain dead concept on the assumption that the brain controls every body function wherefore death must occur immediately after a total brain failure[14]. However, instead of consequently criticizing the conventional practices of organ donation, the commission deemed it necessary to build up a new justification—not because the scientists were convinced of the brain death concept per se but because they saw the necessity for discussing the ambivalence of the brain death concept in light of the problem of organ shortage.[15]

A second argument states that there are new techniques in functional imaging which are able to measuring brain activity even after brain death has—seemingly clearly—been diagnosed. Correspondingly, cases are known in established literature which, through the use of technical diagnostics, blood supply to the brain could be shown in patients who had been clinically diagnosed as brain dead. These cases provide medical evidence on the issue of why brain dead patients often show reactions during organ removal, which are normally explained as pain and defensive responses when they are observed in other unconscious patients: blood pressure and heart rate escalate, the face turns red, sweat beads appear, and arms and legs move. For this reason, organ donors are anaesthetized before organ harvesting in some countries (for example, Switzerland and Great Britain). In Germany, this is not practiced because to administer analgesics would mean to accept that a brain dead person is not a dead human being, but a seriously ill and dying patient.

In any case, it is well known that brain dead patients show certain signs of life, like moving their arms and legs. Such movements are usually described as *spi-*

[12] Shewmon (1998a).

[13] See President's Commission (2008, p. 42).

[14] For the conventional justification and its critic see Byrne ed. (2009).

[15] See President's Commission (2008); Müller (2011).

nal reflexes or *Lazarus signs*. According to DSO, these signs can be observed in 75 % of brain dead patients. In DSO's point of view however, these are not signs of life but signs of death, and therefore DSO recommends the deactivation of the vegetative nervous system during organ removal "in order to optimize the surgical intervention" (DSO 2013). But, an important problem of this procedure is that only the movements and physical reactions of the organ donor are suppressed, but not necessarily his or her pain. Thus, this measure is supposed to calm the nurses and other personnel assisting in the operation. After all, a brain dead patient still appears to be a living human being and to watch his or her movements and vital signs is hardly bearable, not only for the nursing personnel and many physicians, but also and especially for the relatives. Brain dead persons have a warm body that is still being supplied with blood, their vital signs are recorded (heart rate, blood pressure, temperature, etc.), they are being nourished and their excretory organs are still active, they may have high temperature, and their wounds still heal. Brain dead children can grow and, up until 2003, ten cases of pregnant brain dead women have been documented who were able to maintain their pregnancy for months until the baby was delivered.[16]

Although these arguments against the concept of brain death are discussed at length among experts all over the world and are known in Germany as well, they have been more or less ignored in both the public discussion and the political debate on the revision of transplantation legislation. The vital necessity of a comprehensive education on this issue has been shown by several studies documenting the sometimes alarming lack of knowledge among experts and laypersons,[17] and from many lectures on this topic I personally know that most people have no idea that there is a difference between a brain dead person and a normal dead body. One frequently asked question, for example, is whether it is true that organs from a deceased person, who has been in the morgue for 48 h, cannot be transplanted. Most people are not aware of the fact that an organ from a dead body would poison the recipient. They also do not realize that there would be no organ shortage at all if it were possible to transplant organs from a dead body—for after all, there is no shortage of normal dead bodies.

12.5 Why the Demand for Organs is Continuously Increasing

The problematic nature of the concept of brain death as such is not the only cause for the chronic supply shortage of patients in transplantation medicine. Other causes arise from transplantation system itself—because the more successful transplantation medicine becomes, the more organs are needed. In the following section, I will discuss some mechanisms inherent to the system, which lead to a continuously *increasing demand* for human organs.

[16] See Müller (2011); Shewmon (1998a, 1998b).

[17] Baureithel and Bergmann (1999); Schweidtmann and Muthny (1997).

Firstly, organ transplantation is considered the most effective therapy for more and more diseases and replaces other therapeutic approaches, for example in the management of acute and chronic hepatic diseases. That is why the waiting list for liver transplants in the Eurotransplant area has more than quadrupled between 1991 and 2011.[18] Secondly, it must be called to mind that—and this is another fact which is almost completely disregarded in the public debate—all organs (from unrelated donors) are, eventually rejected by the new host. Moreover, patients who have suffered a transplant rejection are then put on the waiting list for re-transplantation and are favored over patients waiting for their first transplantation. Though this practice might be understandable from an ethical point of view, it also means that the re-transplantation rate is increasing continuously. For example, a single patient can be provided with a new kidney *four or more times* during his or her lifetime. The total demand for organs is multiplied by this. Thirdly, the number of *multiple organ transplantations* is also rising continuously: For example, patients with type-1 diabetes often receive a new pancreas *and* a new kidney at the same time because this procedure allows for a better chance of recovery.

Last but not least, there are organizational reasons for the ever-increasing demand for organs. Hospitals that specialize in transplantation, for example, must carry out a minimum number of transplantations because otherwise they would run the risk of losing the right to perform transplantations. The recent scandals at the hospitals *Rechts der Isar* and *Großhadern* in Munich have made it abundantly clear that the prevailing criteria for the urgency of a transplantation procedure are not always taken into account. In 2013, the public prosecutor's office was investigating transplant physicians who were responsible for liver transplantations in patients who, at the time of the surgery, were not in urgent need of a new organ. Beside the ethical question this practice raises, the complication arose that one of the patients died from a transplant rejection after short time—a patient to whom an organ transplantation was not really necessary at that time.

In summary, it can be stated that the demand for organs will increase the more successful and expansive transplantation medicine is. The gap between the supply of and the demand for organs will continue to widen.[19] Hence, there will emerge more and more practices which shift the boundary between life and death to an earlier point to gain vital organs prior to the moment of total brain failure, as the following chapter shows.

12.6 Beyond Brain Dead: Disturbing Practices of Acquiring Organs

How the boundary between life and death has been shifted for the benefit of organ procurement can already be observed in other countries. In Great Britain, vital organs are harvested directly after *brainstem death,* which takes place before a total brain failure. In Germany, this practice is not allowed because it cannot be ruled out

[18] See Eurotransplant Foundation (2014).

[19] A problem which is more and more seen and is problematized by transplant physicians as well. See http://www.freiepresse.de/NACHRICHTEN/DEUTSCHLAND/Wissenschaftler-setzen-auf-Alternativen-zur-Organspende-artikel8987550.php.

that patients in this condition are still conscious. Patients suffering from so-called *locked-in syndrome*, e.g., are completely paralysed, due to the failure of some part of the brain stem, but with adequate technical support, they are able to answer questions, read, watch TV, etc.[20]

Harvesting organs immediately after cardiac death is another practice where the boundary between life and death is shifted to an earlier point of live for the purpose of organ procurement. It means to obtain vital organs from a dying patient *before* he or she suffers a total brain failure. In accordance with the "Maastricht protocol" (an EU directive which rules the harvesting of organs after cardiac death in Europe since 1995) these donors are called "Non-heart-beating-donors" (NHBDs) whereas patients who suffer a partly or total brain failure are called "Heart-beating-donors" (HBDs).[21] To date, the transplant organization *Eurotransplant* has not been successful in establishing this practice in Germany although they have tried to do so more than once. However, in other countries that are also part of the *Eurotransplant* network, this has become common practice for quite some time. In Austria, Belgium, Switzerland, the Netherlands and the USA, for example, organs may be harvested directly after cardiac arrest. According to current German law those patients would not be considered as being dead—which means the removal of the organs *is ultimately responsible for the death of these patients*. The fundamental ethical problem of this practice is evident: even if these patients have definitely begun the process of dying, harvesting their organs in such an early time means terminating their lives for the purpose of a third person. This practice cannot even being grasped as euthanasia since a possible benefit for the dying patient is not taken into consideration at all.

However, it is not only those patients whose hearts have already stopped beating due to a sickness or an accident that are eligible for organ harvesting after cardiac death, but also seriously ill patients with an unfavorable prognosis are used as organ donors. In these cases, a procedure can be conducted which is called *controlled Donation after Cardiac Death (controlled DCD)* or *physician-assisted suicide*, a procedure which has been legal in the USA since the early 1990s and has also been performed in Belgium since 2005: seriously ill patients who have agreed to the procedure are put to death in an operating room and their organs are removed as soon as they are officially declared dead. From the point of view of transplantation medicine, this method offers special benefits: since all medical examinations of the organs necessary for transplantation can be performed while the patient is still alive, it is possible to greatly reduce the ischemia time of the organs (which is the time while the organs are extracorporeal and lack blood supply. The longer this time lasts the more harmful the graft will be for the recipient).[22]

Whereas in Germany this practice is regarded as an act of euthanasia, in highly esteemed international journals it is emphatically appreciated as a new source of organ procurement, e.g., by the internationally renowned bioethicist and philosopher

[20] Geisler (2010).

[21] See Chaib (2008); Holznienkemper (2005).

[22] Keller (2011).

Julian Savulescu.[23] Savulescu—and amongst others the German bioethicist Dieter Birnbacher, a longstanding member of the ethics board of the *German Medical Association*—want the *dead donor rule*, according to which a human being has to be dead before vital organs may be harvested, to be given up.[24] Instead of holding on to the concept of brain death despite the lack of empirical evidence, we should instead admit that a brain dead person is a dying person anyway. Hence, we should admit that for years it has been common practice worldwide to harvest organs from dying human beings (HBDs) and, by doing so, put an end to their lives. From this perspective, "Euthanasia for Organ Donation" (Wilkinson and Savulescu 2010), as Savulescu calls this practice, appears to be nothing more than a logical consequence and the continuation of the common practice to obtain organs from HBDs.

At present, all those procedures of organ procurement (harvesting after brain stem death, after cardiac death, and after death through euthanasia) are still illegal in Germany. Moreover, in 2011, the *German Medical Association* asserted that "killing is not part of the business of physicians" and that in order to create a relationship of trust between patients and doctors it is absolutely essential for the patients to be sure that they are treated solely for their own benefit and not for the benefit of others. This is an important statement because one thing is true for all of these suggestions: Whether with or without consent from the organ donor, the overall aim of acquiring organs from dying or seriously ill human beings is for the benefit of third parties, not for the patient himself.

12.7 Conclusion: The Demand for Organs Must Be Reduced and Alternatives to Transplantation Medicine Must Be Promoted

To summarize: I have shown that the so called organ shortage is a systematic and inherent problem of the transplantation system itself and does not result from the lack of willingness of the general population to donate organs. Even if each and every citizen would hold a donor card there would never be enough donor organs for all needy patients because—in contrary to what is constantly claimed—organs from dead people cannot be used for transplantation. Moreover, if transplantation medicine continues to expand, the demand for organs will continue to increase. As a result, more and more attempts will be made to acquire viable organs from healthy human beings (living donation) and from seriously ill and dying patients—not to mention illegal or (as in Iran) legal organ trafficking. From an ethical viewpoint we have to ask, whether we should keep on supporting this medical technology—strongly and almost exclusively—which in the long run has such unavoidable and undesired consequences.

---

23 Wilkinson and Savulescu (2010).

24 Birnbacher (2007).

Instead of spending more and more resources on transplantation medicine—without even asking whether this medical system is being able to take good care of its patients—it would be necessary *to reduce the demand for organs and to promote alternative therapies*. Therefore the problem of organ shortage must—firstly—be better labeled as *inadequate supply or supply shortage of patients* than as organ shortage. Because, the term "organ shortage" restricts the search for solutions only to the procedure of organ replacement. In contrast, talking about an *inadequate supply* or *supply shortage of patients* in transplantation medicine widens the view also for alternative therapies which do not require vital organs from living human beings. As a second step, a variety of measures could be discussed to accomplish this goal—in the field of prevention as well as in (interventional) curative care.

In the field of prevention: Since a significant amount of illnesses which are currently being treated by organ replacement are the result of diseases of civilization, such as diabetes, obesity, cardiovascular diseases, substance abuse diseases, etc. Measures to prevent these basic diseases could be targeted both at the level of healthcare, labor, and social policies (by improving the conditions of life, work and environment) and at the level of people's individual behavior. Another important aspect is that organ damage is often caused by the adverse side effects of medication, which in particular for chronically ill patients poses a serious problem, for example patients suffering from rheumatism. It would be necessary to ensure that political regulations like discount agreements (in other words, the price) are not the main criterion for prescription, but instead the patients' tolerance.

Issues related to curative care could also be addressed in a number of ways in that organ replacement is not the only form of therapy which is available to modern medicine. On the one hand, there are alternative (bio)technological therapies like tissue engineering or the use of artificial hearts which should be promoted.[25] On another note, *pharmacological therapies* as well as *complementary and alternative medical therapies* (CAM), which do not involve organ replacement but are aimed at the (self-)healing of the body, should be promoted even further. Which options are reasonable and available in this context should be determined in the course of a broad expert discussion involving not only representatives from medicine, the pharmaceutical industry, and patient associations, but also health and nursing scientists and politicians responsible for labour and health care politics. This discussion could, for example, be organized in the form of a *concerted action in health care*.

Last but not least, it must be ensured that organ transplantation is subject to the same quality controls as other medical therapies. For example, it could be evaluated by institutions like (in Germany) the *Institute for Quality and Efficiency in Health Care* (IQuWiG = *Institut für Qualität und Wirtschaftlichkeit im Gesundheitswesen*), the *Office for Technology Assessment of the German Federal Parliament* (TAB = *Büro für Technikfolgenabschätzung im Bundestag*), or others. It is fair to note that any technological innovation outside of the health care system would be taken off the market at a moment's notice if it were as inefficient and unlikely to

[25] Meanwhile, there are prestigious physicians and scientists who are postulating this suggestion, too. See footnote 19.

provide long-term solutions to existing problems as transplantation medicine does. Due to the global orientation of transplantation medicine and the lack of alternative therapies currently, this is—of course—not yet possible. In the long run, however, nothing speaks against the development of therapies which are not based on the exploitation of a patient's fellow human beings. Until then, transplantation medicine would possess the status of a *bridging technology*, which in the long run will be replaced more and more by other procedures.[26]

References

Baureithel, Ulrike, and Anna Bergmann. 1999. *Herzloser Tod. Das Dilemma der Organspende*. Stuttgart: Klett-Cotta Verlag.

Birnbacher, Dieter. 2007. Der Hirntod—eine pragmatische Verteidigung. *Jahrb Recht Ethik* 15:459–477.

Byrne, Paul A., ed. 2009. *Finis vitae. Is „brain death" true death?* Oregon: Life Guardian Foundation.

Chaib, E. 2008. Non heart-beating donors in England. *CLINICS* 63 (1): 121–134.

Deutsches Ärzteblatt. 1998. 95. Heft 30. 24. Juli 1998 (53), A–1861.

DSO. 2013. http://www.dso.de/fachinformation/organentnahme.html. Accessed 18 March 2014.

EFiD. 2013. Evangelische Frauen in Deutschland. Organtransplantation. Ein Positionspapier. In: http://www.evangelischefrauen-deutschland.de/publikationen/positionspapiere/649. Accessed 18 March 2014.

Eurotransplant Foundation. 2014. https://www.eurotransplant.org/cms. Accessed 18 March 2014.

Förderreuther, S., and H. Angstwurm. 2003. Organspende in Deutschland. *Dtsch med Wochenschr* 128:2437–2440.

Geisler, Linus S. 2010. Die Lebenden und die Toten. *Universitas* 65 (763): 4–13.

Holznienkemper, Thomas. 2005. *Organspende und Transplantation und ihre Rezension in der Ethik der abrahamitischen Religionen* (62 ff.). Münster: LIT-Verlag.

Jonas, Hans. 1974. *Against the stream: Comments on the definition and redefinition of death*. Prentice-Hall.

Keller, Martina. 2011. Carine, 43, lässt sich töten. *DIE ZEIT*, 20 October 2011, Nr. 43.

Manzei, Alexandra. 2003. *Körper, Technik, Grenzen. Kritische Anthropologie am Beispiel der Transplantationsmedizin*. Münster: LIT-Verlag.

Müller, Sabine. 2011. Wie tot sind Hirntote? *APuZ* 20/21:3–9.

Ohm, J., et al. 2001. Organspende: Wie viele potentielle Organspender gibt es? *Intensivmed* 38:118–123.

Presidents commission on Bioethics. 2008. https://bioethicsarchive.georgetown.edu/pcbe/reports/death. Accessed 18 March 2014.

Schweidtmann, W., and F. A. Muthny. 1997. Einstellung von Ärzten zur Organtransplantation. Ergebnisse einer empirischen Studie. *Transplantationsmedizin* 9 (1): 2–7.

Shewmon, Alan D. 1998a. Chronic "brain death": Meta-analysis and conceptual consequences. *Neurology* 51:1538–1545.

Shewmon, Alan D. 1998b. "Brainstem death", "Brain death" and Death: A critical re-evaluation of the purpoted equivalence. *Issues in Law and Medicine* 14 (2): 125–145.

Wesslau, C., et al. 2007. How large is the organ donor potential in Germany? *Transplant International* 20:147–155.

Wilkinson, Dominic, and Julian Savulescu. 2010. Should we allow organ donation euthanasia? *Bioethics*. doi:10.1111/j.1467–8519.2010.01811.x.

---

[26] Cf. Müller (2011).

Prof. Dr. Alexandra Manzei is Professor for Sociology with the focus on Health Sociology at the Faculty of Philosophy and Social Sciences of Augsburg University, Germany. Her research interests lie in the fields of medical ethics, science and technology studies and social anthropology. Before her studies, she worked as a nurse in an intensive care unit where she cared for brain-dead and comatose patients.

Chapter 13
Donation and Devolution: The Human Transplantation (Wales) Act 2013

Tom Hayes

13.1 Introduction

Since it first became possible to replace defective organs with healthy organs from other persons, including from the recently deceased, it has become possible to think in terms of a certain need for organs for transplantation. Where this need outstrips the numbers of organs available it has become possible to speak of an *organ shortage*. The extent of the organ shortage can be illustrated through the numbers of patients registered on the transplant waiting list.[1] Currently there are 118,184 people on the US waiting list,[2] 15,500 people registered on the Eurotransplant waiting list,[3] 7,636 patients on the UK waiting list,[4] around 300 of whom are Welsh[5] residents (Griffiths 2012, para. 5). The seriousness of the organ shortage problem is shown by the fact that every year people who are registered on the waiting lists die for want of a transplant.

[1] It is possible that the numbers on this waiting list do not represent the total number of those who might benefit from a transplant operation, as not everyone in need may be on the waiting list.

[2] http://www.organdonor.gov/index.html, accessed 17th May 2013.

[3] http://www.eurotransplant.org/cms/, accessed 10th January 2013, NB: the Eurotransplant area includes a number of European countries.

[4] In March 2012. A further 2880 were temporarily suspended from the waiting list at this time: NHSBT (2012, p. 2).

[5] Wales is a part of the United Kingdom, inhabited by 3.1 m people (4.9 % of the UK population), which through a process of devolution that began in 1997, now has a semi-autonomous status insofar as it has the power to create its own binding legislation in certain legislative areas through the NAW. Healthcare is one area of legislative competence and it is this area of legislative competence which is relied upon in the creation of the current Bill under discussion.

T. Hayes (✉)
Cardiff Law School, Cardiff University, Cardiff, UK
e-mail: Hayestp@cardiff.ac.uk

R. J. Jox et al. (eds.), *Organ Transplantation in Times of Donor Shortage*,
International Library of Ethics, Law, and the New Medicine 59,
DOI 10.1007/978-3-319-16441-0_13

Organs can be supplied inter vivos (which is increasingly popular in the UK: see Jackson (2010, p. 595)), but this carries risks for the donor, which means that it is largely seen as an act of extraordinary generosity. As such, this mode of donation cannot be relied upon as the sole or primary source of organs. By contrast, cadaveric donation is generally seen as a less ethically problematic form of donation, because there are no ongoing clinical risks for the donor and it retains the same potential benefits for those in need of organ transplantation. However, there do remain ethical concerns relating to the proper and dignified treatment of corpses (see Feinberg 1985, pp. 72–77) and this is reflected by the current law in England and Wales[6] which protects the body of the deceased by inter alia prohibiting the removal of organs for transplantation without prior patient consent, without the consent of an appointed proxy (on the rare occasions when a proxy is appointed: see NAWHSCC (2013, para. 180) (Dr Alan Clamp)), or the consent of someone in a "qualifying relationship" (s 54(9) Human Tissue Act 2004 (HT Act)). As express consent is required in these cases, cadaveric donation is still seen as a genuine form of donation, but one which is less onerous for the giver than living donation. Hence it is the promotion of cadaveric donation that is considered the most appropriate strategy for increasing the overall rate of donation ahead of some of the more contentious options.[7]

The very ability to transplant organs from the recently deceased and thereby save lives generates a tremendous normative pull towards increasing cadaveric donation. And, as the state has an interest in promoting the health of its population (Foucault 2004, p. 242), the state must be concerned with increasing donation rates. But, in liberal societies, there is also a demand on government to minimise its interventions in order to maximise freedoms (Rose 1993, pp. 290–292). Thus there is a compromise to be made between the extreme of the compulsory confiscation of organs and making absolutely no intervention on organ donation. In the UK, that compromise has been arrived at by maintaining express and informed consent as the cornerstone of the donor system, but by simultaneously maintaining a place for people to record their wishes to become a donor (i.e. the Organ Donor Register (ODR)), promoting donation through advertisements, and allowing a fairly high level of persuasion (i.e. anything which does not 'overbear the will': *U v Centre for Reproductive Medicine* [2002] EWCA Civ 565) to encourage donation. Indeed, governments within the European Union are required to actively promote organ donation (Directive 2010/45/EU). Additionally, a blind eye is turned to the low possibility of making a meaningful capacity assessment at the point of registration on the ODR, as consent can be granted by ticking a box on a form without being in the presence of another (See Rithalia et al. 2009, p. 3). Notwithstanding these measures, the Welsh government believed that the normative case for increasing organ donation provided adequate justification for going still further, by legislating for an opt out system of consent.

[6] As well as the other countries of the UK i.e. Scotland and Northern Ireland under separate legislation specific to those places. See Human Tissue Act (Scotland) 2006.

[7] E.g. xenotransplantation, dispensing with the 'dead donor rule', or, at the most extreme, ending people's lives deliberately and at random in order that their organs could be distributed to eliminate the organ shortage as John Harris hypothesised in the Survival Lottery (1975).

The question of moving to an opt out system (i.e. one in which people will be presumed to have consented unless they give an explicit refusal) was considered in 2008 in the light of the UK's comparatively poor rate of organ donation at the time (ODT 2008b, p. 1.5).[8] Such a move would have brought the UK in line with countries with higher donation rates (see ODT 2008a, p. 10). The theory behind such a move is consistent with the popular policy strategy of 'nudging' people through the normative manipulation, in order to routinise cadaveric donation (Thaler and Sunstein 2008, pp. 175–182). However, the Organ Donation Taskforce (ODT), established by the UK government, rejected this option. It did so mainly on the grounds that opt out systems may violate the European Convention on Human Rights (ECHR) (ODT 2008a, p. 12), that the potential for an adverse public reaction may even cause a reduction in the rates of donation as happened in Brazil (see ODT 2008a, p. 23), that the public support for opt out systems found in opinion polls might not offer a genuine reflection of public opinion and that, fundamentally, whatever the problems with the ethical safeguards of the present system, inferring an active consent from a failure to object is logically and ethically dubious (ODT 2008a, p. 15).

13.2 Consent as a Barrier to Organ Donation?

Notwithstanding the conclusions of the ODT, the Welsh government viewed the opt in system as an impediment to organ donation, as it believed that changing the law to an opt out (or *deemed consent)* system, as it has, would result in an increase in available organs. Some commentators, such as John Harris (1975), have suggested taking a more radical approach and dispensing with any consent requirements (see Price 2010, p. 44). However, such a move would be highly controversial given the considerable importance afforded to the doctrine of informed consent in the UK. In recognition of this, the National Assembly for Wales (NAW) have sought to arrive at a position which balances the competing deontological interests pertaining to autonomy with the utilitarian, community interest reducing the organ shortage.

Even so, serious concerns were raised that such a system would change the nature of organ donation from an act of altruism, into an act made under obligation. Under opt in systems (i.e. those which require express consent), those who do not donate might simply be regarded as being less generous than others, but under an opt out system, those people might be viewed as being selfish or antisocial. Potentially those who choose not to become donors may experience a degree of shame, even if there is no requirement to make their decision public. It is questionable whether it is legitimate to expose people, who may have a strong conscientious or

[8] Even though there had already been significant improvements in donation rates by this point. For instance the number of kidney donations increased by 93 % between 2000 and 2006 (ODT 2008b, p. 1.9).

religious objection to donating their organs,[9] to this kind of shame (even indirectly) in these circumstances.

John Fabre has also argued that moving to a system of deemed consent would "degrade the ethical framework of our society" (Devlin 2008) as it goes against the central post-war medical norm of express and informed consent as the basis for medical intervention.[10] On this point, it would be unfair to suggest that presumed consent precludes the possibility of informed consent, as it is possible for the absence of a decision to opt out to be well-considered and informed. It would also be misleading to pretend that all instances of express consent are meaningfully well-considered and informed (see O'Neill 2002, pp. 42–44). However, under an opt in system, steps can be taken to ensure that sufficient information is made available prior to the decision to consent. Under an opt out system, by contrast, there is no guarantee that those who fail to opt out are doing so having had a real opportunity to become so informed. Furthermore, under an opt out system, there is no way of knowing that the donor directed their mind to the question of donation, whereas this is at least minimally indicated in opt in systems through the expression of consent itself.

Some of these concerns may be assuaged if it were clear that the change would increase donation rates. The NAW relied on research from Abadie and Gay, which suggests that opt out systems are associated with a 25–30 % increase in the rate of organ donation (Griffiths 2012, para. 103). If this is realised it will provide 15 extra organ donors in Wales and with an average donation of three organs per donor, there would be an additional 45 organs made available for transplantation. The NAW use this estimate to project this increase in donors to result in a net saving of £ 148 m over ten years (see Griffiths 2012, para. 124) based on the Quality Adjusted Life Years (QALYs) gained and the reduction in the need for costly chronic treatments, such as dialysis.

However, not all studies project an increase of this magnitude and although opt out systems may be correlative with higher rates of donation (Boyarski et al. 2012), a clear causal link between opt out systems and increases in rates of donation has not been established (Rithalia et al. 2009, p. 20; Rudge and Buggins 2011). Establishing this causal link would require the examination and control of a much larger number of variables than the system of consent alone. In particular, the differences in the systems and infrastructure which surround organ donation are also considered to be highly important (see e.g. Hitchen 2008; see Fabre et al. 2010). This is a point which ought to resonate strongly in the UK which has "the lowest number of critical care beds in Europe" and is thereby limited in the number of transplants that can be performed (NAWHSCC 2013, paras. 100–101) (Dr Peter Matthews). Moreover, in Wales, the only transplant operations which can be performed are kidney and pancreas transplants and therefore Wales is reliant on the services and infrastructure

[9] Although most major religions do not prohibit organ donation: NHSBT 2005. http://www.organdonation.nhs.uk/how_to_become_a_donor/religious_perspectives/leaflets/summary_leaflet.asp accessed 6th June 2013.

[10] The Nuremburg Code 1947: principle 1 http://www.bmj.com/content/313/7070/1448.1, accessed 25th March 2012 and Chester v Afshar [2004] UKHL 41 [14].

in England for all other transplant operations (Griffiths 2012, para. 54). Thus, there are plainly alternative ways of improving the rate of donation without resorting to modifying the associated consent requirements.

However, in the event that the Human Transplantation (Wales) Act 2013 (HTWA) does precipitate an increase in organ donation once it comes into force (in December 2015), the rest of the UK beyond Wales will also benefit. This is because, only around 30 % of organs donated by people in Wales are currently provided to people in Wales (Griffiths 2012, para. 129). If this trend were to continue, the positive effect of the legal change will be diluted for Welsh citizens.

Adding to the doubts over the likely efficacy of the legislation, the director of the *Organización Nacional de Trasplantes* in Spain (the system to which Wales implicitly aspires in its new legislation) is even reported to have said that concentrating on the legal framework and overestimating its power to bring about changes in practice would be 'dangerous' (See also Devlin 2008). Indeed Spain itself provides a good example of the importance of addressing factors beyond consent. It moved to an opt out system of consent in 1979, but it was only when the specialist training, infrastructure and the systems for coordinating donation processes were developed in the 1990s that a significant increase in the number of donations and transplantations was achieved (Fabre et al. 2010 and see also NHSBT (2008)). Furthermore, in practice, it is reported that Spain does not strictly enforce its presumed consent law (Rithalia et al. 2009, p. 11) and therefore it is rather disingenuous to present it as an exemplar for presumed consent, per se, boosting rates of donation.

Still more troubling than underestimating the potential increase, is the possibility that there could be a decrease in the rate of donation if public trust in the system is lost. There is precedent for this scenario in Brazil, where, after the system of consent was changed to an opt out system, opponents decided to opt out en masse and ultimately forced the system to be reversed (Csillag 1998). Indeed, suspicions of a public backlash have already been raised following the release of statistics which indicate a 22 % year-on-year decline in the number of organ donations taking place in Wales since commencement of the legislative process for the HTWA[11] NHSBT 2013). The NAW minister responsible for the Bill was quick to downplay any link between the decrease and the passage of the legislation,[12] but the figures must be a matter of concern considering that the other four nations of the UK experienced increases in their rates of donation over the same period (see NHSBT 2013).

Such concerns chime with some recent experiences in which public confidence in the medical system has been shaken. For example, in the aftermath of Andrew Wakefield's discredited report suggesting a link between the Measles Mumps and Rubella (MMR) vaccine and autism there has been a marked reduction in the rate of vaccination among children (who were therefore exposed to the risk of serious

[11] Which was known as the Human Transplantation (Wales) Bill 2012 (HTWB) prior to its enactment.

[12] http://www.bbc.co.uk/news/uk-wales-22104275, accessed 8th May 2013.

illness).[13] The scandals in the UK at Bristol (see Kennedy 2001) and Alder Hey (see Redfern 2001) damaged public confidence in the medical profession and led to a strengthening in the informed consent requirements when dealing with human tissue and organs which the HT Act emphasises. More recently, Germany suffered an 18 % reduction in the rate of organ donation[14] following a scandal concerning the allocation of donated organs.[15] Such is the importance of public confidence in the medical profession and the corrosive consequences of its loss.

Notably some patient groups expressed concern during the passage of the the Human Transplantation (Wales) Act 2013 (HTWA) through the Welsh legislature. The Patients Association argued that consent is fundamental to modern medical practice and that "[p]resumed consent is no consent" (2011). This point was echoed by 92 % of respondents to the consultation on the Bill[16] questioned whether it was possible to speak of deemed consent, without undermining consent as a concept (Welsh Government Consultation 2012, p. 5). Another group, Patient Concern, argued along similar lines and drew attention to the fact that a system of presumed consent had been considered a number of times previously and had been rejected and branded the proposed opt out system as "dishonest, disrespectful and unethical" (2011, p. 1). And although the British Medical Association (BMA)[17] currently supports a move to an opt out system (BMA 2012), it is at least possible that there will be medical professionals who might have a conscionable objection to an involvement in the transplantation of organs under a system of presumed consent, if they consider such a system to lack ethical legitimacy.

In spite of these concerns, there was a popular mandate for the change in Wales, as the Welsh Labour Party made a manifesto pledge to introduce an opt out system in Wales in the 2011 NAW elections (2001, p. 53) and since being elected to government have made good on that pledge by through legislation. Furthermore there have been surveys that suggest a high level of support for the principle of opt out legislation (i.e. 63 % of those questioned: BBC/ICM 2012). However, reliance on this poll is somewhat questionable, as the respondents were asked their opinion on *organ donation* (Q4), whereas the HTWA speaks of the donation of *relevant material* meaning: "material, other than gametes, which consists of or includes human cells" (s 18(1)).

The distinction is significant, because it is likely that some people who would like to consent to their kidneys or liver being explanted after their death, but who might not be willing for their hands, face or uterus[18] to be removed and transplanted.

---

[13] The uptake level was 92 % in 1995 and fell to 80 % in 2003/2004: See http://www.hpa.org.uk/Topics/InfectiousDiseases/InfectionsAZ/MMR/GeneralInformation/, accessed 6th June 2013.

[14] http://www.sueddeutsche.de/gesundheit/sinkende-spendebereitschaft-organspenden-brechen-um-prozent-ein-1.1657743, accessed 6th June 2013.

[15] >http://www.sueddeutsche.de/thema/Organspende-Skandal, accessed 6th June 2013.

[16] i.e. 2657 of 2891 respondents.

[17] The professional representative body and trade union for doctors in the UK.

[18] This happened recently in Turkey, and the recipient is currently pregnant: http://www.guardian.co.uk/uk/2013/may/03/womb-transplant; see also: http://www.bbc.co.uk/news/world-europe-19637156, accessed 8th May 2013.

This is possible to request under the current opt in system,[19] but both the HTWA its explanatory note and the explanatory memorandum which accompanied the Bill are silent on the question of whether a person may refuse to donate certain organs but not others. As a matter of legal logic, this should be possible, but whether this would take place in practice would depend on instituting a system that could deal with such wishes. But, before anyone could render such a refusal to donate certain organs, they would need to know which organs would be the subject of deemed consent; a point which is currently unclear because while there are plans to introduce regulations (under s 7(2) HTWA) about what kinds of tissue could be explanted under the deemed consent provisions, excluding novel forms of transplantation (Griffiths 2012, para. 20), precisely what will be excluded remains a further point of obscurity until specific Regulations are created.[20]

13.3 The New Legislation in Wales

Much of the HTWA replicates, or approximates to, the current law governing both England and Wales through the HT Act, particularly as regards consent to living organ donation (HTWA s 4(3)) and the establishment of certain criminal offences for acting without valid consent (ss 10–11). While this has the advantage of keeping much of the relevant law on organ donation within the same legislative document, it has made the Act more complex and laboured than was necessary to effect the changes sought. One example is where HTWA refers to those cases in which the donor is both adult and alive. The HTWA states that on such occasions express consent is required.[21] Unhelpfully, express consent is defined simply as: "The person's consent" (s 4(3)). The major point of divergence is the mode by which consent to cadaveric donation is established.

The HTWA makes clear that in respect of adults, regard must be had to any express wishes of the deceased during their lifetime, whether for or against becoming a donor (ss 4(2)–(3)). If no such wishes are in evidence, and if that person has not appointed another to act as a proxy to give consent on their behalf (which rarely happens under the HT Act (NAWHSCC 2013, para. 180)(Dr Alan Clamp) on the matter, consent can be *deemed* subject to limited grounds of objection from persons in a *qualifying relationship* to the deceased (ss 4(4) and 19(3) HTWA).[22]

[19] See https://www.organdonation.nhs.uk/how_to_become_a_donor/registration/registration_form.asp (step 2), accessed 14th Jan 2013.

[20] The Health Minister has indicated that "limbs and face transplants" will be excluded (Saul 2013).

[21] Draft Regulations, under the title "The Human Transplantation (Excluded Relevant Material) (Wales) Regulations 2015" have now been created for the approval of the National Assembly for Wales. English law takes the same position on this point (s 3(2) HT Act).

[22] NB The HT Act operates in the opposite direction to this: i.e. it is possible for those in a qualifying relationship to grant consent on behalf of the deceased in respect of certain matters s 3(6)(c) HT Act.

Voluntariness is therefore respected through the fact that those who do not wish to have their organs removed will be able to prevent this by registering their refusal[23] and, in addition, those in a *qualifying relationship* to the deceased (i.e. relatives and long-standing friends) may also prevent the removal of organs by claiming that the deceased would have objected (s 4(4)(b) HTWA).

13.3.1 Objections from Those in a Qualifying Relationship

The fact that those in a qualifying relationship (see s 19(3) HTWA) will acquire a limited legal right to refuse *transplantation activities* (s 3(2) HTWA) (if they can show that the deceased would not have wanted their organs or tissue to be explanted) represents a technical change from the current law. Presently this right of refusal does not exist under the HT Act, but in practice if those in a qualifying relationship express a strong objection, the organs of the deceased will not be removed (even, in around 6 % of cases in 2010/2011, where the deceased themselves had consented: BMA 2012, pp. 11–12; Griffiths 2012, paras. 41–42). It is thought that avoiding the need to ask the family for permission will precipitate an increase in explantations. Theoretically, it will be harder psychologically for the family to refuse consent if the norm is to give consent as a matter of course and thus requires no action on their part.[24]

This ability for the family to prevent explantation is an ethical safeguard against the idea that organs could be confiscated by the state.[25] In the UK, where the scandals at Bristol (See Kennedy 2001) and Alder Hey (see Redfern 2001) involving inter alia the retention of organs without the knowledge of the family were strong informers of the HT Act (for critical discussion see Liddell and Hall (2005) esp. pp. 207–208), there is a particular sensitivity to the way that the bodies of the deceased are treated and therefore it is entirely understandable that such a safeguard should be included in the HTWA. However, it is possible that this new limited right of refusal could significantly hamper the attempt to increase the rate of organ donation. This is because, in the UK, the most recent empirical evidence (in respect of the 2011/2012 tax year) suggests this familial rate of refusal was aprox. 36 % overall. Where the deceased had made a clear expression of their wishes to become a donor this refusal rate dropped to aprox. 7 %, but the absence of such an expression that figure rose to 52 % (see Murphy and Allen 2012). This will be of concern to an opt out system which operates on the basis of silence being equated with consent,

[23] The Nuffield Council on Bioethics has recommended that people in the rest of the UK should also have the right to register an objection to becoming a donor on the ODR as well as a wish to become a donor (2011,Para, 6.55)

[24] This form of norm-adjusting legislation is in line with the influential policy movement based around the concept of the 'nudge' which is designed to operate within liberal systems of government to adjust choice frameworks in order to shape choices (Thaler and Sunstein 2008).

[25] This is sometimes referred to as a system of "conscription" (see Price 2010, p. 44).

because those who wish to become organ donors may well decide that they do not need to register on the ODR in the expectation that their organs will be explanted after their death. While this is technically correct, the family may not feel confident that their relative genuinely wanted to become a donor rather than simply failing to give the matter any thought. Of course, the changes to the system of consent will be accompanied by an advertising campaign, informing people of the importance of discussing cadaveric organ donation with their families, but the effectiveness of such a campaign remains to be seen. It is, however, unlikely that such an assumption of knowledge would satisfy family members in the same way as a positive expression of the wish to become an organ donor. And even if this is insufficient to ground a legal right to refusal, it will put medical teams in the invidious position of having to decide whether to explant organs (in accordance with their legal entitlement) or to respect family wishes. Moreover, the very granting of this legal right may run counter to the objective of avoiding confronting the relatives with the question of donation while their relative is dying, because responsible relatives would naturally want to give proper thought to the question of whether their relative would really have wanted for their organs to be explanted.

13.3.2 Cases in Which Deemed Consent does not Apply

The deemed consent provisions of the HTWA will only apply to adults who have not suffered from a *lack of capacity* for a significant part of their lifetime and who are Welsh residents. It is important to consider how each of these requirements is defined. While there are sound ethico-legal reasons for having such exclusions, they may also create practical problems.

13.3.2.1 Children

Children are defined as persons under the age of 18 and will be excluded from the deemed consent provisions (s 19(1) HTWA). However, children will be able to express a wish to become a donor before the age of 18 (s 6(3) HTWA).

This restriction is important, because it prevents organs being taken from the bodies of those unable to understand what will happen following their death (see Price 2010, p. 152), but it simultaneously restricts the ability of the HTWA to address the organ shortage in respect of children, for whom there are special considerations for making donations to add to any matching criteria in terms of size and development.

13.3.2.2 Non-Residents

Anyone who has not been "ordinarily resident in Wales for a period of at least 12 months immediately before dying" (HTWA s 5(3)(a)) is classed as an excepted adult to whom the deemed consent provisions do not apply. The explanatory memorandum to the HTWB envisaged that the test of ordinary residency will be predicated on asking whether the person's current address is in Wales and whether that is the place that where they reside for the majority of the time (Griffiths 2012, para. 25). Deemed consent will therefore include people who may not consider themselves Welsh e.g. temporary workers and students (see Griffiths 2012, para. 25). Even acknowledging the general principle that "ignorance of the law is no defence", the breadth of this provision in the HTWA could foreseeably prove controversial, as people may unwittingly fall into the category of "residents".[26]

13.3.2.3 Adults who Lacked Capacity

Those who "lacked capacity to understand the notion that consent to transplantation activities can be deemed to be given" for "a significant period before dying" are also excluded from the opt out provisions of the Act (s 5(3)(b)). The aim is to ensure that those who fail to express a refusal would have had a real opportunity to do so, having had both the time and capacity to make their choice. While this is a crucial ethical safeguard promoting voluntariness, it leaves entirely unanswered the question as to how a *significant period* will be defined.

The explanatory memorandum offers scant elucidation, stating that a *significant period* means "a sufficiently long period before dying so as to lead a reasonable person to conclude that it would be inappropriate for consent to be deemed" (Griffiths 2012, para. 38). This definition will afford a considerable interpretative leeway to the courts and therefore it will have to be tested. However, in determining what will amount to a significant period it would be incumbent on the reasonable person to establish some sense of how often people direct their minds to the question of becoming an organ donor. In the absence of reliable empirical evidence, it is an entirely moot point.

In more general terms, when considering the question of mental capacity it becomes apparent that deemed consent does not sit well with the ethos of the Mental Capacity Act 2005 (MCA). This is because the MCA gives a presumption of capacity that may only be negated if capacity is found to be lacking upon assessment. Importantly, such assessments of capacity must relate to a specific decision made at a specific time (s 2(1) MCA). On this basis, it is problematic that the deemed consent provisions invite us to believe that all those who fail to register an objection to donating their organs have directed their minds to the question of organ donation, because it leaves unanswered the question of precisely when the decision

---

[26] Although the explantation of organs may still be prevented for persons classified as residents under s 4(4)(b) HTWA.

was (supposedly) made. Without knowing this, it would be almost impossible to make a meaningful investigation of mental capacity without using the mechanism in s 5(3)(b) HTWA.[27] Furthermore, it is difficult to understand how capacity is to be assessed in the temporally generalised terms of s 5(3)(b) HTWA, particularly considering that the MCA states that people are not to be adjudged as lacking capacity merely because of a mental disorder, or their behaviour or appearance (MCA s 2(3)).

13.4 Effect on Other Parts of the UK

Though the HTWA is a Welsh piece of legislation, it will also have an effect on the rest of the other parts of the UK. As Wales lacks comprehensive transplant facilities, the HT Act will need to be modified so that organs can be removed under the deemed provisions of the HTWA in Wales and transported to England for lawful transplantation (Griffiths 2012, p. 53). Furthermore, medical staff, and particularly Specialist Nurses for Organ donation (SNODs), will require training in both systems of consent in order that they can operate within the applicable law and communicate effectively with families, having identified which legal framework applies (HTA 2013, p. 32, 51). The British Medical Association (BMA)[28] has urged for the new rules to be made clear as possible on behalf of the doctors it represents, who may risk criminal sanctions under the HT Act (e.g. s 5) or the HTWA (s 10). Codes of practice will need to be drafted in order to assist doctors to know precisely what steps they must take to satisfy themselves of the correct legal regime before proceeding.

One of the areas where there is perhaps most potential for confusion relates to the removal of organs for research or storage (or another scheduled purpose under s 1 HT Act), which is an activity which will not be regulated under the HTWA, but under the HT Act. In fact, the HTWA only concerns *transplantation activities* (s 3(2) HTWA) so there could be occasions where medics want to explant some of the organs or tissue from the donor for the purposes of transplantation and some other material for research, whereupon the medical team would have to apply different tests of consent to the same body. This could also be a regrettable matter of confusion for the family of the deceased.

Additionally, a publicity campaign will be needed for the non-Welsh UK population to explain the new rules in Wales and how they will be affected in order that people will not fall under false apprehensions, such as assuming that the HTWA will

[27] The current opt-in system might be criticised for lacking the possibility of making a meaningful and timely assessment of mental capacity, but as there is a presumption of capacity, the burden lies on the party seeking to prove that capacity was lacking. By contrast, under the HTWA, the reasonable person must consider whether the potential donor would have been assessed as having capacity at a point in time when they are imagined to have considered the question of becoming an organ donor. This test contradicts a central principle of the MCA.

[28] http://bma.org.uk/news-views-analysis/news/2013/april/opt-out-organ, accessed 6th June 2013.

apply to the whole of the UK (see HTA 2013, p. 68). The new ODR in Wales will also have to be integrated with the ODR system in the rest of the UK.

13.5 Conclusion

It has been argued that however worthy the objective of saving and improving lives through alleviating the organ shortage, the particular means by which the NAW are attempting to achieve this are flawed and unjustified. As there is no established causal connection between opt out systems and the rate of donation, there is no guarantee that the rate of donation will increase with a change in the law and there is a possibility that the rate will decrease; particularly if the change leads to a loss of public confidence in the transplant system. Consequently, in a liberal society where strong concerns have been voiced over the change, there is insufficient justification for increasing the level of state intervention in the matter by creating a presumption of consent in law.

This conclusion is supported by the fact that improvements of a technical and logistical nature could be made to the transplant system which would not intervene directly in the lives of citizens and which could increase donation rates. This has been most recently evidenced by the 50 % increase in the rate of donation the UK has achieved in the past five years through such measures without resorting changing the system of consent (see NHSBT 2013).

In addition, changing the system of consent within a nation state will also make for a more confusing legal landscape for citizens and healthcare professionals alike. This may give rise to delays and litigation at a time-sensitive period through the requirements to determine residency and the absence of a significant period of incapacity. Moreover, Welsh citizens who wish to become organ donors will still have to register on the ODR if there believe they might die in another part of the UK.

Acknowledgments An earlier version of this work was presented at the Ludwig-Maximilians Universität München at an Interdisciplinary Workshop on Organ Donation. I wish to thank the organisers and to all those who attended the workshop for their helpful comments and questions and especially to Katherine Mendis and Nathan Emmerich for acting as discussants on this paper. An earlier version of this work was also presented in Bristol at the Centre for Ethics in Medicine as part of the seminar series there and I extend my thanks to all those who attended and contributed to that session especially Richard Huxtable. I am also grateful to Manon George for discussing some aspects of Welsh law with me. I am responsible for any errors.

References

BBC/ICM. 2012. BBC Wales poll February 2012. http://www.icmresearch.com/bbc-wales-poll-february-2012. Accessed 14 Jan 2013.

Boyarsky, Brian J., Erin C. Hall, Neha A. Deshpande, Lorie R. Ros, Robert A. Montgomery, Donald M. Steinwachs, and Dorry L. Segev. 2012. Potential limitations of presumed consent legislation. *Transplantation* 93 (2): 136–140.

British Medical Association (BMA). 2012. Building on progress: Where next for organ donation policy in the UK? http://bma.org.uk/news-views-analysis/news/2013/april/opt-out-organ. Accessed 6 June 2013.

Csillag, C. 1998. Brazil abolishes "presumed consent" in organ donation. *The Lancet* 352:1367.

Devlin, K. 2008. Presumed consent "will not increase organ donations". The Daily Telegraph, September 5, 2008. http://www.telegraph.co.uk/health/2688160/Presumed-consent. Accessed 8 May 2013.

Fabre, J., P. Murphy, and R. Matesanz. 2010. Presumed consent: A distraction in the quest for increasing rates of organ donation. *British Medical Journal* 341 (2): c4973–c4973.

Feinberg, J. 1985. *Harm to others: The moral limits of criminal law*. vol. 2. Oxford: Oxford University Press.

Foucault, M. 2004. In *Society Must Be Defended: Lectures at the Collège De France*, 1975–1976, ed Mauro Bertani, Alessandro Fontana, and David Macey (tr). London: Penguin.

Griffiths, L. 2012. Human transplantation (Wales) bill draft explanatory memorandum incorporating the regulatory impact assessment and explanatory notes. http://www.senedd.assemblywales.org/mgIssueHistoryHome.aspx?IId=5178. Accessed 4 May 2013.

Harris, J. 1975. The survival lottery. *Philosophy* 50 (19): 81–87.

Hitchen, L. 2008. No evidence that presumed consent increases organ donation *British Medical Journal* 337:a1614.

Human Tissue Authority (HTA). 2012. Written evidence submitted by the human tissue authority. Welsh affairs committee—Sixth special report proposed legislative competence orders relating to organ donation and cycle paths. http://www.publications.parliament.uk/pa/cm201011/cmselect/cmwelaf/896/896vw18.htm. Accessed 6 June 2013.

Jackson, E. 2010. *Medical law: Text, cases and materials.* 2nd ed. Oxford: Oxford University Press.

Kennedy, I. 2001. The report of the public inquiry into children's heart surgery at the Bristol Royal Infirmary 1984–1995: Learning from Bristol. http://webarchive.nationalarchives.gov.uk/+/www.dh.gov.uk/en/Publicationsandstatistics/Publications/PublicationsPolicyAndGuidance/DH_4005620. Accessed 6 June 2013.

Liddell, K., and A. Hall 2005. Beyond Bristol and Alder Hey: The future regulation of human tissue. *Medical Law Review* 13:170–223.

Murphy, C., and J. Allen 2012. Potential donor audit: Summary report for the 12 month period 1 April 2011–31 March 2012. http://www.organdonation.nhs.uk/statistics/potential_donor_audit/. Accessed 6 June 2013.

National Assembly for Wales Health and Social Care Committee. 2013. Human Transplantation (Wales) Bill: Stage 1—Evidence Session 4. (Wednesday, 30 January 2013). Accessed 6 June 2013.

National Health Service Blood and Transplant (NHSBT). 2005. General leaflet on religious viewpoints. http://www.organdonation.nhs.uk/how_to_become_a_donor/religious_perspectives/leaflets/summary_leaflet.asp. Accessed 6 June 2013.

NHSBT. 2008 National Health service blood and transplant opt in or opt out. http://www.organdonation.nhs.uk/newsroom/statements_and_stances/statements/opt_in_or_out.asp. Accessed 14 Jan 2013.

NHSBT. 2012. Organ donation activity report 2011/2012. http://www.organdonation.nhs.uk/statistics/transplant_activity_report/. Accessed 6 June 2013.

NHSBT. 2013. National health service blood and transplant NHS achieves ground breaking 50% increase in deceased organ donors. http://www.nhsbt.nhs.uk/news/2013/newsrelease110413.html. Accessed 14 Jan 2013.

Nuffield Council on Bioethics. 2011. Human bodies: Donation for medicine and research. http://www.nuffieldbioethics.org/donation. Accessed 6 June 2013.

O'Neill, Onora. 2002. Autonomy and trust in bioethics: The Gifford lectures, University of Edinburgh, 2001. Cambridge: Cambridge University Press.

Organ Donation Taskforce (ODT). 2008a. The potential impact of an opt out system for organ donation in the UK: An independent report from the Organ Donation Taskforce. http://webarchive.nationalarchives.gov.uk/20130107105354/http://www.dh.gov.uk/en/Publicationsandstatistics/Publications/PublicationsPolicyAndGuidance/DH_090312. Accessed 14 Jan 2013.

Organ Donation Taskforce (ODT). 2008b. Organs for transplants: A report from the Organ Donation Taskforce. http://www.bts.org.uk/MBR/Clinical/Publications/Member/Clinical/Publications.aspx?hkey=0bca99a9-40c2-4d40-bb9f-510e30d769b9. Accessed 14 Jan 2013.

Patient Concern. 2011. Written evidence submitted by Patient Concern. Welsh Affairs Committee—Sixth special report proposed legislative competence orders relating to organ donation and cycle paths. http://www.publications.parliament.uk/pa/cm201011/cmselect/cmwelaf/896/896vw05.htm. Accessed 6 June 2013.

Price, D. 2010. Legal and ethical aspects of organ transplantation. Cambridge: Cambridge University Press.

Redfern, M. 2001. The royal liverpool children's inquiry. http://www.official-documents.gov.uk/document/hc0001/hc00/0012/0012_ii.asp. Accessed 14 Jan 2013.

Rithalia, A., McDaid, C., Suekarran, S., Norman, G., Myers, L., and Sowden, A. 2009. A systematic review of presumed consent systems for deceased organ donation. *Health Technology Assessment* 13 (26): 1–95.

Rose, N. 1993. Government, authority and expertise in advanced liberalism. *Economy and Society* 22 (3): 283–299.

Rudge, C. J., and E. Buggins. 2011. How to increase organ donation. Transplantation 93 (2): 141–144.

Saul, H. 2013. Opt-out scheme for organ donation given go-ahead in Wales. http://www.independent.co.uk/news/uk/home-news/optout-scheme-for-organ-donation-given-goahead-in-wales-8684984.html. Accessed 3 July 2013.

Thaler, R. H., and C. R. Sunstein 2008. *Nudge: improving decisions about health, wealth and happiness*. Michigan: Yale University Press.

The Lancet. 2013. Crisis in Germany's organ transplantation system. *The Lancet* 381 (9862): 178.

The Nuremberg Code. 1947. http://www.bmj.com/content/313/7070/1448.1. Accessed 14 Jan 2013.

The Patient's Association. 2011. Written evidence submitted by The Patient's Association. Welsh Affairs Committee—Sixth Special Report Proposed Legislative Competence Orders relating to Organ Donation and Cycle Paths. http://www.publications.parliament.uk/pa/cm201011/cmselect/cmwelaf/896/896vw08.htm. Accessed 6 June 2013.

Welsh Government Consultation. 2012. Summary of responses: Draft Human Transplantation (Wales) Bill and Explanatory Memorandum: Consent to organ and tissue donation in Wales. http://cymru.gov.uk/consultations/healthsocialcare/organbill/?lang=en. Accessed 6 June 2013.

Welsh Labour Manifesto. 2011. Standing Up for Wales. www.welshlabour.org.uk/. Accessed 14 Jan 2013.

Online Sources

http://www.bbc.co.uk/news/uk-wales-22104275. Accessed 8 May 2013.

http://www.bbc.co.uk/news/world-europe-19637156. Accessed 8 May 2013.

http://bma.org.uk/news-views-analysis/news/2013/april/opt-out-organ. Accessed 6 June 2013.

http://www.eurotransplant.org/cms/. Accessed 10 Jan 2013.

http://www.organdonor.gov/index.html. Accessed 17 May 2013.

https://www.organdonation.nhs.uk/how_to_become_a_donor/registration/registration_form.asp (step 2). Accessed 14 Jan 2013.

http://www.publicinquiries.org/inquiries/1990-1999/the_royal_liverpool_childrens_inquiry. Accessed 6 June 2013.

http://www.senedd.assemblywales.org/documents/s14202/30%20January%202013.html?CT=2. Accessed 6 June 2013.

http://www.sueddeutsche.de/gesundheit/sinkende-spendebereitschaft-organspenden-brechen-um-prozent-ein-1.1657743. Accessed 6 June 2013.

http://www.sueddeutsche.de/thema/Organspende-Skandal. Accessed 6 June 2013

The Nuremburg Code 1947: principle 1 http://www.bmj.com/content/313/7070/1448.1. Accessed 25.
http://www.guardian.co.uk/uk/2013/may/03/womb-transplant. Accessed 8 May 2013.

Cases and Legislation

U v Centre for Reproductive Medicine [2002] EWCA Civ 565.
Chester v Afshar [2004] UKHL 41 (HL).
Convention for the Protection of Human Rights and Fundamental Freedoms (European Convention on Human Rights as amended) (ECHR).
Directive 2010/45/EU of the European Parliament and the Council of 7 July 2010 on standards of quality and safety of human organs intended for transplantation.
Human Tissue Act 2004 c. 30 (HT Act).
Human Tissue Act (Scotland) 2006 asp 4 (HTSAct).
Human Transplantation (Wales) Bill 2012 (HTWB).
Human Transplantation (Wales) Act 2013 anaw 5.

Tom Hayes is a Lecturer in law in Cardiff Law School with an LLB (Law) and an MSc (Socio-Legal Studies) from the University of Bristol. Tom's research interests are in medical law and ethics, particularly regarding advance decision-making and end-of-life decision-making, and in social and political theory. He is currently writing his doctoral thesis, which examines the development of advance decisions to refuse medical treatment using Michel Foucault's work on governmentality.

Chapter 14
Advance Commitment: Rethinking The Family Veto Problem in Organ Procurement

Jurgen De Wispelaere and Lindsay Stirton

14.1 Introduction

It is a well-known fact that the demand for transplant surgery significantly outstrips the supply of available organs. In the UK alone, 506 patients died in 2007–2008 awaiting a transplant, while many more patients continue to suffer significant loss of quality of life for lack of a much-needed organ transplant.[1] In an attempt to increase the number of available organs, many countries have begun to rethink their approach to cadaveric donation. Controversial proposals include the use of financial incentives or advancing the case for compulsory organ donation.[2] More practically, a number of countries (e.g., Belgium and Sweden) have recently switched their organ procurement policy from a system of opt-in (informed) consent to a system of opt-out (presumed) consent, which sanctions posthumous organ removal unless the donor has explicitly objected. The precise benefits of presumed consent remains in doubt, however: there would likely still be a significant shortage of organs even if

Reproduced from [Journal of Medical Ethics, Advance commitment: an alternative approach to the family veto problem in organ procurement, Jurgen De Wispelaere/Lindsay Stirton, Volume 36, Issue 3, p. 180–183, 2010] with permission from BMJ Publishing Group Ltd.

[1] NHS Blood and Transplant (2007-2008).

[2] Erin and Harris (2003); Taylor (2005); Fabre (2006); Wisnewsky (2008); Delaney and Hershenov (2009).

J. De Wispelaere (✉)
Institute for Health and Social Policy, McGill University, Montreal, Canada
e-mail: Jurgen.dewispelaere@gmail.com

L. Stirton
Sussex Law School, University of Sussex, Brighton, UK

R. J. Jox et al. (eds.), *Organ Transplantation in Times of Donor Shortage*,
International Library of Ethics, Law, and the New Medicine 59,
DOI 10.1007/978-3-319-16441-0_14

we accept optimistic estimates that a move towards presumed consent laws would lead to an increase of around 25–30% in donation rates.[3]

With family members reportedly blocking about half of the available donations, we believe the key to increasing the availability of cadaveric organs lies in effectively addressing the *family veto*.[4] In contrast with proposals that aim to restrict the impact of family members on donation, we outline a scheme which gives families a positive role in the decision-making process, provided the donor values their involvement. Under our scheme, donors would appoint a designated second consenter (DSC), in most cases likely to be a family member, who would as part of the organ donor registration process signal their *advance commitment* to uphold the donor's decision after the death of the latter. Our proposal gives moral weight to the distress caused to family members (and medical staff) in seeking permission for organ harvesting at a time of sorrow, while at the same time respecting the autonomy of donors and the needs of patients awaiting a transplant. We should make it clear from the outset that, under our proposal, the right of the family to veto organ donation would not be indefeasible. It does however offer donors and families the opportunity of a *deliberative space* in which the decision to donate can be taken at a moment which is likely to be less distressing and more conducive to the making of a genuinely informed decision.[5] Our proposal has a number of pragmatic advantages that should appeal to those who disagree on ethical grounds with an approach that affords validity to the claims of family members.[6] In particular, disregarding the views of donors' families, even if morally defensible, would be politically unpalatable and could lead to a significant decrease in organ donors. Our proposal, by contrast, is politically feasible and effective in increasing the number of available organs for transplant.

14.2 Family Veto Matters

The existence of a widespread family veto may seem puzzling given that families typically have no real legal right to a say, once the deceased has validly expressed her intention to donate. In the UK, for example, the Human Tissue Authority Code of Practice on Consent advises clinicians to encourage family members and others close to the deceased to accept the wishes of the deceased, emphasising that they have no legal right to veto or overrule those wishes.[7] Any reluctance to proceed with cadaveric organ removal against the wishes of the family may be due less to fear of legal liability than to an understandable reluctance on the part of medical practitioners to add to the distress of grieving family members. Medical staff routinely

[3] Abadie and Gay (2006).

[4] Klassen AC and Klassen DK (1996); Wilkinson (2005, 2007).

[5] Sque et al. (2005, 2008).

[6] Klassen AC and Klassen DK (1996); Wilkinson (2005, 2007).

[7] Human Tissue Authority (2006).

acknowledge the added distress or loss of control of family members confronted with requests to remove body parts from a recently diseased spouse, child or parent.[8]

The belief that requests to approve organ donation may cause distress to grieving families explains not only reluctance on the part of transplant staff to *proceed* with organ harvesting without explicit consent by next-of-kin, but similarly reluctance on behalf of medical staff to even *approach* families at this difficult time. Unfortunately, delay is problematic because the chances of a successful organ transplant decrease significantly as the period from the time of the donor's death increases. While some commentators believe medical staff should be held under a required request obligation to enquire routinely about possible organ donation, it is also acknowledged that this puts staff under considerable emotional pressure.[9] Needless to say, the combined effects of reluctance by medical staff to *request* family consent and reluctance by next-of-kin to *give* consent has a deleterious effect on the supply of cadaveric organs.

One obvious solution would be to proceed with a policy of routine salvaging or the compulsory removal of donor organs independent of family's objections.[10] In some cases this may involve a subtle policy of distinguishing between *informing* family members of harvesting but not actively *requiring their consent.*[11] While there is some evidence that such a policy could improve organ supply, it remains unclear how one would deal with families that persist in their objection. The proposal of allowing next-of-kin to register their objection while nevertheless proceeding with harvesting smacks of cheap symbolism and will likely contribute to families' feelings of disrespect and loss of control. Ignoring the complex emotional dimension associated with cadaveric organ donation is also likely to backfire on the supply of organs. This was vividly illustrated when, in February 2007 in Singapore, the kidneys and corneas of Sim Tee Hua were harvested against the family's explicit objections. Because Sim had not signed a statement refusing to donate his organs, the hospital decided to go ahead with organ removal and ended up having to restrain the distressed family members by force while whisking away Sim's body for harvesting. The Sim case caused a massive public outcry and resulted in a significant subsequent drop in potential donors.[12]

If ignoring family distress—either by instituting required request policies or by ignoring the family perspective altogether—amounts to bad policy (as well as, perhaps, poor ethics), are there any alternatives that take the family veto seriously whilst also addressing the organ deficit? In the next section we outline one such alternative, based on a weak form of *advance commitment.*

---

[8] Sque et al. (2000).

[9] Caplan (1984).

[10] Fabre (2006); Wisnewsky (2008); Delaney and Hershenov (2009).

[11] Peters (1986); May et al. (2000).

[12] Xin (2007).

14.3 Advance Commitment As an Organ Procurement Policy

Suppose you wish to donate your organs. You sign onto the organ donor register and make a declaration of intent that your organs may be posthumously removed and used for transplant purposes. In our proposal, however, you are also asked to nominate a *designated second consenter* (DSC), who will be notified of your decision to become a donor and asked to register her agreement to allow your organs to be harvested upon death. While there is a superficial similarity between our proposed DSC and the nominated representatives envisaged under S.4 of the UK's Human Tissue Act 2004, there are also crucial differences.[13] When the DSC agrees to undertake this responsibility she receives an explicit request to support the posthumous removal of the donor's organs, under the conditions stipulated by the donor (if any). Importantly, in view of ensuring donor autonomy, the DSC cannot add or alter any of the stipulations of the donor's consent.

After being fully informed and ideally having discussed key aspects of the decision with the donor, the DSC next registers a statement of intent to agree to organ removal upon the event of the donor's death. The DSC may of course refuse to do so after having reflected on the request, in which case the donor would be entitled to designate another person to fulfill this role. Similarly, if the DSC first agrees but then later on formally rescinds her decision, again the donor is informed and may choose to reassign the DSC responsibility to another person.

Upon the death of the suitable donor, the local donor coordinator would normally inform the DSC. In most cases, we envisage that it would then be straightforward to proceed with organ removal, and less harrowing for both medical personnel and family members than under current arrangements. In the event that it is not possible to contact the DSC, the fact that advance commitment has been obtained would be a *prima facie* reason to proceed with organ removal. Another possibility is that the DSC raises an objection to organ removal *after the death of the donor*, perhaps under pressure from the immediate family in the hospital. Under our scheme the local donor coordinator would have to accept that decision and abort the process of organ removal. It is true that this would, in some sense, violate the wishes of the donor as well as ignore the impact of this decision on the organ recipient. Our proposal in this sense offers only a weak form of commitment. Although it is possible to envisage a scheme in which the DSC's assent, once given, would be difficult or impossible to revoke, this may be self-defeating if it discourages second consenters and perhaps even donors from signing up in the first place. Alternatively, we might consider combining the scheme outlined here with the use of financial incentives for those signing up to the scheme. Elsewhere we propose that such incentives could take the form of an *organ transplant tax credit*.

The introduction of a DSC into the organ donation process raises a number of concerns, however. From the perspective of respecting donor autonomy an impor-

[13] Human Tissue Authority (2006).

tant question concerns the freedom of the donor to choose her DSC as she pleases. We envisage that in most cases, most donors would opt for a family member, and that the exercise of this choice would be relatively uncontentious. Nonetheless, leaving aside children and others who do not have the full capacity to give consent, it is important for the donor to retain the power to choose for a number of reasons. Most straightforwardly, a donor who rightly anticipates that, say, her mother would be distressed by the *mere responsibility* of having to agree on this matter—independent of whether she believes donation is the right or wrong course of action—surely has the right (perhaps even a weak obligation) to assign someone less burdened to this task. More controversially, in some cases the donor might not have a close relation with any of her relatives, and might want to assign a friend or even colleague who would in those circumstances be much better placed to exercise a trusteeship function than family members. In other cases, there might be a problem where the law does not recognize certain intimate relations as full partnerships—as is the case for gay couples in many countries—and this way the donor ensures the partner's status in this decision.

Quite a different sort of reason in favour of donor's right to assign their DSC is when she feels some of her close relatives would manifestly refuse to assent to the removal of organs for transplant. For a donor who is committed to have her organs used for transplant purposes to know that this will be vetoed by her family surely constitutes a level of ante-mortem distress that we would like to avoid if we could. In such cases it is conceivable, even likely, that some or all family members would find themselves in dispute with the expressed wishes of the donor and by extension with the commitment given by the DSC. The donor's choice of DSC may not be decisive in securing her wish to donate, since the DSC may ultimately give way in the face of sustained family objections. Nonetheless, the presence in such cases of the DSC as a *living advocate* for the donor's wishes, would surely shift the balance towards the side of donor autonomy. Moreover, while there is no easy solution to such hard cases, the DSC would in most cases be best placed to balance the competing considerations of the donor's expressed wishes, and the likely effects on the family.

Another issue in relation to the role of the DSC concerns whether donors should be restricted in nominating a single person as DSC or instead be allowed to nominate several individuals to undertake this important role? Presently, under the Human Tissue Act 2004, an individual may nominate more than one person to give consent on her behalf after death, jointly and severally.[14] A case could be made for a scheme based on a single nominated DSC, since that role is essentially to merely ratify the wishes already conveyed by the donor, lessening the imperative of obtaining permission again after the death of the donor. This would weaken the case for appointing several people in order to make sure at least one of them can be reached in time at the crucial moment of organ removal. Furthermore, family disputes may also be less likely to impede organ removal if a single individual were designated. On the other hand, donors are in a good position to know their own family dynamics, and presumably would in most cases not choose more than one DSC without

[14] Human Tissue Authority (2006).

good reason. Even if this more permissive approach were to create complications in exceptional cases, it might be a price worth paying for maintaining a *minimally presumptuous* approach.

14.4 The Advantages of Advance Commitment

We discern four reasons for thinking the weak advance commitment scheme outlined in the previous section would constitute good organ procurement policy: respect for autonomy, better informed consent, accommodation of emotional distress of both next-of-kin and medical staff, and a significant increase in the supply of cadaveric organs.

First, we believe our proposed scheme significantly improves the autonomy of the donor in terms of influencing what happens to her organs after death. The scheme robustly secures donors' negative right not to have their organs taken without their consent: on this dimension, it is fully at a par with current informed consent policies and significantly improves on presumed consent policies.[15] But in addition, our proposal offers considerable advantages in terms of respecting donors' positive claims to determine what happens to their body after death.[16] By allowing donors to substantially influence who amongst the next-of-kin (or even outside of the circle of family relations) will have the power to posthumously veto their preferences on organ donation, they influence what happens to their body after death. One significant advantage of our advanced commitment scheme that the DSC is not put into a position of having to give a substituted judgement as to what he or she *thinks* the donor *might* have wanted. One aim of our scheme is precisely to reduce as much as possible *epistemic uncertainty* about donor preferences.

Second, our scheme significantly improves the informed aspect of organ donor decision-making, both in terms of donor and next-of-kin. Despite numerous campaigns to raise public awareness about organ donation, the level of disinformation remains quite staggering. In fact one of the main worries with the two leading alternatives to current organ donation policy—presumed consent and mandated choice—is that they seem to allow many potential donors to *consent* on the basis of information that scarcely qualifies as such.[17] At present incentives to inform oneself are weak at best. By contrast, the combination of having both donor and a member of the family sign onto a national register may improve both the active seeking of information as well as genuine deliberation afterwards, presumably even discussion amongst various members of the family. All of this seems conducive to boosting informed consent not only by the donor, but particularly by the family who under current arrangements are typically ill-informed when asked to reflect on organ removal

[15] Wilkinson (2005, 2007); Siminoff et al. (1995).

[16] Caplan (1984); Peters (1986); McGuinness and Brazier (2008); Siminoff et al. (1995).

[17] Siminoff et al. (1995); Chouhan and Draper (2003); Spital (1996).

requests immediately after the death of the donor.[18] Note that the improved quality of informed consent also applies to those who *refuse* to agree to the harvesting of their loved-ones organs: it is reasonable to assume that the proportion of people who make such a decision in our scheme will be better informed compared to alternative policies simply because opportunities to become informed and deliberate are disconnected from the distressing event of death.

Third, in line with one of the major reasons why we should take family vetoes seriously, we argue that our proposal will in the majority of cases significantly decrease the additional distress incurred by family members as well as medical staff at, and immediately after, the death of the donor. This is most obviously the case for family members to the extent that much of the required decisions have been taken well before death, relieving the next-of-kin of the added emotional pressure related to such decisions. Moreover, the reduction in epistemic uncertainty, discussed earlier in this section, would be expected to make the DSC's decision to abide by her earlier assent easier. It has been suggested that any argument in favour of taking the distress of the family seriously would imply removing the family veto altogether.[19] However, this argument fails to take into account distress associated with loss of control and (perceived) lack of respect by the family, and we maintain that an advanced commitment scheme that removes the decision process from the time of bereavement remains the better option. In our scheme, all that is required is that the DSC and other family are informed of organ removal: to many family members the fact that the person did register as a donor, and that the family is genuinely represented in the decision process through the DSC, may be sufficient reason to not further engage with the organ donation process. This is certainly the case where the whole immediate family was fully involved in the advance commitment process and a genuine joint agreement was reached.

One immediate objection to the last point is to suggest that advance commitment in fact *increases* distress when families disagree with the DSC. It is hard to deny that in some cases this may turn a serene period of bereavement into one of internal strife and struggle. However, we suggest that the proportion of families who experience this more acrimonious engagement with the donor process is likely to be much smaller than under the current system for two reasons. On the one hand, in many cases a good number of family members will have been involved in the decision process well in advance, improving the chances to reach a collective decision. On the other hand, those who were not involved may have less trouble agreeing with *one of their own* rather than having to deal with a representative of the transplant team. As mentioned before, it is often the loss of control and what is regularly perceived as insensitivity of medical staff broaching the topic of organ donation that distresses the next-of-kin.[20] The advance commitment scheme would address this aspect of the problem outright. As for the remaining cases where families quarrel amongst themselves, or where the donor chooses someone outside of the family

[18] Sque et al. (2005, 2008).

[19] Wilkinson (2007).

[20] Sque et al. (2005, 2008).

group to act as a DSC, in our view it cannot be an objection to our scheme that we cannot fully resolve internal division in *all* families since any scheme that involves individuals having to collectively agree on a delicate issue will encounter the same problem. Under our scheme at least the donor has granted one or more persons the authority to impose a decision on the family if conflict cannot be resolved. Even where family disputes cannot be resolved, it is still surely desirable to have some form of binding settlement, in order to limit the duration of family conflict.

Next, we must consider the important point of relieving medical staff from some of the distress associated with having to juggle the moral commitment to saving lives through organ donation with the acknowledgement of family members' emotional distress.[21] In this respect our proposal has two major advantages. The fact that a DSC has already agreed considerably shortens the amount of time and effort to be spent on trying to *convince* next-of-kin to consent, including being torn between either failing the family or failing the potential recipient in need of a transplant organ. Further, the fact that legitimate consent pre-exists allows for a low-distress approach to organ removal even where some family members object, as medical staff can proceed knowing the family perspective has not been entirely disregarded. Compared to alternative proposals advance commitment can make a plausible claim to decrease distress on all parties.

Finally, we believe our proposed scheme has the potential to significantly boost the current supply of cadaveric organs. This is in large part because of the three advantages discussed above. If current estimates that family vetoes effectively block roughly half of potential donor organs are correct, we should expect to seriously increase this supply when the autonomy of donors is respected. Similarly, more information should positively affect the supply of organs if much current objection to organ donation is based on donors and family being ill-informed. A further interesting side-effect is that family members who are asked to become a DSC of course immediately will be reflecting on their own reasons for (not) becoming a donor. Finally, respect for family distress will affect the supply in at least three ways: by making it easier for encouraging family members to agree to organ removal; by encouraging greater numbers of donors to sign up with the reassurance that their families will not experience an unnecessarily distressing process of request consent; and by transplant staff more routinely proceeding with organ removal. One important reason tied in with this last point is that in cases where the next-of-kin cannot be reached in time, despite good-faith effort to reach them, transplant staff can go ahead with organ removal in the knowledge that family consent has already been obtained. This would imply a sizeable reduction in the number of organs currently going to waste because family cannot be reached in time.

Acknowledgements A previous version of this paper was presented at the 2009 annual conference of the Association for Social and Legal Philosophy, University of Edinburgh, and at departmental seminars at the University of Manchester, Université de Montréal and Queen's University Belfast. We are grateful to the audiences at those events for probing questions and in particular to Charles Erin, Nir Eyal, Matthew Hunt, David Hunter and Ruth Stirton for pertinent suggestions.

[21] Sque et al. (2000).

References

Abadie, A., and S. Gay. 2006. The impact of presumed consent legislation on cadaveric organ donation: A cross-country study. *Journal of Health Economics* 25 (4): 599–620.

Caplan, A. 1984. Ethical and policy issues in the procurement of cadaver organs for transplantation. *New England Journal of Medicine* 311 (15): 981–893.

Chouhan, P., and H. Draper. 2003. Modified mandated choice for organ procurement. *Journal of Medical Ethics* 29 (3): 157–162.

Delaney, J., and D. B. Hershenov. 2009. Why consent may not be needed for organ procurement. *The American Journal of Bioethics* 9 (8): 3–10.

Erin, C. A., and J. Harris. 2003. An ethical market in human organs. *Journal of Medical Ethics* 29 (3): 137–138.

Fabre, C. 2006. *Whose body is it anyway? Justice and the integrity of the person.* Oxford: Clarendon.

Human Tissue Authority. July 2006. Code of Practice—Consent.

Klassen, A.C., and D. K. Klassen. 1996. Who are the donors in organ donation? The family's perspective in mandated choice. *Annals of Internal Medicine* 125 (1): 70–73.

May, T., M. P. Aulisio, and M. A. DeVita. 2000. Patients, families, and organ donation: Who should decide? *Millbank Quarterly* 78 (2): 323–336.

McGuinness, S., and M. Brazier. 2008. Respecting the living means respecting the dead too. *Oxford Journal of Legal Studies* 28 (2): 297–316.

McLean, S. 1996. Transplantation and the 'nearly dead': The case of elective ventilation. In *Contemporary issues in law, medicine and ethics*, ed. S. McLean, 143–161, 146. Aldershot: Dartmouth.

NHS Blood and Transplant. 2007–2008. Transplant activity in the UK. 2008, 4.

Peters, D. A. 1986. Protecting autonomy in organ procurement procedures: Some overlooked issues. *Millbank Quarterly* 64 (2): 241–270.

Siminoff, L. A., R. M. Arnold, A. L. Caplan, and B. A. Virnig. 1995. Public policy governing organ and tissue procurement in the United States. *Annals of Internal Medicine* 123 (1): 10–17.

Spital, A. 1996. Mandated choice for organ donation: Time to give it a try. *Annals of Internal Medicine* 125 (1): 66–69.

Sque, M., S. Payneb, and J. Vlachonikolisa. 2000. Cadaveric donotransplantation: Nurses' attitudes, knowledge and behaviour. *Social Science & Medicine* 50 (4): 541–552.

Sque, M., T. Long, and S. Payne. 2005. Organ donation: Key factors influencing families' decision-making. *Transplantation Proceedings* 37 (2): 543–546.

Sque, M., T. Long, S. Payne, and D. Allardyce. 2008. Why relatives do not donate organs for transplants: 'Sacrifice' or 'gift of life'? *Journal of Advanced Nursing* 61 (2): 134–144.

Taylor, J. S. 2005. *Stakes and kidneys: Why markets in human body parts are morally imperative.* Aldershot: Ashgate.

Veatch, R. M., and J. B. Pitt. 1995. The myth of presumed consent: Ethical problems in new organ procurement strategies. *Transplantation Proceedings* 27 (2): 1888–1892.

Wilkinson, T. M. 2005. Individual and family consent to organ and tissue donation: Is the current position coherent? *Journal of Medical Ethics* 31 (10): 587–590.

Wilkinson, T. M. 2007. Individual and family decisions about organ donation. *Journal of Applied Philosophy* 24 (1): 26–40.

Wisnewsky, J. 2008. When the dead do not consent: A defense of non-consensual organ use. *Public Affairs Quarterly* 22 (3): 289–309.

Xin, L. April 3, 2007. Forced organ removal in Singapore raises concerns. The epoch times. http://en.epochtimes.com/news/7-4-3/53670.html.

Jurgen De Wispelaere is a Researcher at the Institute for Health and Social Policy, McGill University. An occupational therapist turned political philosopher, he holds degrees in occupational therapy and moral sciences. Previously, he held positions at the University of Montreal (CREUM), Trinity College Dublin and University College Dublin. His main research is in the philosophical aspects of social policy and institutional design, with specific application to unconditional basic income, disability policy, parenting, and public health and health policy. He has a strong interest in the ethical and policy implications of family objections to posthumous organ donation.

Lindsay Stirton is Professor of Public Law at the University of Sussex. He has previously held academic positions at the University of Sheffield, the University of Manchester, University of East Anglia, the London School of Economics and Political Science and the University of the West Indies. His research interests span public administration and public law, and his recently published work covers competition in health services, the implementation of basic income policies, comparative legal history, regulation of utility services in transition and developing countries. He holds a PhD from the University of London. His doctoral dissertation examined the regulation of health services in the United Kingdom since the 1980s.

Chapter 15
Power of Legal Concepts to Increase Organ Quantity

Ulrich Schroth and Karin Bruckmüller

15.1 Introduction[1]

The legal preconditions for and limits of organ transplantation as well as the interpretation and implementation of these framework conditions in practice significantly affect the willingness to donate an organ and subsequently the quantity of organs available. When generating innovative concepts to increase the quantity of organs, the legal provisions of the individual countries cannot be disregarded. Therefore, where alterations to current systems are discussed, also legislative suggestions for modification have to be presented.

Concerning post-mortem organ removal, the effects of the respective legal concept on the quantity of organs available become impressively apparent. This is conveyed by the German and Austrian legal situation. Regarding post-mortem and especially living organ donation it can, moreover, be shown that also interpretation and implementation of the law in legal and medical practice in the two countries can strongly influence organ quantity.

[1] Parts of this article are in Schroth 2012, and Schroth 2013. The authors thank Mag. Katrin Forstner and Dominika Peter for their support with this article.

K. Bruckmüller (✉)
Faculty of Law, LMU Munich, Munich, Germany and Faculty of Law, JKU Linz, Linz, Austria
e-mail: karin.bruckmueller@jura.uni-muenchen.de, karin.bruckmueller@jku.at

U. Schroth
Faculty of Law, LMU Munich, Munich, Germany
e-mail: ulrich.schroth@jura.uni-muenchen.de

R. J. Jox et al. (eds.), *Organ Transplantation in Times of Donor Shortage*,
International Library of Ethics, Law, and the New Medicine 59,
DOI 10.1007/978-3-319-16441-0_15

15.2 Diverging Willingness of the Population to Agree to Post-mortem Removal…

In Germany, post-mortem organ donation is—in contrast to Austria—not a success story. Germany, with regards to organ quantity, does not even meet the European average. In Germany, 15–16 persons per one million inhabitants (Deutsche Stiftung Organtransplantation)[2] donate their organs post-mortem. Therefore, the number of organs obtained from corpses does not nearly suffice to supply the seriously ill. This has a significant, unfortunate consequence: two to three seriously ill patients on the wait list in need of organs die on a daily basis in Germany because of a shortage of donor organs.

Austria, however, as well as e.g. Belgium, counts 29–30 donors per one million inhabitants. In Spain, organs from 35–36 persons per one million inhabitants (Gesundheit Österreich 2013)[3] are obtained for transplantation post-mortem, thus making Spain the only European country able to amply provide its citizens with organs.[4]

15.3 … Due to Different Legal Models

In both countries, the diverging quantity of organs can be ascribed to the different legal systems which the legislators chose. In Germany, the so-called "decision solution" ("*Entscheidungslösung*", a form of opt-in solution)[5] is in force. This is a system of organ donation whereby the potential donor has to explicitly express a wish to become a donor. The Austrian legislator has continually[6] decided in favour of the so-called "dissent solution" ("*Widerspruchslösung*", an opt-out solution)[7]. This means that, in principle, everybody is an organ donor unless she or he stated or registered that he or she is not willing to donate.

The different approaches of the two countries, which are essentially comparable in terms of social, cultural, and legal situation, lie perhaps in the different (legal) traditions[8] with regards to post-mortem personality rights. Both legal systems have in common that the event of total brain death is the precondition for post-mortem organ removal. This means—from a legal perspective—that the body as an integrated

[2] See www.dso.de (still on the opt-in solution without information).

[3] There you also can find data on other European countries.

[4] For more details Schroth (2010b).

[5] For details see 15.4.1.

[6] It had already been ruled in the so-called Act on Hospitals and Sanatoria (Kranken- und Kuranstaltengesetz—KaKuG) and has been adopted without changes for the Act on Organ Transplantations (Organtransplantationsgesetz—Austrian OTPG) (§§ 5 et seq.), which has been enforced December 2012. See to the new act Heissenberger (2013).

[7] Also known as "presumed consent"; for details see 15.4.1.

[8] See infra 15.5.1.

biological organism does not exist any longer and the person per se is ultimately lost and unrecoverable.[9]

The differences become apparent in the level of protection of the potential donor's autonomy. Whereas in Germany there has to be consent to post-mortem organ removal—the post-mortem personality right is highly valued—in Austria, in general, everybody is a post-mortem organ donor and has to object in order to prevent the removal.[10] The Austrian legislator clearly decides that the protection of the living is more important than the protection of the deceased and their post-mortem personality right.

15.4 Opt-In Solution in Germany

15.4.1 Legal Provisions

In Germany, an agreement has been reached on the so-called "decision solution".[11] It is an extended opt-in solution because the potential donors are encouraged to declare to donate by receiving preceding information on transplantation. The declaration is then registered on their health card. However, there is no obligation to make a declaration.

According to the decision solution, post-mortem organ removal is permitted if the potential donor has given his consent during his lifetime. This means that a potential donor's active act of deciding is necessary. In order to be able to make this decision accordingly and subsequently deliver a statement, the health insurance companies provide adequate information to the citizens. This is absolutely necessary, because the donor's autonomy can only be taken seriously if the citizens have been sufficiently informed about the possibility to donate organs, as well as the alternatives.

In case the deceased did not consent during lifetime, removal is still legitimated if a person associated with the organ donor has consented to the organ removal after his death. In doing so, the relative has to take into account the donor's presumed will. The person authorised to consent only has a right to do so if the will of the deceased cannot be determined.[12] According to law, a formalistic approach has to be taken regarding the order of relatives authorised to consent. Spouses and civil

[9] In detail Schroth (2010a); see also the corresponding recommendations of the Austrian so-called Obersten Sanitätsrat. http://www.austrotransplant.at/download/Hirntod_2005.pdf.

[10] It is to be questioned if in the case of the opt-out solution it can be referred to donors in the narrower sense.

[11] See § 2 German Act on Transplantation (Transplantationsgesetz—German TPG).

[12] Cf. Schroth (2005). The option of relatives consenting to an organ removal does not exist if a legally effective dissent of the potential organ donor exists. Every citizen who has reached the age of 14—and therefore the religious majority—is entitled to legally binding dissent to organ removal after his death. The legally binding permission to consent is obtained when reaching the age of 16. (§ 2 Paragraph 2 Sentence 3 German TPG).

partners rank first, children who are of full legal age second, followed by parents, siblings of full legal age, and finally grandparents. The relatives are, however, only authorised to consent if they have been in personal contact with the potential donor during the last 2 years prior to the organ donor's death.[13]

It is the aim of this legal model to allow the potential donor to make an informed decision on the handling of his corpse and at the same time the best possible way to protect his autonomy, as well as guarantee maximum post-mortem protection of personality rights. These provisions are protected by criminal law. Whoever removes an organ following brain death without the person concerned having consented during his or her lifetime, or a relative having consented after the respective person's death, is liable to prosecution under the Act on Transplantation.[14]

15.4.2 Hardly any Declarations on Organ Transplantation—Low Organ Quantity

There exists hardly any consent on organ donation. Only 9 % of the citizens suitable to be an organ donor make a decision on whether or not they want to donate.[15] Albeit there was hope that the introduction of the "decision solution" in 2012, prior to which only the so-called "consent solution" (an opt-in solution without any preceding information for potential donors) had been in force, would increase the number of statements in favour of organ donation; this has not been the case.

This means that in 91 % of cases the relatives decide whether the brain-dead patient is an organ donor or not. As of now it is not clear to what extent the relatives' decisions orientate themselves on the presumed will; relatives in many cases presumably are making the decision according to their own beliefs since a presumed will often cannot be determined.

Ultimately, as has already been said above, in Germany only 15–16 persons per one million inhabitants are post-mortem organ donors.

15.5 Opt-Out Solution in Austria

15.5.1 Legal Provisions

Austria has codified the so-called "dissent solution".[16] According to this opt-out solution, it is legitimate, as long as the potential donor did not object during life-

[13] See § 1a Paragraph 5 German TPG.

[14] See § 19 Paragraph 2 German TPG.

[15] See data source: www.dso.de.

[16] In Europe, the opt-out solution is in force inter alia in Belgium, France, the Scandinavian countries, and, as has already been mentioned, in Spain. The regulation of the Austrian OTPG is ap-

time, to explant single organs or organ parts of a deceased person in order to save another's life or restore his health by way of transplantation.[17]

Therefore, the removal is only prohibited if a declaration (either in writing or recorded in the dissent register) exists stating that the deceased, or his legal representative, has explicitly objected to organ donation[18] prior to his death. It is, in principle, the duty of the patient or his legal representative to arrange for the doctor to gain knowledge of this declaration. The doctor does not have an obligation to make comprehensive enquiries. It can, however, be demanded that the doctor has to check whether or not a respective declaration exists within the domain of the hospital.[19] In any case, an obligation[20] to enquire with the Austrian Institute for Health Care[21], which manages the Austrian-wide dissent register exists.[22] Everybody, from age 14 onwards, can give his dissent to the removal of organs, or certain organs respectively, by way of declaration.

In practice, doctors usually only explant an organ after consultation with the deceased's relatives. Therefore, a so-called extended dissent solution is practised, according to which the relatives can object to organ removal, with the consequence that organ removal is not performed.[23] It is the aim of these rules to balance the two legal goods standing in opposition to each other, namely rescue of human life and restoration of health, respectively, and post-mortem personality right and dignity. Ultimately, the superiority of life and health has been legally determined.[24]

That the living persons' interests are valued higher than those of the dead becomes apparent in a long (legal) tradition in Austria concerning the provisions on autopsy. Rules on autopsy had already been established during the reign of Emperor Joseph II,[25] and regulation has continued until today. Nowadays, an autopsy cannot only be ordered for reasons of security and criminal procedure, but also in order to preserve other public or scientific interests.[26] The law mentions particular diagnostic ambiguities of the case or performed surgical interventions as reasons. Due to the use of the word *particular* it is clear that autopsies may be performed also for other reasons, for example out of sheer scientific interest or curiosity, perhaps in order to

plicable independently of the in Austria deceased potential organ donor's nationality or residency. This results from Art. 49 of the Austrian Constitution, which stipulates the territorially validity of the Austrian legal provisions.

[17] §§ 5 etseq. Austrian OTPG.

[18] The dissent can also only apply to a specific organ.

[19] Possibilities would include examination of personal belongings, especially clothing and wallet, or of the patient's room. Cf. Bruckmüller and Schumann (2010); of the same opinion Radner et al. (2000).

[20] § 7 Austrian OTPG.

[21] Cf. Gesundheit Österreich GmbH.

[22] Cf. Aigner (1994). On registration and query, see http://www.goeg.at/de/Widerspruchsregister.

[23] On the legal situation and practice in detail, see Dujmovits (2013); Bruckmüller and Schumann (2010); Barta et al. (1999); Kopetzki (1988).

[24] This is, however, attenuated by the relatives' possibility to decide.

[25] Autopsies were already legally defined for scientific purposes in 1749.

[26] § 25 Austrian KaKuG.

get results that would be of interest to the living. This principle *mors auxilium vitae* (The dead shall serve the living)[27] is also evident in the legal conception of post-mortem donation.

Maintaining the status quo as potential organ donor, i.e. staying passive during lifetime, is—due to the long tradition—most probably regarded as being sufficient in protecting post-mortem personality rights by the legislator.

An additional safeguard is legally provided by way of ruling that the removal may not lead to a deformation of the corpse, which would be violating its dignity. Therefore, permitted explantations should be restricted to single organs or organ parts.[28] By way of also including relatives in decisions on explantation in practice, their sense of dignity is taken into consideration as well. Infringements are punishable under so-called administrative criminal law.

15.5.2 Hardly any Opposition to Organ Removal—High Organ Quantity

As of December 31, 2012, 28,875 people were registered in the dissent register, 25,056 of those were residents of Austria. This corresponds with 0.29 % of the resident population. Among the other registered people, 3505 were from Germany. Another 111 originated from Slovenia, 98 from Switzerland, 32 from the Netherlands, 18 from France, ten from Spain, and small numbers from other countries.[29] The organs of the remaining resident population are—with the exception of where the relatives object—at disposal for removal. Therefore, the organ quantity in Austria is relatively high, about twice as high as in Germany, namely 29–30 donors per one million inhabitants.

15.6 Opt-Out Solution Increases Organ Quantity

All statistical data evidently show that organ quantity is significantly higher in countries, which apply the opt-out solution than in countries with the opt-in solution. A comparison between Austria, Belgium, or Spain and Germany shows that in the former 40 % or even 100 % more post-mortem organ donors are available than in Germany.[30] In light of the fact that three to four seriously ill patients on the waiting list die, the advantage of the opt-out solution becomes obvious.[31]

---

[27] Signs depicting this sentence can still bc found in Austrian pathologies.

[28] In 2012, an average of 3.6 organs was removed from every organ donor and transplanted. Gesundheit Österreich (2013).

[29] Gesundheit Österreich (2013).

[30] On recent data, see www.dso.de.

[31] On the arguments pro and contra to the opt-out solution, see Gutmann (2006) with further references.

15.7 Legal Framework Conditions Influence Decisions and Organ Quantity

Findings within the *Behavioral Law and Economics*-studies[32] distinctly show that the respective legal framework conditions determining the realisation of the right of self-determination significantly influence the willingness to donate organs. Therefore, the individual's autonomous decision on whether or not he wants to be an organ donor is dependent on the legal framework conditions.

The behavioural-economic research calls this phenomenon *Framing-Effect*.[33] Depending on the scope of the depiction of the problem (so-called *framing*), depending on the alternatives provided (so-called *default rules*[34]), and depending on the fashion in which the decision maker is conveyed the risks, differences in the development of preferences and selection decisions exists. It must, based on the empirical knowledge of behavioural economics, be stated that people decidedly do not make decisions according to stable and clear preferences. On the contrary, their decisions are influenced by weaknesses of will and cognition; they require a stimulus for their decision-making behaviour. It therefore appears that the opt-out solution is understood as a regulation in which the State shows its positive approach towards organ donation. This *attitude* of the State or the legal tradition respectively is, as it is in Austria, an impulse for a decision to permit the removal of organs after death.

The experiment conducted by Johnson and Goldstein[35] as described by Thaler and Sunstein in their Monography "Nudge—Improving decisions about Wealth, Health and Happiness" shows the same results (Thaler and Sunstein 2009). Three groups of subjects were asked in an online-questionnaire in diverging settings whether they wanted to become organ donors. The subjects of the first group were told they moved to a country in which they had not been registered as an organ donor. They now had, however, the possibility to agree to being a donor, or to confirm their status as a non-donor. The second group was told that they were automatically registered as organ donors in their new residence area. However, they had the possibility to object to this status as a donor, or maintain it. The subjects of the third group were told that they had to make a decision pro or contra their status as an organ donor. In all three settings, the subjects could make their decision with one click only. The result was impressive. Whereas in the first group, which basically was a simulation of the opt-in solution, only 42 % opted for registration as an organ donor, 82 % of the second group, in which the opt-out solution was simulated, maintained their status as organ donors.[36] Surprisingly, of the members of the third group, in which the participants were forced to make a decision, 79 % consented to being organ donors.

---

[32] See e.g. the anthology Engel et al. (2007).

[33] The Nobel Prize winner Kahneman's research has to be mentioned as fundamental in this context, see e.g. Kahneman et al. (1982); Kahneman and Tversky (2000).

[34] Such as, for example, the different models of post-mortem organ donation.

[35] See Johnson and Goldstein (2003).

[36] In Austria, an active act is not even necessary, as was also the case in the project.

15.8 Implementation of the Law and Organ Quantity

Adequate interpretation and implementation of the law is also required in order to increase the organ quantity. This accounts for every legal concept on post-mortem organ donation and is evident in practice of living organ donation in Germany and Austria.

15.8.1 Organising the Practice of Post-mortem Donation

Some German federal states were already able to obtain a higher quantity of organ donors due to a superior organisation in practice. It is said that the number of reports of total brain death have increased. Also in Austria, an enhanced report system of brain death diagnosis could further increase organ quantity. Additionally, appropriate spatial and technical resources and therefore ultimately financial resources have to be provided for in both countries.

A model example once again is Spain. In some parts of the country, for example in the region surrounding Barcelona, organ donation is especially well organised. In this region, a particularly high number of organs is obtained, which does not find its match anywhere else, especially not in any part of Germany.

15.8.2 Legal Interpretation and Practice of Living Organ Donation

On the example of living organ donation in Germany[37] and Austria,[38] it can be demonstrated that the interpretation of the law may lead to a reduction or increase of potentially available organs. The restriction of the donor pool is chosen as an example.

In Germany, the law states that only persons related to or otherwise closely associated with the recipient are potential living organ donors for transplantations of a kidney, parts of the liver or other non-regenerating organs. This provision is heavily disputed in theory[39], among other things, because it restricts the autonomy of potential donors who do not belong to the named group of people, but also because it subsequently constitutes a barrier for increasing the organ quantity. In Austrian law—the corresponding criminal law[40] and the new Act on Organ Transplantation, which has been enforced since the end of 2012, there are no restrictions as to the

---

[37] See § 8 German TPG.

[38] See § 8 Austrian OTPG.

[39] See Schroth (2010c) with further references to the discussion.

[40] The corresponding rules in the Austrian Criminal Code are §§ 83 et seq. (acts against limb) and § 90 (consent).

pool of donors. Strictly speaking, this means that in theory organ donation to the benefit of everyone is permitted.

Theory in Austria, however, views this as controversial. By way of interpreting corresponding provisions of the Criminal Code, limits are set. One opinion qualifies the removal of an organ from a person not closely associated as a criminal offence against life and limb.[41] Besides, the German restriction of the donor pool has been adopted in a directive of the Austrian Advisory Committee on Transplantation. Although this directive only has the character of a recommendation, practice at large adheres to it; the guideline seems to provide a certain security for doctors' decisions.

Albeit donations to strangers are possible in Austria, theory and practice keep it at bay and by doing so decrease the potential organ quantity. It remains to be seen whether the legislator's decision not to make any restrictions on the part of the donor pool in the new separate Act on Organ Transplantation will lead to changes in practice. One formulation in the explanatory comment on the law gives occasion to such hopes. It makes it clear that "consent can only be given with regards to a certain person." It can be perused, that a donor can make his organ available to a person who is a stranger, as well. It would probably be a misinterpretation or even an inconsistency with the valuation of legal goods if theory and practice were to continue to—contra the legislator's historical will—restrict the pool of donors.

15.9 Conclusion

It is shown that the legislator has the *power* to increase the organ quantity through legal provisions, and the interpretation and implementation of these play a significant role in this respect. Therefore, also from the perspective of being able to save lives or enhance the physical condition of many people—with consideration to cultural and religious principles—the opt-out solution has to be given priority.[42] For people living in countries with the opt-out solution, it facilitates the decision on the removal of body parts after death or not changing the status as potential organ donor. Moreover, it implicates relief for the doctors when talking to relatives so that also they can finally consent to removal.

Due to the possibility of dissent, the potential donor's autonomy and post-mortem personality right is given sufficient consideration. This should be maintained by an extensive obligation to inform—e.g. mainly by the health insurance companies—in order to guarantee that a self-determined decision can be made against removal as well.[43] It would, of course, be reasonable for all legal concepts dealing

[41] See discussion in Burgstaller and Schütz (2010) and Bruckmüller and Schumann (2010).

[42] Interestingly—because of cultural and religious issues—there are no preferences in the EU directives 2010/45/EU of 7 July 2010 on standards of quality and safety of human organs. See Bruckmüller and Schumann (2010a).

[43] It is questionable, whether the Austrian population is informed in a comprehensive way. Is it enough that there is information on the opt-out solution on corresponding homepages and refer-

with post-mortem donation to grant the potential donor the right to determine that certain organs be transplanted primarily to persons of the donor's own choice. This concept of helping a certain person is capable of positively influencing the attitude towards post-mortem organ donation and enhancing the willingness to donate.

In addition to the legal situation, the organisation of the transplantation process has to be improved. In particular, respective provisions have to be made to ensure brain-dead patients are reported,[44] since the quantity of post-mortem available organs primarily depends on this information. Finally, also theory and practice should be stimulated to corresponding interpretation encouraging organ removal, naturally within the limits of the right of self-determination.

References

Aigner G. 1994. Organentnahmen bei Verstorbenen zu Transplantationszwecken gemäß § 62 a KAG; Widerspruchsregister. RdM (Recht der Medizin), 119.

Barta, H., G. Kalchschmid, C. Kopetzki, and E. Dujmovits. 1999. *Rechtspolitische Aspekte des Transplantationsrechts*. Wien: Hanz

Bruckmüller, K., and S. Schumann. 2010. Die Heilbehandlung im österreichischen Strafrecht. In *Handbuch des Medizinstrafrechts*, ed. C. Roxin and U. Schroth. 4th ed., 847. Stuttgart: Boorberg.

Bruckmüller, K., and S. Schumann. 2010a. *Organmangel und Organspende—Europarechtliche Rechtsetzung und nationaler Anpassungsbedarf, Jahrbuch Gesundheitsrecht*. Wien: NWV Verlag.

Burgstaller H., and H., Schütz. 2010. In *Wiener Kommentar zum Strafgesetzbuch*. 2nd ed., ed. Ratz Höpfel. Wien: Manz Verlag.

Deutsche Stiftung Organtransplantation, Statistiken. www.dso.de.

Dujmovits, J. 2013. Organtransplantation. In *Handbuch Medizinrecht für die Praxis (Loseblattsammlung)*, ed. Kletečka Aigner and M. Kletečka-Pulker, et al. Wien: Manz Verlag.

Engel, C., M. Englerth, J. Lüdemann, and I. Spiecker., eds. 2007. *Recht und Verhalten: Beiträge zu Behavioral Law and Economics*. 1st ed. Tübingen: Mohr Siebeck.

Gesundheit Österreich GmbH—Geschäftsbereich ÖBIG. 2013. ÖBIG-Transplant. Jahresbericht 2012, 2013.

Gutmann, T. 2006. *Für ein neues Transplantationsgesetz. Eine Bestandsaufnahme des Novellierungsbedarfs im Recht der Transplantationsmedizin*, 155. Berlin: Springer.

Heissenberger W. 2013. *Das Bundesgesetz über die Transplantation menschlicher Organe und dessen wesentliche Neuerungen*. RdM (Recht der Medizin), 50. Wien: Manz Verlag.

Johnson, E. J., and D. Goldstein. 2003. Do defaults save lives? *Science* 302:1338.

Kahneman, D., and A. Tversky. 2000. *Choices, values and frames*. Cambridge: Cambridge University Press.

Kahneman, D., P. Slovic, and A. Tversky. 1982. *Judgement under uncertainty: Heuristics and biases*. Cambridge: Cambridge University Press.

Kopetzki, C. 1988. *Organgewinnung zu Zwecken der Transplantation: Eine systematische Analyse des geltenden Rechts*. New York: Springer.

ences can frequently be found in newspaper articles, including daily newspapers for the general public?

[44] § 11 Paragraph 4 German TPG.

Radner, A., A. Haslinger, and P. Reinberg. 2000. *Krankenanstaltenrecht*. 1st ed. Austria: Trauner Verlag.

Schroth, U. 2005. § 16 Richtlinien zum Stand der Erkenntnisse der med. Wissenschaft. In *Transplantationsgesetz. Kommentar*, ed. U. Schroth, P. König, T. Gutmann, and F. Oduncu. München: C.H. Beck.

Schroth, U. 2010a. Die postmortale Organ- und Gewebespende. In *Handbuch des Medizinstrafrechts*, ed. Schroth Roxin, 4th ed., 448. Stuttgart: Boorberg.

Schroth, U. 2010b. Kritische Einführung in die Rechtslage der postmortalen Organtransplantation sowie der Lebendorgantransplantation in Deutschland. In *Recht am Krankenbett—Zur Kommerzialisierung des Gesundheitssystems*, ed. Dochow Duttge and Weber Waschkewitz, 3. Göttingen: Universitätsverlag Göttingen.

Schroth, U. 2010c. Die strafrechtlichen Grenzen der Organlebendspende. In *Handbuch des Medizinstrafrechts*, ed. Schroth Roxin, 4th ed., 466. Stuttgart: Boorberg.

Schroth, U. 2012. Postmortale Transplantation und Autonomie. Zur Debatte 2:36.

Schroth, U. 2013. Die strafrechtliche Beurteilung der Manipulation bei der Leberallokation. NStZ (Neue Zeitschrift für Strafrecht) 437.

Thaler, R. H., and C. R. Sunstein. 2009. *Nudge—Wie man kluge Entscheidungen anstößt*. 2nd ed., 244. Berlin: Econ.

Ulrich Schroth is professor for criminal law, criminal procedure law, legal philosophy and sociology of law at the Ludwig-Maximilians-University Munich. His research focuses on topics within medical criminal law and bioethical law. He is also chairman of a committee for living organ donation.

Karin Bruckmüller is researcher and lecturer in criminal law and criminal procedure law at the Ludwig-Maximilians-University Munich and the University of Linz. Her research focuses on medical-criminal law and ethics as well as victims' rights. She is expert for the European Union and the United Nations.

Chapter 16
Legal Consequences of Organ Transplantation Malpractice

Ruth Rissing-van Saan

16.1 Introduction

Transplantation medicine assumes and calls for the availability of donor organs. The Federal Republic of Germany as well as seven other countries[1] have joined the *Eurotransplant* procuration organization in Leiden, Netherlands, in order to increase a chronically ill and waiting patient's chances of receiving a donor organ, for him to receive the most immunologically suitable organ, or to transplant this organ as quickly as possible in acute life-threatening situations by implementing a collective donor-alert system.

As of January 1, 2013, there were 11,233 patients on the main Eurotransplant wait list, 6713 of which had just recently registered in 2012. In 2012, the small sum of 4042 procurable organs from deceased donors were actually transplanted.[2] Thus, this process of procuring donor organs represents the distribution of scarce goods among numerous interested parties. This is an ethical and legal challenge, in that one donor organ has many chronically ill potential takers, who either receive a new chance at life through the allocation of this organ or whose body will fail in the case of non-consideration.

Medicine has always been confronted with the prevalent problematic of accommodating and saving numerous injured or ill individuals and the issue of sensibly distributing scarce resources for their treatment, whether that meant treating an endless number of injured individuals in times of war, helping hundreds of fatalities or injuries after natural catastrophes, or treating injuries after multiple-vehicle collisions on the highway or Autobahn. A generally valid set of rules, which can be used to justly and effectively distribute and implement the rather scarce medical and

[1] Belgium, the Netherlands, Croatia, Luxemburg, Austria, Slovenia, and Hungary.

[2] www.eurotransplant.org/index php?page=pat_germany.

R. Rissing-van Saan (✉)
Bochum, Germany
e-mail: r.rissing@t-online.de

R. J. Jox et al. (eds.), *Organ Transplantation in Times of Donor Shortage*,
International Library of Ethics, Law, and the New Medicine 59,
DOI 10.1007/978-3-319-16441-0_16

human resources that are needed to treat and save that many people, will always be necessary in order to find an acceptable solution to this recurring problematic. Thus, certain criteria have to be established that are the same for all affected individuals and define a priority plan of action that applies to everyone as is the case in the so-called *Triage*, which, among other things, goes by the principle of accommodation according to necessity, meaning: those that can wait must wait!

16.2 Legal Principles of Organ Transplantation in Germany

Organ transplantation is not immune from German law, but instead falls under the realm of the transplantation law (TPG), which has been in place since December 1, 1997[3] and which was significantly amended and has recently been reformed on July 12, 2012[4] and July 21, 2012[5]. The law explicates the medical and legal premises for organ donation and controls the coordination of the extraction of the organ or tissue from the donor and the transfer of procurable organs to a specific recipient. It provides the basis for the organization of the organ transplantation, separating the responsibilities for the extraction of organs and tissues (§ 11 TPG), and getting the procurable, eligible organs to the potential recipient (§ 12 TPG). The institution that holds the position that is responsible for organ*retrieval* and procurement preparation is reserved for a so-called coordinating center (§ 11 Paragraph 1 TPG), which in Germany is the German Organ Transplantation Foundation (German: Deutsche Stiftung Organtransplantation (DSO)). The procurement itself is carried out by a medical board, health insurance providers, and a financially and organizationally independent procurement committee within each respective hospital (§ 12 Paragraph 1 TPG). The procurement agency responsible for the German transplantation centers (German: Transplantationszentren (TPZ)) is, as mentioned above, Eurotransplant. They are responsible for procuring the organs to a proper recipient by following a set of rules, which adhere to contemporary findings in the medical sciences and which adequately ensure that the transplantation is for the benefit of the patient and takes the urgency of the need for an organ transplant into consideration (§ 12 Paragraph 3 Sentence 1 TPG).

The transplantation law requires that all the wait lists from various transplantation centers be treated as one collective wait list (§ 12 Paragraph 3 Sentence 2 TPG). The regulation stating that patients from each individual transplant center register collectively on *one wait list* guarantees that patients registered in Germany all have an equal chance of getting a donor organ. In general, standard procedure requires

[3] German law on organ donation, retrieval, and transfer (German Transplantation Law=TPG), Federal Law Gazette (BGBl.) (1997 I, pp. 2631–2639).

[4] German law regulating the decision-making process and solution in the transplantation law BGBl. (2012 I, pp. 1504–1506).

[5] Amendment to the German Transplantation Law BGBl. (2012 I, pp. 1601–1612).

that an organ be allocated to *one specific patient* as opposed to allocating or offering it to a transplant center. However, there are exceptions (for example, resource allocations), which have certain guidelines regarding their prerequisites, which will not be elaborated on here.

Decisions regarding which guidelines should be used for the procurement of organs in coherence with modern medical research, is not determined by law, but instead commissions the German Medical Association with this task, as can be seen in § 16 TPG. The German Medical Association makes its decisions according to a *set of guidelines*, which vary with the different phases of the organ transplantation process: starting with rules that verify the donor's death, the measures taken for organ retrieval, guidelines for the process of organ procurement, and assuring that the organ is qualitatively adequate. The transplantation law connects the guidelines from § 16 Paragraph 1 Sentence 2 TPG with important *legal consequences*: if these guidelines are followed then, according to statutory presumption, the transplantation was carried out in compliance with modern medical standards and knowledge, and it was performed according to set rules, which signifies that the procurement and transplantation of the organ were performed legally and thus, cannot be disputed.

The German Medical Association has fulfilled this legal task and has provided a set of guidelines for all procurable and transplantable organs, including the liver, heart, and kidneys. Further details concerning each of these guidelines will not be discussed in detail here. Exemplary are the (general) guidelines for wait lists and organ procurement, especially the guidelines used for liver transplants, which consist of the so-called MELD-Score (Model End-Stage Liver Disease) that requires three lab results (creatinine, bilirubin, and INR) as its defining parameter, and which plays an important role in estimating the severity of the patient's liver disease. It permits the prognosis of whether or not a patient with a specific liver disease will die within a timeframe of 3 months if he does not receive a new organ. A patient's MELD-Score directly determines the urgency of the liver transplant.

16.3 Malpractice and the Possible Legal Consequences

If one keeps in mind that all the patients registered on the wait list for one specific organ are chronically ill—given they are in different stages of their illness—and do not have a chance at survival or more quality of life if they do not receive a new organ, then it becomes clear that it could be tempting for their doctors to make the patient appear to be worse off than he actually is, for example by manipulating the blood test results in the MELD-Score, in order for him to move up on the wait list. This would give the patient a better chance of receiving the organ that he needs in a shorter amount of time than the severity of his illness would normally require. Thus, the doctor would be helping his patient get the replacement organ that he needs even though, if the general guidelines would have been followed, it would have been distributed to another patient, who was thus denied the organ, leading to an increased threat to his health and the risk of him passing away due to an extended waiting period. This type of manipulative behavior by a doctor can also be motivated by factors other than concern for the patient, as well, such as keeping one's job by demonstrating a high number of cases or also personal entitlement.

The transplantation law has certain penal provisions for deliberate and negligent violations against adhering to the prerequisites for the retrieval of organs from both living and deceased donors (§ 19 Paragraph 1 and 2 TPG) and punishes organ trafficking by law (§§ 17, 18 TPG).[6] However, there are no standardized legal consequences for intentionally defying the allocation rules and thus, also the organ procurement and transplantation guidelines nor for manipulating the required results necessary for allocation. One can only speculate about the possible reasons for this. Perhaps, before these accusations were made public, it never occurred to the responsible parties in some, admittedly few, of the transplantation centers, which also includes lawmakers and medical boards, that this type of scenario would ever happen. If this is the case, then they, unfortunately, were wrong.

Nevertheless, this type of misconduct generally cannot go unpunished. Common law applies even within the field of transplantation medicine including, for example the German Civil Code (German: Bürgerliches Gesetzbuch (BGB)) and its laws governing compensation for damages (§§ 823 ff. BGB), as well as the penal code (German: Strafgesetzbuch (StGB)) and its elements of offense.[7] According to the elements of offense in §§ 211, 212 StGB a person will be punished if he (deliberately) kills another person. However, the law does not dictate *how* the offense has to occur or *what* counts as a kill operation in order to prosecute someone on account of predetermined, deliberate murder. Put simply, the death of one person must be directly attributable to the behavior or action by another person.

This type of behavior, which puts the other patients on the wait list at a definite disadvantage, can be seen for example in a patient's higher MELD-Score achieved by manipulating the relevant lab results or by stretching the truth and stating that the patient has received multiple dialyses. This type of behavior, which leads to the allocation of an organ to this particular patient due to his high MELD-Score, has the consequence that at least one of the other patients that actually ranked higher on the wait list and who normally would have received this organ, is exposed to a higher risk of death and may possibly die before receiving an organ, which was given to someone else. Even the question of cause and effect, or rather the question of whether the manipulation of the test results was responsible for the death of the patient, can only truly be answered in very few cases. However, the charge of attempted murder would be feasible if were able to prove if and how many patients ranked higher on the wait list than the patient who was favorably treated (using an anonymized wait list). The manipulating doctor, having ample experience in the field of transplantation medicine, knows that higher-ranking patients with a high MELD-Score are at risk of death and could die because they did not receive the available organ. These doctors know this and *accept it as fact*, which is why lawmakers have proscribed this type of deliberate behavior in the willful intent section

[6] Schroth in Roxin and Schroth (2010, p. 444, 462 ff.); Oglakcioglu (2012 (8), pp. 381–388).

[7] Kudlich NJW (2013 (13), pp. 917–920).

of the law. It does not matter to him that another patient (whom he does not know) will die as a result of his actions. In German law, this counts as contingent deliberate murder. The doctor knew and decided in favor of his own patient, despite knowing that another person, who would have received the organ had it not been for his manipulation of the lab results and whose identity he does not need to know, will die as a result.

In addition to the legal consequences that result from this type of malpractice, the question also remains whether the doctor, who consciously manipulated the required results for the procurement of the organ in his patient's favor, should have to face job-related consequences as well, prior even to the legal consequences. It should also be questioned whether the hospital in which this doctor was able to go about his work without being checked on or supervised, should also be held accountable and reminded of its responsibilities in conforming to the rules concerning the overall organization and process of organ transplantation. These decisions are to be made by the German Medical Association and the respective Ministry of State.

16.4 Organizational and Structural Measures

Lastly, all responsible parties must make it a priority to resolve the issue of what we can or must do in order to avoid these types of incidents from occurring in the future and to ensure a warrantable transplantation system, which is fair and which gives every patient an equal opportunity at life. In my opinion, this should include regular as well as sporadic inspections of the transplantation centers. The motto here should be: Trust, but verify.

This has been the credo followed by lawmakers in the past, as well, and has thus given the German Medical Association, amongst others, the obligation of taking on the task of supervision and control (§ 11 Paragraph 3 TPG and § 12 Paragraph 5 TPG), which has been implemented in the form of an Assessment and Supervisory Commission that has recently, due to the current incidents, been reinforced by special investigators. The coordinating center (German Organ Transplantation Foundation), as well as the procurement organization (Eurotransplant), and all of the transplantation centers in Germany are inspected and assessed on a regular basis. The inspection of the transplantation centers has been intensified, due to recent irregularities with liver transplantations that have been made public. Since the summer of 2012, the visits and inspections at each individual center have focused on the liver transplantation program. Once these assessments have been completed, the transplantation programs for all procurable organs and the execution of these programs in each transplantation center will also be systematically reviewed.

After noticing that the general hospital hierarchy, as well as other structural aspects within individual transplantation centers, can obstruct the level of transparency of the procedures of organ transplantations, the German Medical Association together with health insurance providers and the hospitals' medical boards decided to implement the independent *Confidential Counseling Committee for transplantation medicine* in November 2012. This committee serves as contact point for reporting situations, either personally or also anonymously, of suspected manipulative behavior. It can also be consulted to report actual or alleged grievances that have to do with organ transplantations. This gives doctors, caregivers, and the entire hospital staff in general the opportunity to reveal and discuss internal knowledge of irregularities for the benefit of the patients and without having to fear for one's job or position in the hospital and one's future career.

Additionally, the committee should give patients, patients' relatives, as well as the general public the opportunity to file personal complaints or to ask questions and receive competent answers, regardless of whether these questions pertain to past transplantations or those which are about to be done or questions on transplantation medicine in general. The committee for transplantation medicine has only been around for a short time, but it has received a generally positive response. During the first 6 months, the committee received over 90 inquiries, complaints, and notifications, which were all individually processed and answered or forwarded to respective experts on the matter, who proceeded to provide answers. In addition, several (anonymous) notifications containing supplementary information led to the re-inspection of a couple of centers or rather certain departments in some of these centers, and their review was deemed incomplete until this inspection was finished.

Hopefully, these measures, combined with an improvement in the general organization of transplantation procedures in hospitals, will contribute to a stronger trust in transplantation medicine by the general public and help facilitate the willingness to donate one's organs.

References

Kudlich, H. 2013. Die strafrechtliche Aufarbeitung des „Organspende-Skandals". *NJW (Neue Juristische Wochenschrift)* 13: 917–920.

Oglakcioglu, M. T. 2012. Aus aktuellem Anlass: Zum strafbaren Handeltreiben mit Organen gemäß §§ 17, 18 TPG, 381–388. In http://www.strafrecht.de/hrr/archiv/12-08/index.php?sz=11.

Schroth, U. 2010. Die postmortale Organ- und Gewebespende. In *Handbuch des Medizinstrafrechts*, eds. C. Roxin, and U. Schroth, 4th. ed., 444–465. Stuttgart: Boorberg.

German Laws

German law on organ donation, retrieval, and transfer (German Transplantation Law = TPG), Federal Law Gazette (BGBl). 1997. I , 2163–2639.

German law regulating the decision-making process and solution in the transplantation law BGBl. 2012. I, 1504–1506.

Insert Author Biography

Ruth Rissing-van Saan J.D. was Supreme Judge for criminal law at the German Federal Court of Justice. After retiring in 2011, she took on a teaching position for criminal law and criminal proceedings at the Ruhr University in Bochum, Germany. Since November 2012, she has been the Director of the German Medical Association's confidentiality and trust committee for transplantation medicine, which deals with questions and concerns that doctors, as well as patients and their relatives have regarding organ transplantation.

Chapter 17
Legal Justice in Organ Allocation. A Legal Perspective on the Failure of the German Organ Allocation System

Bijan Fateh-Moghadam

17.1 Introduction: Redistributing Survival Chances—The Current Transplantation Scandals

The German organ allocation system is out of joint. In July 2012, the medical community as well as the broader public got alarmed by several high-profile transplantation scandals.[1] Several physicians at different university hospitals have been accused of altering data related to their patients to make them appear sicker than they actually were in order to place them in front of other patients that were on the waiting list for liver donations. In the case of Göttingen University Hospital, a senior transplant surgeon is currently facing a criminal trial on account of manslaughter in eleven cases because of allegedly manipulating liver allocations. The prosecution argues that by unduly privileging his own patients, the physician intentionally accepted that other patients on the waiting list might die, however the prosecution—so far—has not been able to provide evidence that a certain patient actually died *because* of the concrete manipulations in question.[2] Regardless of the outcome of the trial, the transplant scandals have already resulted in a significant decrease in the number of organ donations in Germany.[3] The reported case raises complex questions concerning the doctrine of criminal law in terms of causation, normative imputation and mens rea (intention). It is highly controversial among commentators

[1] Stafford (2013). German transplant group fights to regain public trust. Stafford (2012). Surgeon is accused of manipulating data to move his patients up organ waiting list; initially reported by Berndt (2012).

[2] E.g. the reasoning of a higher regional court upholding an arrest warrant against the accused transplantation surgeon, OLG Braunschweig, Beschl. v. 20.03.2013, Az. Ws 49/03.

[3] DSO (2013).

B. Fateh-Moghadam (✉)
Cluster of Excellence 'Religion and Politics', University of Münster, Münster, Germany
e-mail: bijan.fateh@uni-muenster.de

R. J. Jox et al. (eds.), *Organ Transplantation in Times of Donor Shortage*,
International Library of Ethics, Law, and the New Medicine 59,
DOI 10.1007/978-3-319-16441-0_17

of the science of criminal law whether the physician can actually be convicted of manslaughter or any other criminal offence.[4]

It is not the criminal law, however, which I am going to focus on in this chapter. What is interesting here is the essential normative dimension of organ allocation. Due to recent scandals, the necessity to make tragic choices in the process of priority setting in transplantation medicine becomes central to public awareness: If doctors *arbitrarily redistribute the chances of survival* for patients on the waiting list, this is not only a problem of respecting certain formal administrative regulations, but also a fundamental problem of *justice in public health*. To move certain patients *up* on organ waiting lists means to move other patients *down*, who might be in even greater need of transplantation therapy. At the core of these allegations, there is an injustice that *could* amount to a criminal wrong in terms of manslaughter because it affects the survival chances of patients. This directs attention to the fundamental normative impact of the established German organ allocation system. The problem with the manipulations in question is not that instead of one needy human being, it is just another needy human being that has been provided with a liver. The problem lies in the fact that the passed-over person is the patient who should have *rightfully*—*ipso jure*—had priority. But what is the significance of *rightfully* and *ipso jure* in the context of the German organ allocation system? To blame physicians, who manipulated organ procurement decisions because they allegedly caused injustice to organ allocation, seems to presuppose that the manipulated allocation system itself meets with the basic demands of justice. This brings us back to the overall question of justice in organ allocation.

From a legal point of view, justice has to be measured primarily by the standard of the rule of law and fundamental rights as defined by the German Basic Law (Grundgesetz). This implies that the statutory framework of organ allocation, as well as the professional guidelines for priority setting have to be in accordance with the basic constitutional demands for the procedural and substantial justification of state-determined allocation orders affecting the basic rights of the people. The kind of justice this article deals with is therefore restricted to what Thomas Osterkamp pre-eminently designated as *legal justice* (juristische Gerechtigkeit).[5] I will argue that the statutory and sub-statutory legal framework for organ allocation provided by the German Transplantation Code (Transplantationsgesetz) and the Guidelines of the German Medical Association (Bundesärztekammer) are not in accordance with the rule of law and are therefore unconstitutional.[6]

[4] Kudlich (2013),NJW 66 (13), pp. 917–920; Schroth (2013), NStZ 33 (8), pp. 437–447; Fateh-Moghadam (2015).

[5] Osterkamp (2004).

[6] For a more detailed exposition of the argument see Gutmann and Fateh-Moghadam (2002), NJW 55 (46), pp. 3365–3372; Gutmann and Fateh-Moghadam (2003, pp. 37–114).

17.2 Who Decides? Deficiencies in the Democratic Justification of Organ Allocation Rules

In German constitutional and administrative law, the intricate problem of allocating scarce resources is discussed under the topic of the *administration of a shortage* (*Verwaltung eines Mangels*).[7] The leading case of the German Federal Constitutional Court (Bundesverfassungsgericht) was concerned with a far less dramatic case of shortage administration, namely the allocation of places at universities. In the so-called *numerus clausus-case*, the court emphasizes the significance of the allocation decision for the prospective *life chances* of university applicants.[8] Therefore, the court decided that it is the duty of the parliament to take responsibility for basic normative allocation decisions.[9] To take responsibility for the basic allocation decisions means, as the court substantiates, that parliament itself has to determine "at least the relevant types of eligibility criteria and the hierarchy between them" (BVerfGE 33, 393 (345 f.)).[10] Determination by the legislator means, as follows from the well-established constitutional law doctrine of the *parliamentary clause* (Parlamentsvorbehalt),[11] determination by way of adequately precise statutory legislation. If this is true for parliamentary decisions which affect life chances in terms of the career opportunities of university applicants, it has to be demanded *a fortiori* for the field of organ allocation, which is literally about life chances in terms of survival. The question is whether the German legislature met the constitutional demands of the parliamentary clause with regard to the allocation of organs for transplantation when enacting the German Transplant Code in 1997.

The relevant statutory clause is Sect. 12, paragraph 3, sentence 1 of the German Transplantation Code.[12] According to the law, organs intended for transplantation have to be procured "by rules, which are consistent with the findings of the medical science, particularly by the criteria of prospect of success and exigency." As follows from the explanatory note to the German Transplantation Code, the legislator wanted to state that organ procurement has to be conducted by "medically justified rules" (Bundestagsdrucksache 13/4355: 26).

What is primarily problematic about this formulation is that it denies the normative nature of allocation decisions in transplantation medicine. The science of medicine is neither qualified nor legitimized to generate normative rules for the prioritization in organ allocation. It is only able to *translate* normative allocation

[7] Badura (1996, pp. 529–543).

[8] BVerfGE 33, 303 (345 f.).

[9] BVerfGE 33, 303 (346).

[10] The Parliament may delegate the power to enact concrete regulations for the allocation process to the universities but not its responsibility for the basic normative decisions.

[11] BVerfGE 33, 125 (158); 33, 303 (337).

[12] Gesetz über die Spende, Entnahme und Übertragung von Organen und Geweben (Transplantationsgesetz – TPG) v. 5. November 1997 in der Fassung der Bekanntmachung vom 4. September 2007 (BGBl. I S. 2206), das durch Artikel 5d des Gesetzes vom 15. Juli 2013 (BGBl. I S. 2423) geändert worden ist.

criteria predetermined by law into medical practice. The science of medicine can specify under which medical circumstances a patient should be declared highly urgent for transplantation. Likewise, the science of medicine and only the science of medicine is qualified to estimate the prospect of success of a certain transplantation therapy for a certain patient. But, what the science of medicine is neither able nor allowed to do is to decide authoritatively whether the exigency and prospect of transplantation outcome are relevant criteria for prioritization and particularly how the criteria of exigency and outcome are related to each other. As the Swiss legislator put it very clearly and in explicit opposition to the German regulatory model: "The thesis, whereas allocation is processed by medical criteria, is insofar wrong: Procurement is carried out on the basis of ethical criteria" (Schweizer Bundesrat 2001, p. 83). That is why Art. 119a paragraph 2 of the Swiss Constitution demands that the criteria for a just organ allocation have to be provided by federal law.

At this point of argumentation a second problem of the cited formulation of the German Transplantation Code in Sect. 12, paragraph 3, sentence 3 has to be addressed. The German Transplantation Code—after all—refers to two criteria, even if this is not supposed to be an exhaustive list, but remains open for further criteria. The two relevant criteria are, as has been mentioned before, prospect of success and exigency. The rather obvious problem with these two criteria is that they are regularly in conflict with each other any time a concrete prioritization decision has to be made; one might even speak of structural contradictory principles, even if there are exceptions.[13] This is particularly true for the case of liver transplantation. Usually this will occur among relatively young patients, who did not wait too long and who are not yet suffering from high co-morbidity, and who are supposed to have the best prospect outcome through transplantation. At the same time, these patients are often times not ill enough to be very urgent cases.[14] Vice versa, liver patients with a high probability to die within the next 3 months without transplantation—this is the perspective of the MELD-Score—are usually very ill. They are often old and suffer from high co-morbidity and other risk factors, so that the prospected success of transplantation—measured in prospected graft survival time—is usually rather low. Of course, there are exceptional cases in which urgency and prospective outcome might run along the same line, like in the case of acute liver failure in a 17 year old patient who ate toxic mushrooms, but this is not a group of patients transplantation centers have to deal with on a daily basis.

The example shows that by establishing the criteria of prospect of success and exigency the German Transplantation Code points out the central conflict of objectives in organ allocation, but fails to even hint at a possible solution. In conclusion, the normative question of how to determine organ procurement decisions is left wide open. The German Transplant Code gives its blessings to a range of possible allocation schemes, even if these schemes are based on normative principles that are basically inconsistent with one another. So, who is it, who *de facto* decides about the normative basis of the process of priority setting in organ allocation and who determines the tangible rules for organ allocation in terms of generally binding law?

[13] Gutmann and Fateh-Moghadam (2003, pp. 46–48).

[14] Dannecker and Streng (2012), JZ 2012, pp. 444–452 (444).

At any rate, as this should have become clear by now, it is not the statutory legislation of the German parliament. This intermediary result alone is enough to conclude that the central statutory norm, which is supposed to determine organ allocation principles is unconstitutional under German basic law, because it does not meet the requirements for creating a democratically legitimized legal framework for the allocation of scarce resources.[15] The constructional flaw of the German Transplantation Code affects the entire German organ allocation system, as can be demonstrated by the example of the guidelines for organ allocation by the German Medical Association, which effectively determine the allocation of organs in Germany today.

17.3 Berlin God Committee: The Guidelines of the German Medical Association

As we have seen, the fundamental conflict of objectives in organ allocation is not solved adequately by the German Transplant Code. The legislature, ignoring constitutional requirements, refused to take responsibility for the inevitable normative allocation decisions. As a consequence, balancing the conflicting criteria of prospect of success and exigency, which means a decision about life and death for certain collectives of patients, is conducted effectively by the *permanent organ transplants commission* of the German Medical Association. The German Transplantation Code, in sentence 16, authorizes the German Medical Association—the exact wording is of special importance here—to determine the state of medical science *for* the rules on organ allocation. The formulation of the statute presupposes that legal rules on organ allocation already exist, which should be operationalized in a way that is consistent with the state of medical science. As this is not the case however,—there simply are no effective legal rules on organ allocation—the German Medical Association decided to take responsibility not only for the scientific task to determine the state of medical science, but also for the fundamental normative task to legislate rules, which determine prioritization in organ allocation in Germany. Notwithstanding the fact that the professional medical association merely closed a fundamental gap of the German Transplant Code, it was neither qualified nor legitimized to do so. The German Medical Association delegated the task of making guidelines for organ allocation to a special body, the permanent commission on organ transplantation, which is not even mentioned by the German Transplant Code.

Against this background, the majority view within German legal science rightly states that the guidelines of the German Medical Association on organ allocation lack democratic legitimacy insofar as they imply normative rules and do not formulate a state of medical science.[16] Moreover, the guideline-making process lacks

[15] Gutmann and Fateh-Moghadam (2002), NJW 55 (46), pp. 3365–3372; Höfling (2007), JZ 62 (10), pp. 481–486 (481); Bader (2010), p. 189 et seq; Dannecker and Streng (2012), JZ 67 (9), pp. 444–452 (445); for a different opinion see: Rosenau (2009), pp. 435–452 (435).

[16] Cf. Gutmann and Fateh-Moghadam (2002), NJW 55 (46), pp. 3365–3372; Höfling (2007), JZ 62 (10), pp. 481–486 (481); Bader (2010, p. 189 et sEq.); Dannecker and Streng (2012), JZ 67 (9),

transparency and is largely uncontrollable. Due to the impossibility to follow the line of normative argumentation of the organ commission, which even denies the normative nature of allocation decisions, the outcome of the guideline-making process appears to be more or less arbitrary.

The arbitrary nature of the current practice can be demonstrated by using the example of the guidelines on liver allocation. Until 2007, these guidelines favored a system primarily orientated at the utilitarian principle of best prospect outcome: two thirds of the livers to be procured were reserved for patients with a low exigency status. In 2007, the guidelines on liver allocation were changed over to the MELD-Score-System, an allocation scheme which clearly gives priority to urgency as the leading determining criteria in liver allocation.[17] In effect, the normative prerequisites of the guidelines on liver allocation—again an issue of life and death—have been reversed to the opposite.

To be sure, there are very good, in my opinion even compelling normative reasons for giving priority to exigency and urgency in liver organ allocation and therefore it was the right thing to introduce the MELD-Score into the German allocation system.[18] It is not the content of the reorganization of the liver organ allocation system in 2007 that is disturbing from an ethical and legal point of view. What is disturbing and basically a declaration of bankruptcy with regard to the effectiveness of the rule of law, is that the normative paradigm change in liver allocation has been heralded by the German Medical Association in the style of an ancient oracle. It does not appear to the public and even to the professional community that there had been any kind of democratically legitimized deliberation of normative reasons that resulted in the new allocation scheme. The normative justification of the MELD-Score system remains fundamentally opaque. This might, incidentally, also be one of the reasons why many transplant physicians do not accept the MELD-Score system as being normatively adequate, as the current transplantation scandals show. Moreover, the recently sparked discussion about a possible reintroduction of outcome-oriented principles in liver allocation reveals that a reversal of the paradigm change might take place in the same autocratic *coup de main*-style that characterizes the history of guideline-making by the German Medical Association.

Summing up, the way in which the German Medical Association legislates normative allocation rules, disguised as the determination of the state of medical science, turns out to be a remainder of what Max Weber called *formally irrational lawmaking* (formell-irrationale Rechtsfindung), a term aiming at the characterization of early forms of law in archaic societies. In the 1960s, it was the arbitrary practice of the so-called *Seattle God Committee*, which initiated the ethical and legal debate about justice in organ failure treatment.[19] Chosen by the local King County Medical Society, seven citizens decided on the allocation of scarce dialysis units to renal patients on the basis of self-defined criteria for prioritization. The *Seattle God*

---

pp. 444–452 (445); for a different opinion see: Rosenau (2009, pp. 435–452 (435)).

[17] For more details see Dannecker and Streng (2012), JZ 67 (9), pp. 444–452 (444).

[18] For substantial critisism however cf. Dannecker and Streng (2012), JZ 67 (9), pp. 444–452.

[19] Rothman (1991, pp. 150).

Committee had to be abandoned after critical public debate on discrimination and justice in public health. As David J. Rothman summarizes in his classic study on the history of bioethics and medical law: "Thus the Seattle experiment taught a second lesson: committees, whatever their makeup, would not necessarily resolve difficult choices. One might well need to construct principles or guidelines to make certain that medical decision making represented more than the accumulated prejudices of a handful of people, whether their training was medical or not" (Rothman 1991, p. 152). Today it is common ground in medical ethics, as well as in medical law that resource allocation is primarily not about *medical* decision making at all, but a *normative* task, which needs legal rules and guidelines provided by democratically legitimized institutions outside of the medical community.

A further formal constitutional problem, which I do not want to elaborate on here, is the assignment of the Eurotransplant International Foundation, which does not meet the constitutional demands for the transfer of sovereign power to private foreign institutions.[20] The central organ procurement institution in the German organ allocation system therefore lacks legitimacy, as well.

17.4 Substantial Justice in Organ Allocation: Constitutional Requirements and Current Practice

The starting point for any substantial regulation of organ allocation is the constitutional presetting that all patients who—from a strictly medical point of view—are in need of an organ have a right to equal access to the available transplantation capacities. Against the background of organ scarcity, this right is not a right to an organ but a right to equality of opportunity with regard to the chance of getting an organ—it is a basic right to *participate* in the organ allocation process based on the principle of equality of opportunity. The constitutional basis for this right to participate are the basic rights to life and bodily integrity (Art. 2 paragraph 2 sentence 1 of the German Grundgesetz), the basic right to equality (Art. 3 paragraph 1 of the German Grundgesetz), and the constitutional principles of the social state and the rule of law following Art. 20 of the German Grundgesetz.[21] As tragic allocation decisions remain inevitable, however, it is necessary to determine adequate or at least acceptable criteria for prioritization under the rule of law.

With regard to the determination of criteria for prioritization, it is vital to recognize that the right to equality of opportunity has to be provided with due respect to the *specific* basic right, which is affected by the priority setting procedure. The quality of a university entrance diploma, to give a simple example, might be a realistic criterion for the selection of university applicants because the selection *only* affects the basic right of a freedom to choose an education granted by Art. 12 of the

[20] Höfling (2007), JZ 62 (10), pp. 481–486 (481).

[21] The structure of the right to participate is developed at length in: Gutmann and Fateh-Moghadam (2003, pp. 60–70); Affirmative: Schulze-Fielitz (2013) Commentary on Art. 2 II.

German Grundgesetz. It is, however, obviously not an adequate criterion for organ allocation in transplant medicine. Organ allocation affects the fundamental right to life and bodily integrity, which is designed as a particularly egalitarian basic right.[22] Not least by learning a lesson from the German history of medicine, where certain groups of particularly vulnerable patients had been labeled as "life-unworthy life" by the Nazi "euthanasia" programs, today the principle of equality of human life, also denoted as indifference with regard to the worth of life (*Lebenswertindifferenz*), is acknowledged as a fundamental element of human dignity (Art. 1 of the German Grundgesetz).[23]

The principle of equality of human life leads to the fact that some of the criteria for prioritization in transplantation medicine, which are discussed in medical ethics, are precluded for constitutional reasons. Absolutely excluded criteria are, inter alia, age, gender, race, social reservations including the willingness to donate organs (reciprocity), actual fault (for example in cases of alcohol abuse). Moreover, the egalitarian nature of the right to life excludes the utilitarian criterion of the prospect transplantation outcome in terms of an inter-personal equation of benefits with the aim to maximize the aggregated benefit of the entire collective of patients (or at least of the transplantation center in question). To deprive patient X from organ transplantation therapy because the prospected statistical graft-survival time is 2 years longer if the available organ is allocated to patient Y violates patient X's right to equal respect of his health interests. Transplantation therapy is no less important to patient X than it is to patient Y, if you take on the view of the individual patient: Most likely it is a question of life and death for both patients and two gained years are not of lesser worth to patient X than four gained years are to patient Y. That is why an inter-personal equation of prospected transplantation outcomes is unacceptable under the rule of the equality of human life. The latter consequence is, however, highly controversial among commentators in medical ethics and medical law and needs further elaboration than can be provided in this chapter.[24]

Until now we have discussed criteria that are forbidden for constitutional reasons because they amount to an undue discrimination of patients. The Constitution, on the other hand, also demands at least one substantial criterion for prioritization to be included in the process of priority setting, namely exigency in terms of the priority of highly urgent patients, who might not survive a longer waiting time. High urgency always advances prospect outcome. In addition to the criterion of urgency the constitutional framework does not demand, but at least it accepts strictly egalitarian criteria for prioritization such as waiting time or lottery, which are forms of priority setting without referring to personal characteristics of the patient and therefore are compatible with the principle of equality.

Finally, under the rule of law certain conditions concerning the practical setting of the allocation procedure have to be taken into consideration. From the basic right to participate in the organ allocation process as outlined above follows firstly, that

[22] BVerfGE 39, 1 (59).

[23] See Gutmann and Fateh-Moghadam (2003, pp. 78–81 with further references).

[24] For an elaborate defence of the prospect of success-criterion see Dannecker and Streng (2012), JZ67 (9), pp. 444–452.

organs have to be procured to individual patients and not to transplant centers (patient orientation against transplant center orientation in organ allocation). Secondly, patient-oriented organ allocation demands that there is a single standard waiting list, which includes all patients who are in need of an organ. Thirdly, the terms which regulate access to the standard waiting list have to be based on strictly medical criteria, indifferent to the problem of rationing. The basic right to equal participation at the available pool of organs is activated invariably when transplantation therapy is medically indicated for the individual patient, regardless of the problem of scarce resources. From this follows a subjective legal right—enforceable by law—to access the waiting list for all patients with a medical indication for transplantation therapy. The waiting list is the gate all patients in need have to pass, to even take part in the process of priority setting. That is why the terms that regulate access to the waiting list must not be abused for anticipated and hidden rationing decisions.

In the German allocation practice, the guidelines of the German Medical Association concerning access to waiting lists are at least partly misused as instruments of discrimination, which operate under the mask of alleged medical contraindications. A particularly prominent example is the absolute exclusion of patients suffering from alcoholic liver disease, if they are not able to prove a period of at least 6 months of complete alcohol abstinence prior to transplantation, as demanded by the guidelines of the German Medical Association.[25] Due to the international state of medical science, there is no medical justification for an invariable period of alcohol abstinence. As a study of the European Association for the Study of the Liver states, "[…] graft and patient survival rates among alcoholics after LT are similar to those seen after transplantation for other aetiologies of liver disease" (European Association for the Study of the Liver 2012, p. 413). It is not even "proven that a set period of 6 months' abstinence prior to transplantation can modify the results" (Pageaux et al. 2009). But even if this would be the case, a modification of the prospected outcome from a legal point of view could be considered—if ever—only by way of benefit-oriented criteria in the process of prioritization, but not as a reason to (literally) terminally exclude patients from this process.[26] A former chairman of the organ transplantation commission of the German Medical Association stated rather bluntly, that the abstinence rule aims at "showing patients quite plainly that they are responsible for a long-term success of the transplantation" (Schreiber and Haverich 2000). The statement reveals that the abstinence guidelines' rationale is educational—not medical. The abstinence guideline therefore amounts to an *ultra vires* action of the German Medical Association that is clearly contrary to the law. Moreover, it misjudges from a medical point of view, as Pageaux et al. rightly stated, that "transplantation is the treatment for the liver disease, not a treatment for alcoholism" (Pageaux et al. 2009). From a legal point of view, on the other hand, there is no such thing as the legal responsibility of the patient for *long-term* transplantation success, which could be turned against the patient by way of mandatory abstinence

[25] Cf. Bundesärztekammer (2013) Richtlinien zur Organtransplantation gem. § 16 Abs. 1 S. 1 Nr. 2 und 5 TPG (Besonderer Teil Leber), p. 12, para 2.1. Alkoholinduzierte Zirrhose.

[26] Cf. Gutmann (2008, pp 113–135 (128)); Dannecker and Streng (2012), JZ 67 (9), pp. 444–452 (451); Schroth (2013), NStZ 33 (8), pp. 437–447 (441).

periods or the opaque criterion of *compliance*.[27] Insofar as the mandatory and invariable abstinence clause precludes even highly urgent patients with alcoholic liver disease from getting access to the waiting list,[28] the guideline is an unlawful attack on the life of these patients, who therefore are entitled to a *right to lie*, if this is the only way to enforce their legal right to access the waiting list. This brings us back to the current transplantation scandal at Göttingen University Hospital. One of two main accusations, which built the basis of an arrest warrant, consists in the case that the transplant surgeon allegedly registered patients with alcoholic liver disease to the waiting list, contravening the six month abstinence guideline of the German Medical Association. From the argumentation above, it can be concluded that the transplantation surgeon might possibly have made a lot of mistakes, but that he did not accept the abstinence guideline is clearly not one of them. The accusation against the surgeon is—at least in this point—fundamentally flawed. The example shows again that there is a strong interdependency between the validity of allegations concerning the injustice of manipulations of the organ allocation system and the lawfulness of the manipulated system itself.

Another problem with legal justice in organ allocation is the establishment of special allocation procedure programs by Eurotransplant and the German Medical Association. Sound medical reasons might exist which justify the establishment of a *Eurotransplant Senior Program* in Kidney allocation (formerly known as *Old-to-Old-Allocation*) and also for the so-called *rescue allocation-procedure*.[29] However, both lack a legal basis in the German Transplant Code. As the public criticism of the extensive use of rescue allocation instead of standard allocation shows, the introduction of legally un-controlled special procedures threatens to violate the principle of patient orientation in organ allocation and the legal requirement of a single standard waiting list.

17.5 Regulated Self-Regulation Versus State Control and Legal Protection

The deficiencies in the legitimacy of the German organ allocation system are exacerbated by the fact that there is virtually no form of state control and supervision over the whole organ procurement process and at the same time effective legal protection is hindered systematically. This is particularly true for the guidelines of the German

---

[27] The German Federal Constitutional Court expressed severe doubts about the legality of the compliance criterion and the legitimacy of the guidelines of the German Medical Association. Cf. BVerfG (2013) v. 28 Jan 2013, Az. 1 BvR 274/12, para 17. http://www.bverfg.de/entscheidungen/rk20130128_1bvr027412.html.

[28] Patients whose hepatitis is not responding to medical therapy are supposed to have a 6 month survival rate of approximately 30 % (Mathurin et al (2011). Early liver transplantation for severe alcoholic hepatitis. New England Journal of Medicine 365(19), pp. 1790–800; for an instructive case report and a summary of the international medical discussion see Umgelter (2013).

[29] For an explanation of the procedure of rescue allocation see Schroth (2013), NStZ 33 (8), pp. 437–447 (439).

Medical Association. There are no statutory rules on the composition of the organ transplant commission, which prepares the guidelines, and there is also no legally defined procedure for the determination of guidelines. Until recently, there was no form of state control on the work of this professional body at all. Since the summer of 2013, the guidelines have to be at least approved by the minister of health, but—due to the indeterminacy of the German Transplant Code—it remains unclear what the legal standard for a serious review by the state authority is. Moreover, the un-transparency of the meshwork of statutory and sub-statutory regulations and guidelines on organ allocation makes it virtually impossible for patients to get legal protection against decisions made by transplantation bureaucracy. Legal experts agree that under the current legal framework nobody knows exactly how to give legal advice to a patient who has been unlawfully barred from access to a waiting list, who has been placed wrongly or who doubts the legitimacy of a certain guideline of the German Medical Association.[30]

17.6 Conclusion

The legal perspective on the current operating system of prioritization in organ allocation revealed several unsolved normative problems. The regulatory framework of organ allocation in Germany is neither compatible with the formal nor with the substantial constitutional requirements for a state organized allocation order, which directly affects the most fundamental rights of patients. There seems to be a lack of political willingness to take responsibility for the basic normative decisions in the process of priority setting in organ allocation, a process that inevitably forces one to make tragic choices. The determination of general binding rules for organ allocation is not a task for the professional self-management of physicians as the current organ procurement practice seems to imply. In fact, it is the responsibility of the legislator and the public health administration, operating within the regulatory framework of the German Grundgesetz. The political failure to take on this responsibility is also one of the reasons why it is difficult to call doctors into account for arbitrarily intervening into an allocation system which fundamentally lacks legitimacy. As long as the normative nature of prioritization decisions is denied and standard criteria for organ allocation are persistently veiled as medical criteria, it will remain illusory to speak of *justice* within organ allocation.

References

Bader, M. 2010. *Organmangel und Organverteilung*. Tübingen: Mohr Siebeck.

Badura, P. 1996. Verteilungsordnung und Zuteilungsverfahren bei der Bewirtschaftung knapper Güter durch die Verwaltung. In *Staat. Wirtschaft. Steuern. Festschrift für Karl Heinrich Friauf*, eds. R. Wendt, W. Höfling, U. Karpen, et al. Heidelberg: C.F. Müller.

[30] Cf. Höfling (2007), JZ 62 (10), pp. 481–486 (482); Gutmann (2008, pp. 113–135).

Berndt, C. 2012. Leber im Angebot. www.sueddeutsche.de/gesundheit/transplantations-skandal-an-goettinger-uni-klinikum-leber-im-angebot-1.1417466. Accessed 25 Sept 2013.

Bundesärztekammer. 2013. Richtlinien zur Organtransplantation gem. § 16 Abs. 1 S. 1 Nr. 2 und 5 TPG (Besonderer Teil Leber), p. 12, para 2.1. Alkoholinduzierte Zirrhose. http://www.bundesaerztekammer.de/downloads/RiliOrgaLeber20130308.pdf. Accessed 25 Sept 2013.

Dannecker, G., and A. F. Streng. 2012. Rechtliche Möglichkeiten und Grenzen einer an den Erfolgsaussichten der Transplantation orientierten Organallokation *JZ* 67: 444–452. (444)

DSO. 2013. Zahl der Organspenden in 2012 dramatisch gesunken. http://www.dso.de/dso-pressemitteilungen/einzelansicht/article/zahl-der-organspenden-in-2012-dramatisch-gesunken-1.html. Accessed 25 Sept 2013.

European Association for the Study of the Liver. 2012. EASL clinical practical guidelines: Management of alcoholic liver disease. *Journal of Hepatology* 57: 399–420. (413)

Fateh-Moghadam, B. 2015. Strafrechtliche Risiken der Organtransplantation. In *Strafrecht der Medizin. Handbuch für Wissenschaft und Praxis*, eds. F. Saliger, and M. Tsambikakis. München: C.H. Beck. [forthcoming]

Gutmann, T. 2008. Allokationsfragen: Aporien und Zweifelsfragen des geltenden Rechts. In: *Die Regulierung der Transplantationsmedizin in Deutschland: Eine kritische Bestandsaufnahme nach 10 Jahren Transplantationsgesetz,* ed. W. Höfling, 113–135. Tübingen: Mohr Siebeck.

Gutmann, T., and B. Fateh-Moghadam. 2002. Rechtsfragen der Organverteilung. Das Transplantationsgesetz, die "Richtlinien" der Bundesärztekammer und die Empfehlungen der Deutschen Gesellschaft für Medizinrecht. *NJW* 55(46): 3365–3372.

Gutmann, T., B. Fateh-Moghadam. 2003. Rechtsfragen der Organverteilung. In *Grundlagen einer gerechten Organverteilung*: eds. T. Gutmann, K. Schneewind, and U. Schroth. Heidelberg: Springer.

Höfling, W. 2007. Verteilungsgerechtigkeit in der Transplantationsmedizin? *JZ* 62 (10): 481–486. (481)

Kudlich, H. 2013. Die strafrechtliche Aufarbeitung des "Organspende-Skandals". NJW 66 (13): 917–920.

Mathurin, P., C. Moreno, D. Samuel, et al. 2011. Early liver transplantation for severe alcoholic hepatitis. *New England Journal of Medicine* 365 (19): 1790–800.

Osterkamp, T. 2004. *Juristische Gerechtigkeit. Rechtswissenschaft jenseits von Positivismus und Naturrecht.* Tübingen: Mohr Siebeck.

Pageaux, G.P., S. Faure, F. Chermak, et al. 2009. Liver transplantation in a patient with alcoholic cirrhosis: discussion about non-abstinence. [French] Gastroenterologie Clinique et Biologique. 33(10–11 Suppl):F44–9, 2009 Oct. [Case Reports. English Abstract. Journal Article] UI:19747790. Cited from MedLine.

Rosenau, H. 2009. Die Setzung von Standards in der Transplantation: Aufgabe und Legitimation der Bundesärztekammer. In *Medizin und Haftung. Festschrift für Erwin Deutsch zum 80. Geburtstag*, eds. H.J. Ahrens, von C. Bar, G. Fischer, A. Spickhoff et al. Heidelberg: Springer.

Rothman, D. J. 1991. *Strangers at the bedside. A History of how law and bioethics transformed medical decision making*. New York: BasicBooks.

Schreiber, H.L., A. Haverich. 2000. Richtlinien für die Warteliste und für die Organvermittlung. *Dtsch Arztebl* 97 (7): A-385/ B-309/ C-289. (commenting on an earlier version of the guidelines.)

Schroth, U. 2013. Die strafrechtliche Beurteilung der Manipulation bei der Leberallokation. *NStZ* 33 (8): 437–447.

Schulze-Fielitz, H. 2013. Commentary on Art. 2 II. In *Grundgesetz-Kommentar*, ed. H. Dreier, 3rd ed. Band 1 Art. 1–19. Tübingen: Mohr Siebeck. (para 1–120 (para 96).)

Schweizer Bundesrat. 2001. Botschaft zum Bundesgesetz über die Transplantation von Organen, Geweben und Zellen (Transplantationsgesetz), p. 83. http://www.admin.ch/opc/de/federal-gazette/2002/29.pdf. Accessed 25 Sept 2013.

Stafford, N. 2012. Surgeon is accused of manipulating data to move his patients up organ waiting list. *BMJ* 345:e5039. doi:10.1136/bmj.e5039.

Stafford, N. 2013. German transplant group fights to regain public trust. *BMJ* 346:f2768. doi:10.1136/bmj.f2768.

Umgelter, A. 2013. Hilfe als Regelverstoß. taz.de (03 April 2013). http://www.taz.de/!113938/. Accessed 25 Sept 2013.

PD Dr. Bijan Fateh-Moghadam is a postdoctoral researcher at the Cluster of Excellence "Religion & Politics" at the University of Münster (sub-project: The religious and ethical neutrality of criminal law). He is also an associate research fellow at the Center for Advanced Studies in Bioethics (Kollegforschergruppe: Normenbegründung in Medizinethik und Biopolitik). Dr. Fateh-Moghadam teaches Medical Criminal Law and Sociology of Law at the University of Münster. His research interests lie at the intersection of comparative criminal law, medical and life-sciences law, sociology of law and legal philosophy.

Chapter 18
In Whose Best Interest? Questions Concerning the Weal and Woe of Transplant Patients

Sibylle Storkebaum

It has become a daily ritual that the topic of organ transplantation shows up in the media. Whether it's the falsely named *organ donation scandal* (it does not concern organ donation, but rather patient selection and procurement), the surveys on the Germans' willingness to donate (everyone approves it, but few actually possess a donor card), or personal stories about happy parents and their terminally ill children whose lives were saved because they received new lungs or a new heart—the touching story of recipient and donor. There are *no* TV-series, *no* mystery series, *no* talk shows that, although in different forms, do not take advantage of the striking drama that these people, who are confronted with life-or-death situations, undergo, as well as the alleged potential temptations that doctors may experience.

What is happening here? Why does this subject matter receive so much attention given that only 1046 transplants took place in 2012? As a comparison, there are approximately 140,000 men and women annually that receive a knee implant. Is this tiny surgical field really curatively significant enough or lucrative enough to make it sufficiently fascinating for the general public to generate attention, criticism, and slight feelings of horror? Consequently, this specialized and highly invasive sector of modern medicine is trivialized through unrelenting bluntness and the inclusion of all-too-human frivolity to ornament the headlines of the local news. Supposedly, with the intention of cleansing one's archaic fear? As purgatory for something that many people still, after all this time, consider to be the devil's work? It might even be in the physicians' interest, and may perhaps be sponsored by the respective foundations, whose cry for more donor organs continues to become louder and that let politicians and health insurance providers publicly advertise for it? Are the good Samaritan image and the money saved the rewards? Yet, for many years, they have all ignored the urgent necessity for transparency. There are far too many questions

S. Storkebaum (✉)
Ludwig-Maximilians-Universität, Transplantationszentrum Großhadern, Munich, Germany
e-mail: s.storkebaum@googlemail.com

R. J. Jox et al. (eds.), *Organ Transplantation in Times of Donor Shortage*,
International Library of Ethics, Law, and the New Medicine 59,
DOI 10.1007/978-3-319-16441-0_18

that still need to be answered before adequate trust can be restored in transplantation medicine.

Who gives the government the right to claim organ donations from its citizens, to proclaim a *social responsibility for organs*? Does something have to be done more frequently just because it is possible to do it? Even the Churches are relatively clear on that and require organ donations. However, they should ask their believers whether organ donation is an imperative act of altruism. Love thy neighbor as yourself: If you love yourself, you should not feel carelessly obliged to care for others in that this type of gift can only be given—and accepted—completely voluntarily and after cautious consideration. This holds true for both living donations as well as post-mortem donations.

What does voluntariness mean in this context? Who knows what kind of physical and psychological complications might await him? Voluntariness requires complete clarification, which would theoretically be possible for the most part, but which cannot be achieved given current conditions in hospitals and which is further distorted by the superficial and not very effective advertisements and public information by the German Organ Transplantation Foundation and the Federal Center for Health Education.

The result is obvious. As soon as the headlines read bad news from the transplantation medicine, the number of donors decreases. A case in point was when a surgeon from Essen, Christoph Broelsch, engrafted organs to patients prematurely, before they had reached the top of the waiting list. They had contributed to his research ambitions. Currently this may have occurred because some hospitals tend to follow the request by their well-staffed board of directors, which may be allured by bonuses to work profitably by implementing diverse modifications in the workflow. Worshipping the golden calf has never been good for humankind.

For many people, the most pressing question concerns the waiting list. Patients, and their relatives even more so, and the general public consider these waiting lists to have a strict sequential structure that needs to be worked off from top to bottom. This is not the case and can never be the case because it contradicts the essence of medical care. Some of the diseases and conditions that call for transplantation as the last therapeutic option tend to worsen quickly. The doctor has to act responsibly and be flexible with his decisions. This seems to be perfect, but remains ambivalent. German courts like the one in Göttingen are called to decide whether illegitimetely prioritizing someone on the waiting list may even constitute a criminal offence up to manslaughter. It is no coincidence that Eurotransplant and other organizations are constantly working on developing fair distribution and procurement criteria. The German Medical Association's permanent working group on organ transplantation continuously issues new additions and omissions, which are currently being discussed once again.

For quite some time, I have not only argued for the principle of voluntary consent, but also the principle that the person who gains the most from transplantation should be favored. Young individuals who have a future, who have attainable goals in life, who have young children, and who show strength should get bonus points. That is the opinion that I support with conviction, even as an elderly individual.

Speaking of age, age was the topic of some of the most frequently asked questions. The older the transplantation physician, the older the acceptable donor tends to be, shows a survey. In the old-for-old program, that procures organs from old donors for old recipients, even an 80-year old donor was deemed acceptable. However, studies show that for example, a heart that has been beating for over 50 years cannot provide the long-term performance that the patient may want. Hospitals may benefit from this practice, but not the patients. Think about the saints Cosmas and Damian in the 3rd century, who are said to have discovered transplantation when they surgically attached the leg from a deceased colored man onto the body of a Roman soldier. It is not without reason that they are the patron saints of doctors, pharmacists, as well as hairdressers, confectioners, and the sick! The Lord had to send them a reconciliation angel later on, because Cosmas resented that his brother Damian accepted an apple from a grateful patient. The two of them had earlier agreed not to accept any payment for their services; they did not want to accept material reward for their cures and treatments.

Ever since Christiaan Barnard, that ideal has become an issue of the past. In my opinion, change has taken place in the past years that has not been for the good of the patient, as we have recently seen in the German cities Göttingen, Regensburg, and Munich (Hospital Rechts der Isar). A new generation of doctors is taking over the hospitals, straight-A students, who probably became doctors or rather medical managers for the purpose of effective profit maximization, not charitable reasons. Apologizing for my generalized prejudice, I must point out that fortunately enough for the patients there are of course also other types of doctors:the type of doctor who is not afraid to use his medical know-how to overrule guidelines or who denounces deficits by going to the authorities, which his own boss accepts and tolerates, but has not asked him for.

Surgeons, anesthesists, or internists who work in the field of transplantation are often versatile and highly competent. These doctors conduct research, teach and are bound by the structures within this niche of high-tech medicine, obliged to document everything and supervised by appointed commissions. They are on duty day and night, they suffer together with their patients, and their natural instinct of self-preservation makes them distance themselves from their own emotions. They portray precisely what goes on in the general field of medicine and the subject matter that is finally being criticized widely. Doctors and hospitals should work in the best interest of the patients. For their very challenging job they should be paid well and receive long-term contracts that provide them with job security and allow them to plan for the future. The most modern technology should be made available to them, but there should also be enough doctors employed to actually allow them enough time to sit and talk with their patients.

Hospitals that are in close proximity to supportive, encouraging relatives are certainly in the best interest of the patient. The transplantation branch of medicine relies on specific competencies, which necessitate different conditions. I am convinced that a reduction and centralization of transplant centers would be in the patients' best interest. It used to be the case that health insurance providers would pay for the relatives' travel expenses. Why is this not the case anymore?

Given the current demand, it is understandable that there is a call for organ donors, but it makes one hesitant when you hear patients talk about the care provided during the long waiting period and even more so concerning follow-up care. There is a decreasing number of experienced employees that have to treat and manage an increasing number of patients, so apparently those in charge consider it logical to make cuts in a medical field that is currently booming. The field of transplantation, however, is very sensitive and needs the *human factor* more than many other fields of medicine—what kind of cynicism does that entail, *human factor*! And here is another ambivalence: Why is there such a drastic increase in the demand for organs? Is it the hospitals' greed that makes them aim to perform a large number of transplantations or is it the pharmaceutical companies striving to make profit? Has death been permanently disposed of? Do people get talked into getting transplants that they actually do not want, just because they are afraid of saying no to the caring man in the white lab coat and their encouraging, loving relatives?

To conclude my point, I have to pose another few urgent questions: What is the most recent development on replacing the brain death criterion with the even more questionable non-heart-beating donor? Who supervises the ethical and humanitarian criteria of the immensely flourishing assist device business instead of heart transplantation? Why is there an increase among living split liver donors when there is a lack of demand for deceased liver donors? And why do in many transplant centers surveys replace consultants, spiritual care providers or psychological assistants?

I would like to clarify my stance on the subject: I am not opposed to transplantation medicine. I have voluntarily chosen to work as a psychologist in transplantation medicine over the past two decades and have tried to use my knowledge and my strength to fight for more humanity in a branch of medicine where people still experience real miracles, which a lot of them view as something divine and sacred. I can spend hours telling true stories about feelings of guilt, remorse, and traumatization. I can also tell hundreds of true stories about heartiness, a mutual improvement of quality of life, or a slight sense of finding meaning in situations where individuals have had to face a premature death. I have spent many days and nights together with transplantation patients and their families and experienced the overwhelming joy, the unbelievable bliss, and the awestruck amazement after a successful transplant, as well as the doubts, fears, and the deep grief that was felt when death, which had been sitting by the bedside all along, found its way even after the doctors did everything in their power to stop it. I shared the feelings of horror, anger, and bewilderment with doctors and nurses and yet, like all of them, I was able to gather enough courage to go to the next patient with a smile on my face, ready to intervene once again, and to motivate him or her to fight. I went to preparatory conversations to encourage patients even though my heart was bleeding and my mind full of reproach. I remained loyal to my patients and their relatives by telling them exactly what the interdisciplinary committee of doctors decided, even though I sometimes disagreed with their decision. I did respect that terminally ill patients, after a profound process of medical and psychological information, decided to go for the transplantation even if I have suggested that they decide against it. This is the psychological consultants' duty: to help his or her patient make a decision that is in their subjective best interest. May the most recent incidents lead to more transparency and have repercussions in all fields of medicine! Perhaps society can still adapt—to act in the best interest of those who are weak and sick and to support them, which really is a true act of altruism, if not a statute of a civil society.

Sibylle Storkebaum has specialized in the treatment of transplant patients. For 20 years, she was the responsible consultant of the Psychosomatic Clinic Rechts der Isar, Technical University Munich, where she still heads the ethical commission for living donation, and sees heart transplant patients, their families and medical teams at Clinic Großhadern, Ludwig-Maximilians-University Munich. The former political journalist is a member of the Academy for Ethics of Medicine and curator of the Evangelische Stadtakademie München. She is a loyal, but critical member of the German Transplantation Society and founder of the psychosomatic work group.

Part III
Alternative Answer to Organ Shortage: Xenotransplantation

While Parts I and II centered on the critical inspection and improvement of ethical, legal and political aspects of human-to-human organ transplantation regimes, Part III leaves this area of reflection and focuses on the analysis of the medical and ethical potential of animal-to-human transplantation. By exploring the capability of xenotransplantation, one of the most controversially discussed responses to the problem of organ shortage is investigated with regard to the advantages and disadvantages of this technology.

The beginning of this section is dedicated to the medical background of xenotransplantation. In their contribution *Bruno Reichart, Sonja Guethoff, Tanja Mayr, Michael Thormann, Stefan Buchholz, Jan-Michael Abicht, Alexander Kind* and *Paolo Brenner* present detailed insights from an ongoing research project aiming to establish xenotransplantation as a medical practice. Their detailed report exemplifies diverse aspects of the actual work of the research consortium: why pigs are best suitable as donor animals for solid organs, what safety problems are posed by cross-species transplantation, which are the first clinical experiences of porcine islet transplantation. Special emphasis is placed on explaining the different forms of rejection and of strategies to overcome these obstacles. As a conclusion, they answer the question of whether the prediction of the great cardiac surgeon Norman Shumway that xenotransplantation will always be the future is still right in a nuanced way, explaining that for different organs different stages of practicability are reached.

In their article, *Galia Assadi, Lara Pourabdolrahim* and *Georg Marckmann* move beyond the borders of medical science and undertake a systematic investigation of the medical and animal ethical issues raised by xenotransplantation in order to assess the potential societal use of this new technology. They argue that, while some of the medico-ethical aspects of xenotransplantation are already very well analyzed, the analysis of animal ethical issues proves to be less theoretically founded and consistent. In order to fill this gap and contribute to a broader discussion of the advantages and disadvantages of xenotransplantation, their article widens the perspective by pointing out some aspects regarding the principles of respect for patient's autonomy and justice and developing an institutional ethics perspective that is not reflected in the literature so far. The final section provides a short summary of the central ideas of four of the most influential theoretical concepts and thereby contributes to a philosophical substantiation of the animal ethical analysis. Furthermore, some concluding reflections are presented on the problem of guaranteeing an adequate consideration of animal welfare against the background of the pluralism of animal ethical theories and attitudes.

Jan-Ole Reichardt takes a different ethical approach and focuses primarily on third person risks, arguing that these represent by far the most important (if not the only important) ethical challenge to xenotransplantation's translational success. Therefore, he discusses a special form of externalities – some uncommon risks that are to be shouldered by uninvolved parties and the public. Reichardt first presents currently available information concerning the probability of xenogeneic infection. Second, he shows that neither benefit optimism nor disaster pessimism are adequate strategies of coping with a situation of informed uncertainty. That is why he advocates a strategy of finding the right balance between risk and cautiousness. Third, he presents suggestions for the continuous assessment of xenotransplant technologies as recommended by the favored interpretation of the precautionary principle and a minimally invasive surveillance of xenotransplant patients to protect them and the public against a sudden lack of funding and the following disruption of post-operative monitoring. He argues that if every transplant would come with a fee attached, which could be interpreted as a contribution to something like a liability insurance fund (in the broadest sense), the necessary funding for an international network of biosecurity experts would seem within reach. Such a network could be established by already existing national and transnational institutions and opened up – in addition to xenotransplantation medicine – to agriculture and farming as well.

Chapter 19
Discordant Cellular and Organ Xenotransplantation—From Bench to Bedside

Bruno Reichart, Sonja Guethoff, Tanja Mayr, Michael Thormann, Stefan Buchholz, Jan-Michael Abicht, Alexander J. Kind and Paolo Brenner

B. Reichart (✉) · S. Guethoff · T. Mayr
Walter Brendel Centre of Experimental Medicine, Ludwig-Maximilians-Universität München, Munich, Germany
e-mail: Bruno.Reichart@med.uni-muenchen.de

S. Guethoff
e-mail: Sonja.Guethoff@med.uni-muenchen.de

T. Mayr
e-mail: Tanja.Mayr@med.uni-muenchen.de

S. Buchholz · P. Brenner
Department of Cardiac Surgery, Ludwig-Maximilians-Universität München, Munich, Germany
e-mail: Sonja.Guethoff@med.uni-muenchen.de

S. Buchholz
e-mail: Stefan.Buchholz@med.uni-muenchen.de

P. Brenner
e-mail: Paolo.Brenner@med.uni-muenchen.de

J. Abicht
Department of Anaesthesiology, Ludwig-Maximilians-Universität München, Munich, Germany
e-mail: Jan.Abicht@med.uni-muenchen.de

A. J. Kind
Chair of Livestock Biotechnology, School of Life Sciences, Weihenstephan, Technische Universität München, Freising, Germany
e-mail: Kind@wzw.tum.de

R. J. Jox et al. (eds.), *Organ Transplantation in Times of Donor Shortage*,
International Library of Ethics, Law, and the New Medicine 59,
DOI 10.1007/978-3-319-16441-0_19

19.1 Introduction

19.1.1 The Clinical Need for Solid Organ Transplantation—the Pig as Preferred Donor

Human allotransplantation has been very successful over the past six decades. Heart and kidney transplantations remain the therapy of choice for end-stage organ failure. Although surgical competence is available in many medical centres around the world, the demand for organs far exceeds the supply from human donors. The consequences for patients waiting for transplants are severe, as can be seen by the following two examples. In Germany, the annual mortality for waiting heart transplant candidates is 18 %.[1] The average waiting time for a cadaveric kidney is five years, which significantly reduces the prospects for patients eventually receiving a donated kidney, because graft survival drops substantially after extended dialysis.[2]

Several alternatives have been suggested to overcome the grave shortage of organs. One possible solution would be clinical xenotransplantation using non-human primates as concordant donors and triple drug immunosuppression, as applied in human allotransplants.[3] However, ethical and logistical considerations preclude this. Apes are endangered species and their use is out of the question, other non-human primates are too small and their growth too slow.

In contrast, discordant species, notably pigs, offer an abundant new source of organs (and cells) for various reasons:

- Similarities in size, anatomy, nutrition and physiology to man
- Short generation intervals (12 months) and high fertility (10–14 offspring per litter)
- Well-established and economic housing and breeding conditions with high hygienic standards
- Availability of advanced reproductive biotechnologies and genetic engineering techniques
- Minor concerns regarding the slaughtering of pigs, at least in western countries, because they are raised for meat production on an industrial scale

Nevertheless, despite these obvious advantages, serious ethical concerns do exist in society regarding the use of pigs as donors, and these have to be allayed.[4]

---

[1] Rahmel (2013).

[2] Meier-Kriesche and Kaplan (2002).

[3] Reichenspurner et al. (1989).

[4] Cozzi et al. (2009).

19.1.2 The Clinical Need for Discordant Cellular Transplantation

There is also clinical need for a huge variety of cell types, some of which are already being investigated as possible xenotransplants, such as liver cells,[5] neurons[6] and corneas[7]. At the moment, there is a particular focus on pancreatic islets.

An epidemic of obesity in Western populations has led to an increasing threat of diabetes mellitus, with the number of patients set to double within the next two decades.[8] Although anti-diabetic therapy is successful for most patients, hypoglycaemia is a life-threatening complication in 5–10 % of cases. At present, allogeneic pancreatic islet cell transplantation offers a solution for type 1 diabetes only and delivers a greatly improved quality of life with relatively low operative risk. Unfortunately, however, a shortage of suitable donors and the extraordinarily high number of islet cells required for each patient severely restricts the availability of treatment. A total of 1400 islet allotransplantations[9] performed worldwide to date stands in striking contrast to the dramatically increasing number of diabetes patients.

Discordant xenogeneic islet transplantation would therefore offer a practical solution. This is supported by the impressive results of porcine islet transplantation into diabetic primate models, using islets from wild-type pigs and immunosuppression of the recipient,[10] encapsulated islets from wild-type pigs,[11] or islets from genetically engineered donor pigs.[12]

19.1.3 The Need for Biological Valve Prostheses for Younger Patients

Another focus of our consortium is on the replacement of heart valves. Approximately 300,000 patients worldwide now carry prosthetic heart valve implants. Current valves are however less than ideal. Mechanical devices necessitate lifelong anticoagulation therapy, incurring serious bleeding side effects with a mortality of one percent per patient year. Biological valves (porcine, bovine) do not need anticoagulation if the patient is in sinus rhythm, but have restricted durability, degenerating quickly in children, adolescents and young adults.[13] Promising new prostheses have been made from decellularised biological heart valve matrices that are revit-

[5] Nagata et al. (2007).

[6] Leveque et al. (2011).

[7] Hara and Cooper (2011).

[8] Hossain et al. (2007).

[9] Collaborative Islet Transplant Registry (2013).

[10] Cardona et al. (2006); Hering et al. (2006).

[11] Sun et al. (1996); Dufrane et al. (2010).

[12] van der Windt et al. (2009).

[13] Kouchoukos et al. (2012).

alised in vivo by cells from the recipient forming a functional epithelium and live interstitium. A decellularised heart valve matrix from wild-type pigs does however attract inflammatory cells and induces platelet activation.[14] Pigs genetically modified to overcome these immune mechanisms may provide a superior source of such materials.

19.2 Safety Issues in Pig-to-Primate Xenotransplantation

The possible transfer of infectious agents to a graft recipient is a major problem in allotransplantation, and risks might be exacerbated with tissue from non-human species. On the other hand, xenotransplantation offers the opportunity to systematically examine the donor for infectious agents before transplantation.[15] To control the infectious burden, donor animals should be raised in a clean environment (*designated pathogen free*, DPF) and xenograft recipients should be monitored post-operatively. Among the numerous infectious agents, porcine endogenous retroviruses (PERV-A, B, C) have received the most attention, because they are integrated in the germ line and transmitted vertically to offspring, and thus cannot be eliminated by raising pigs in a DPF facility. Initial studies showed the human-tropic potential of PERV in vitro[16] and revealed their predisposition for retroviral recombination.[17] Recombined PERV-A/C has higher infectious potential than PERV-C.[18] But most importantly, there was no evidence of cross-species transmission in the first clinical trials of islet xenotransplantation.[19] Regarding safety issues, the International Xenotransplantation Association (IXA) and the WHO have defined and regularly update their conditions for xenotransplantation[20] (current update on the 2nd International Conference on Clinical Islet Xenotransplantation, August 2014, San Francisco, USA, current unpublished).

19.3 Immunological Barriers and Strategies to Overcome them

Xenotransplantation would undoubtedly provide substantial advantages for human regenerative medicine. The main problems arise from disparities between swine and primates resulting from approximately 90 million years of evolutionary divergence, which can affect important protein-protein and other biochemical interac-

[14] Kasimir et al. (2006).

[15] Mueller et al. (2011); Scobie and Takeuchi (2009).

[16] Le Tissier et al. (1997).

[17] Klymiuk et al. (2002); Oldmixon et al. (2002).

[18] Bartosch et al. (2004).

[19] Garkavenko et al. (2008a, b); Wynyard et al. (2014).

[20] Denner et al. (2009); WHO summaries (2008, 2011); Fishmann et al. (2011).

tions. Considerable immunological and physiological incompatibilities must therefore be overcome before xenogeneic grafts can be clinically effective. Fortunately, our understanding of these barriers is increasing rapidly and rational strategies are being developed to overcome them. Humoral rejection from preformed antibodies and the blood coagulation system present the immediate obstacles, in the longer term the greatest challenge comes from the adaptive immune response.

19.4 Humoral Responses in Vascularised Organs

An unmodified porcine organ transplanted into a human or primate recipient is confronted with a series of rejection responses. The first is hyperacute rejection (HAR), followed by acute humoral xenograft rejection (AHXR), also known as acute vascular or delayed xenograft reaction. Both HAR and AHXR are ultimately the result of antibodies binding to cell surface antigens on the graft endothelium.

19.4.1 Hyperacute Rejection

Pre-existing antibodies[21] in human blood against the α1,3-galactosyl-galactose (α-Gal) epitope on porcine vessel walls cause the rapid formation of an antigen-antibody complex that immediately activates the host complement system. This causes cell disruption and lysis of donor endothelium, which in turn activates the blood coagulation cascade. The result is extensive haemorrhage, oedema and thrombosis of small blood vessels, leading to death of the graft within hours. Old-world primates (including humans) lack α-Gal epitopes, due to an inactive α-1,3-galactosyltransferase (GGTA1) gene. Therefore, a suitable solution would be to disable or *knock out* the orthologous porcine gene. Homozygous GGTA1 deficient pigs have been generated[22] and several independent herds established. Organs from these pigs have been tested in numerous pig-to-baboon organ transplantation studies[23] and revealed a maximum survival of three month for kidneys[24] and of over 800 days for beating but non-working hearts[25].

---

[21] Galili (2013).

[22] Phelps et al. (2003).

[23] Ekser et al. (2011).

[24] Yamada et al. (2005).

[25] Kuwaki et al. (2005); Mohiuddin et al. (2014, and personal communication 2015).

19.4.2 *Acute (Delayed) Humoral Rejection, Thrombotic Microangiopathy*

Once HAR is overcome, AHXR presents the next immunological obstacle. Hearts from GGTA1-KO pigs transplanted into baboons were found to exhibit widespread thrombotic microangiopathy, ischemia, focal haemorrhage and necrosis as a consequence of progressive humoral rejection and disordered thromboregulation.[26] The underlying mechanisms are not completely understood, but are thought to involve changes to the porcine endothelium following transplantation that lead to a procoagulant state. Antibodies to antigens other than α-Gal (non-Gal) epitopes also seem to play a major role in AHXR.[27] However, the number and diversity of non-Gal antigens precludes their removal by gene targeting. The preferred strategy is thus to prevent a complement-mediated destruction of the xenograft. Various transgenic pigs expressing human complement regulators[28] on the vascular endothelium have been generated, combined with GGTA1-KO animals, and tested in pig-to-baboon transplantation experiments. Transgenes that modulate endothelial activation, such as heme oxygenase 1 (HO-1), are also thought to be beneficial.[29]

In addition to the antibody-mediated activation of the xenograft endothelium, incompatibilities in the coagulation components in the human blood stream and the porcine vessel wall might also contribute to the formation of microthrombi.[30] One example: Porcine thrombomodulin binds weakly to primate thrombin, leading to insufficient levels of activated protein C to interrupt coagulation.[31] This effect might be overcome by expressing human thrombomodulin in the porcine donor.[32]

19.5 Cell-Mediated Rejection

As with allogeneic procedures, cellular reactions should be expected following xenogeneic transplantations. Since the time of the intervention is known in advance, the bone marrow (and therefore antibody production) is suppressed prior to transplantation using anti-CD20 to destroy B-cells, bortezomib in combination with cortisone to destroy plasma cells, and cyclophosphamide for myeloablation.[33] Extracorporeal immunoadsorption is used to remove pre-existing α-Gal and non-Gal antibodies and any antibodies formed postoperatively. Maintenance immunosup-

[26] Ezzelarab et al. (2009); Shimizu et al. (2008).

[27] Byrne et al. (2011); Diswall et al. (2010).

[28] Pierson et al (2009), Ekser et al. (2011).

[29] Petersen et al. (2011).

[30] Cowan et al. (2009); Pierson et al (2009).

[31] Roussel et al. (2008).

[32] Peterson et al. (2009); Wünsch et al. (2014).

[33] Palumbo and Anderson (2011).

pression is provided by tacrolimus, mycophenolate and cortisone; antithymocyte globulin induction therapy is also applied.

Additional immunosuppressive treatment will clearly be necessary to overcome the consistently delayed humoral rejection reaction, such as total thoracic lymph node irradiation with 6-7 Gray,[34] or co-stimulation blockade with CD40, CD40 L antibodies.[35] A useful genetic approach is to express a T-cell co-stimulation blocker such as the improved form of CTLA4-Ig, LEA29Y, on transplanted cells or organs. This has been successfully demonstrated by researchers within our consortium, who transplanted transgenic pig islets into humanised immunodeficient mice.[36]

19.6 The Future of Xenotransplantation—is the Shumway Paradigm Still Valid?

The great cardiac surgeon Norman Shumway, who developed allogeneic heart transplantation in the sixties, used to say, "Xenotransplantation is the future, and always will be!" Fortunately, this pessimistic view is no longer true. In a recent review, Ekser and colleagues[37] listed the longest survival times reported for xenografted porcine cells and organs. Micro-encapsulated pancreatic islets from wild-type animals survived more than 800 days.[38] Non-encapsulated islets transgenic for the human-complement regulatory protein CD46 survived almost 400 days.[39] Abdominally placed heterotopic (non-working) triple genetically-modified (GGTA1-KO, CD46, hTM) hearts beat for up to 800 days,[40] hearts placed heterotopically within the thorax beat for up to 50 days and orthotopically for 57 days.[41] Transplanted CTLA4-Ig transgenic neuronal cells to treat Parkinson's disease, and wild-type decellularised corneas were also successful for hundreds of days.[42] Whole kidneys from CD55 transgenic animals survived for 90 days,[43] although porcine renal erythropoietin is not recognised by primate recipients and must be replaced. Liver and lung transplants do however stand in contrast, surviving only eight and five days, respectively.[44]

Since porcine islet transplantation will be the first to be introduced in clinics, its success will be crucial for further organ procedures with hearts and kidneys.

---

[34] Heinzelmann et al. (2008).

[35] Hering et al. (2006); Kenyon et al. (1999); Corcoran et al. (2010).

[36] Klymiuk et al. (2012).

[37] Ekser et al. (2012).

[38] Dufrane et al. (2010).

[39] Van der Windt et al. (2009).

[40] Mohiuddin et al. (2012, 2014, and personal communication)

[41] Bauer et al. (2010); McGregor et al. (2009).

[42] Badin et al. (2010); Choi et al. (2011).

[43] Baldan et al. (2004).

[44] Ramirez et al. (2000); Cantu et al. (2007).

19.7 First Clinical Experiences in Porcine Islet Transplantation

Porcine insulin is itself recognised and functional in primate recipients, however without immunosuppression, unmodified porcine insulin producing cells succumb to early graft loss known as the *immediate blood-mediated inflammatory reaction* driven by preformed antibodies, complement and excessive coagulation. The need for immunosuppressive drugs can however be obviated by encapsulation, in which islets are surrounded with a porous biopolymer composed mainly of alginate.[45] The pores are large enough for small molecules like water, glucose, oxygen and most importantly insulin to permeate, but exclude cells and larger molecules such as antibodies. However, it is not known how long these capsules can maintain their function in vivo, since loss of integrity or occlusion of the pores would be problematic.

The New Zealand company Living Cell Technologies is a pioneer in the field, having treated more than twenty diabetic patients suffering from frequent episodes of unaware hypoglycaemia to date.[46]A dose-finding and safety study showed improvement in some treated patients, for example through reduced glycated haemoglobin levels. Most importantly however, there was no evidence of zoonoses and no sign of the activation of porcine endogenous retroviruses,[47] a theoretical risk that has long been recognised. The genetically unmodified donor animals were from a DPF herd that originated from a feral breed from the sub-Antarctic Auckland Island, where they had essentially no contact with other animals or humans for approximately 150 years, since English sailors left them.

A German study using macroencapsulated immobilized islets (Beta-O2 Technologies, Israel),[48] has been conducted - this will also provide an useful opportunity to address the legal and ethical issues related to xenotransplantation.

References

Badin, R.A., A. Padoan, and M. Vadori, et al. 2010. Long-term clinical recovery in parkinsonian monkey recipients of CTLA4-Ig transgenic porcine neural precursors. *Transplantation* 90 (Suppl 2): 47.

Baldan, N., P. Rigotti, and F. Calabrese, et al. 2004. Ureteral stenosis in hDAF pig-to-primate renal xenotransplantation: A phenomenon related to immunological events? *American Journal of Transplantation* 4 (4): 475–481.

Bartosch, B., D. Stefanidis, and R. Myers, et al. 2004. Evidence and consequence of porcine endogenous retrovirus recombination. *Journal of Virology* 78 (24): 13880–13890.

Bauer, A., J. Postrach, and M. Thormann, et al. 2010. First experience with heterotopic thoracic pig-to-baboon cardiac xenotransplantation. *Xenotransplantation* 17 (3): 243–249.

[45] Calafiore et al. (2004).

[46] Elliot et al. (2011, and personal communication).

[47] Wynyard et al. (2014).

[48] Ludwig et al. (2012), Ludwig et al. (2013).

Byrne, G. W., P. G. Stalboerger, and Z. Du, et al. 2011. Identification of new carbohydrate and membrane protein antigens in cardiac xenotransplantation. *Transplantation* 91 (3): 287–292.

Calafiore, R., G. Basta, and G. Luca, et al. 2004. Grafts of microencapsulated pancreatic islet cells for the therapy of diabetes mellitus in non-immunosuppressed animals. *Biotechnology and Applied Biochemistry* 39(Pt 2): 159–164.

Cantu, E., K. R. Balsara, and B. Li, et al. 2007. Prolonged function of macrophage, von Willibrand factor-deficient porcine pulmonary xenografts. *American Journal of Transplantation* 7 (1): 66–75.

Cardona, K., G. S. Korbutt, and Z. Milas, et al. 2006. Long-term survival of neonatal porcine islets in nonhuman primates by targeting costimulation pathways. *Nature Medicine* 12 (3): 304–306.

Choi, H. J., M. K. Kim, and H. J. Lee, et al. 2011. Efficacy of pig-to-rhesus lamellar corneal xenotransplantation. *Investigative Ophthalmology and Visual Science* 52 (9): 6643–6650.

Collaborative Islet Transplant Registry. 2013. www.citeregistry.org. Accessed 6 June 2015.

Corcoran, P. C., K. A. Horvath, and A. K. Singh, et al. 2010. Surgical and nonsurgical complications of a pig to baboon heterotopic heart transplantation model. *Transplantation Proceedings* 42 (6): 2149–2151.

Cowan, P. J., J. C. Roussel, and A. J. d'Apice. 2009. The vascular and coagulation issues in xenotransplantation. *Current Opinion Organ Transplantation* 14 (2): 161–167.

Cozzi, E., M. Tallacchini, and E. B. Flanagan, et al. 2009. The International Xenotransplantation Association consensus statement on conditions for undertaking clinical trials of porcine islet products in type 1 diabetes. Chapter 1: Key ethical requirements and progress toward the definition of an international regulatory framework. *Xenotransplantation* 16 (4): 203–214.

Denner, J., H. J. Schuurman, and C. Patience. 2009. The International Xenotransplantation Association consensus statement on conditions for undertaking clinical trials of porcine islet products in type 1 diabetes. Chapter 5: Strategies to prevent transmission of porcine endogenous retroviruses. *Xenotransplantation* 16 (4): 239–248.

Diswall, M., J. Angstrom, and H. Karlsson, et al. 2010. Structural characterization of alpha1,3-galactosyltransferase knockout pig heart and kidney glycolipids and their reactivity with human and baboon antibodies. *Xenotransplantation* 17 (1): 48–60.

Dufrane, D., R. M. Goebbels, P. Gianello. 2010. Alginate macroencapsulation of pig islets allows correction of streptozotocin-induced diabetes in primates up to 6 months without immunosuppression. *Transplantation* 90 (10): 1054–1062.

Ekser, B., G. Kumar, M. Veroux, and D. K. Cooper. 2011. Therapeutic issues in the treatment of vascularized xenotransplants using gal-knockout donors in nonhuman primates. *Current Opinion Organ Transplantation* 16 (2): 222–230.

Ekser, B., M. Ezzelarab, and H. Hara, et al. 2012. Clinical xenotransplantation: The next medical revolution? *Lancet* 379 (9816): 672–83.

Elliott, R. B. 2011. Living cell technologies. Towards xenotransplantation of pig islets in the clinic. *Current Opinion Organ Transplantation* 16 (2): 195–200.

Ezzelarab, M., B. Garcia, and A. Azimzadeh, et al. 2009. The innate immune response and activation of coagulation in alpha1,3-galactosyltransferase gene-knockout xenograft recipients. Transplantation 87 (6): 805–812.

Fishmann, J. A., S. Scobie, and Y. Takeuchi. 2011. Annex 4. Xenotransplantation-associated infectious risk: A background paper for the second WHO global consultation on regulatory requirements for Xenotransplantation clinical trials. Geneva, Switzerland, 17–19 October 2011. http://www.who.int/transplantation/xeno/en/. Accessed 20 April 2015.

Galili, U. 2013. Discovery of the natural anti-Gal antibody and its past and future relevance to medicine. *Xenotransplantation* 20 (3): 138–147.

Garkavenko, O., B. Dieckhoff, and S. Wynyard, et al. 2008a. Absence of transmission of potentially xenotic viruses in a prospective pig to primate islet xenotransplantation study. *Journal of Medical Virology* 80 (11): 2046–2052.

Garkavenko, O., S. Wynyard, and D. Nathu, et al. 2008b. Porcine endogenous retrovirus (PERV) and its transmission characteristics: A study of the New Zealand designated pathogen-free herd. *Cell Transplantation* 17 (12): 1381–1388.

Hara H, and Cooper, D. K. 2011. Xenotransplantation—The future of corneal transplantation? *Cornea* 30 (4): 371–378.

Heinzelmann, F., P. J. Lang, and H. Ottinger, et al. 2008. Immunosuppressive total lymphoid irradiation-based reconditioning regimens enable engraftment after graft rejection or graft failure in patients treated with allogeneic hematopoietic stem cell transplantation. *International Journal of Radiation Oncology, Biology, Physics* 70 (2): 523–528.

Hering, B. J., M. Wijkstrom, and M. L. Graham, et al. 2006. Prolonged diabetes reversal after intraportal xenotransplantation of wild-type porcine islets in immunosuppressed nonhuman primates. *Nature Medicine* 12 (3): 301–303.

Hossain, P., B. Kawar, and M. El Nahas. 2007. Obesity and diabetes in the developing world—A growing challenge. *The New England Journal of Medicine* 356 (3): 213–215.

Kasimir, M. T., E. Rieder, and G. Seebacher, et al. 2006. Decellularization does not eliminate thrombogenicity and inflammatory stimulation in tissue-engineered porcine heart valves. *Journal of Heart Valve Disease* 15 (2): 278–286.

Kenyon, N. S., M. Chatzipetrou, and M. Masetti, et al. 1999. Long-term survival and function of intrahepatic islet allografts in rhesus monkeys treated with humanized anti-CD154. *Proceedings of National Academy of Sciences United States of America* 96 (14): 8132–8137.

Klymiuk, N., M. Muller, G. Brem, and B. Aigner. 2002. Characterization of porcine endogenous retrovirus gamma pro-pol nucleotide sequences. *Journal of Virology* 76 (22): 11738–11743.

Klymiuk, N., L. van Buerck, and A. Bähr, et al. 2012. Xenografted islet cell clusters from INSLEA29Y transgenic pigs rescue diabetes and prevent immune rejection. *Diabetes*. 61 (6):1527–1532.

Kouchoukos, N. T., E. H. Blackstone, F. L. Hanley, J. K. Kirlin, J. Kirklin, und B. Barratt-Boyes. 2012. *Cardiac surgery.* 4th ed. Churchill Livingstone, Elsevier, Oxford. 619–620.

Kuwaki, K., Y. L. Tseng, and F. J. Dor, et al. 2005. Heart transplantation in baboons using alpha1,3-galactosyltransferase gene-knockout pigs as donors:Iinitial experience. *Nature Medicine* 11 (1): 29–31.

Le Tissier, P., J. P. Stoye, Y. Takeuchi, C. Patience, and R. A. Weiss. 1997. Two sets of human-tropic pig retrovirus. *Nature* 389 (6652): 681–682.

Leveque, X., E. Cozzi, P. Naveilhan, and I. Neveu. 2011. Intracerebral xenotransplantation: Recent findings and perspectives for local immunosuppression. *Current Opinion Organ Transplantation* 16 (2): 190–194.

Ludwig, B., A. Rotem, and J. Schmid et al. 2012. Improvement of islet function in a bioartificial pancreas by enhanced oxygen supply and growth hormone releasing hormone agonist. *Proceedings of National Academy of Sciences United States of America* 109 (13): 5022–5027.

Ludwig, B., A. Reichel, and A. Steffen et al. 2013. Transplantation of human islets without immunosuppression. *Proceedings of National Academy of Sciences United States of America* 110 (47): 19054–19058

McGregor, C. G., G. W. Byrne, and M. Vlasin, et al. 2009. Early cardiac function and gene expression after orthotopic cardiac xenotransplantation. *Xenotransplantation* 16: 356.

Meier-Kriesche, H. U., and B. Kaplan. 2002. Waiting time on dialysis as the strongest modifiable risk factor for renal transplant outcomes: A paired donor kidney analysis. *Transplantation* 74 (10): 1377–1381.

Mohiuddin, M. M., P. C. Corcoran, and A. K. Singh, et al. 2012. T-Cell depletion extends the survival of GTkO/hCD 46 Tg pig heart xenografts in baboons for up to 8 months. *American Journal of Transplantation* 12 (3): 763–771.

Mohiuddin, M. M., A. K. Singh, and P. C. Corcoran et al. 2014. Genetically engineered pigs and target-specific immunomodulation provide significant graft survival and hope for clinical cardiac xenotransplantation. *The Journal of Thoracic and Cardiovascular Surgery* 148 (3): 1106–1113.

Mueller, N. J., Y. Takeuchi, G. Mattiuzzo, and L. Scobie. 2011. Microbial safety in xenotransplantation. *Current Opinion Organ Transplantation* 16 (2): 201–206.

Nagata, H., R. Nishitai, and C. Shirota, et al. 2007. Prolonged survival of porcine hepatocytes in cynomolgus monkeys. *Gastroenterology* 132 (1): 321–329.

Oldmixon, B. A., J. C. Wood, and T. A. Ericsson, et al. 2002. Porcine endogenous retrovirus transmission characteristics of an inbred herd of miniature swine. *Journal of Virology* 76 (6): 3045–3048.

Palumbo, A., and K. Anderson. 2011. Multiple myeloma. *The New England Journal of Medicine* 364 (11): 1046–1060.

Petersen, B., W. Ramackers, and A. Tiede, et al. 2009. Pigs transgenic for human thrombomodulin have elevated production of activated protein C. *Xenotransplantation* 16 (6): 486–495.

Petersen, B., W. Ramackers, and A. Lucas-Hahn, et al. 2011. Transgenic expression of human heme oxygenase-1 in pigs confers resistance against xenograft rejection during ex vivo perfusion of porcine kidneys. *Xenotransplantation* 18 (6): 355–368.

Phelps, C. J., C. Koike, and T. D. Vaught, et al. 2003. Production of alpha 1,3-galactosyltransferase-deficient pigs. *Science* 299 (5605): 411–414.

Pierson, R. N., III. 2009. Antibody-mediated xenograft injury: Mechanisms and protective strategies. *Transplant Immunology* 21: 65–69.

Rahmel, A. 2013. Eurotransplant International Foundation. Annual Report.

Ramirez, P., R. Chavez, and M. Majado, et al. 2000. Life-supporting human complement regulator decay accelerating factor transgenic pig liver xenograft maintains the metabolic function and coagulation in the nonhuman primate for up to 8 days. *Transplantation* 70: 989–998.

Reichenspurner, H., P. A. Human, and D. H. Boehm, et al. 1989. Optimalization of immunosuppression after xenogeneic heart transplantation in primates. *Journal of Heart Transplantation* 8 (3): 200–207.

Roussel, J. C., C. J. Moran, and E. J. Salvaris, et al. 2008. Pig thrombomodulin binds human thrombin but is a poor cofactor for activation of human protein C and TAFI. *American Journal of Transplantation* 8 (6): 1101–1112.

Scobie, L., and Y. Takeuchi. 2009. Porcine endogenous retrovirus and other viruses in xenotransplantation. *Current Opinion Organ Transplantation* 14 (2): 175–179.

Shimizu, A., Y. Hisashi, and K. Kuwaki, et al. 2008. Thrombotic microangiopathy associated with humoral rejection of cardiac xenografts from alpha1,3-galactosyltransferase gene-knockout pigs in baboons. *American Journal of Pathology* 172 (6): 1471–1481.

Sun, Y., X. Ma, and D. Zhou, et al. 1996. Normalization of diabetes in spontaneously diabetic cynomologus monkeys by xenografts of microencapsulated porcine islets without immunosuppression. *Journal of Clinical Investigation* 98 (6): 1417–1422.

Van der Windt, D. J., R. Bottino, and A. Casu, et al. 2009. Long-term controlled normoglycemia in diabetic non-human primates after transplantation with hCD46 transgenic porcine islets. *American Journal of Transplantation* 9 (12): 2716–2726.

WHO, First World Health Organization Global Consultation on Regulatory Requirements for Xenotransplantation Clinical Trials: Changsha, China, 19–21 November 2008. The Changsha Communique. Xenotransplantation;16:61-3., and Second World Health Organization Global Consultation on Regulatory Requirements for Xenotransplantation Clinical Trials: Geneva, Switzerland, 17-19 October 2011. http://www.who.int/transplantation/xeno/en/. Accessed 6 June 2015.

WHO global consultations on regulatory requirements for xenotransplantation clinical trials. Changsha, China. November 19–21, 2008; Geneva, Switzerland, October 17–19, 2011. http://www.who.int/transplantation/xeno/en/.

Wolf, E. et al. Unpublished.

Wuensch, A., A. Baehr, and A. K. Bongoni et al. 2014. Regulatory sequences of the porcine THBD gene facilitate endothelial-specific expression of bioactive human thrombomodulin in single- and multitransgenic pigs. *Transplantation* 97 (2): 138–147.

Wynyard, S., D. Nathu, O. Garkavenko, J. Denner J, and R. Elliott. 2014. Microbiological safety of the first clinical pig islet xenotransplantation trial in New Zealand. *Xenotransplantation* 21 (4): 309–323.

Yamada, K., K. Yazawa, and A. Shimizu, et al. 2005. Marked prolongation of porcine renal xenograft survival in baboons through the use of alpha1,3-galactosyltransferase gene-knockout donors and the cotransplantation of vascularized thymic tissue. *Nature Medicine* 11 (1): 32–34.

Bruno Reichart is a German heart surgeon and former Director of the Department of Cardiovascular Surgery, Ludwig-Maximilians-Universität München (LMU). For many years, he has worked in the various fields of thoracic transplantations, both clinical and experimental. Since 2012, he is the Speaker of the Collaborative Research Center (SFB/Transregio) 127: "Biology of xenogeneic cell, tissue and organ transplantation—from bench to bedside" of the German Research Foundation (DFG). Within the Consortium, he covers legal and ethical aspects as well as cardiac transplantation.

Sonja Guethoff was a resident physician at the Department of Cardiac Surgery, Ludwig-Maximilians-Universität München (LMU, Director Prof. B. Reichart/Prof. C. Hagl) from 2010 to 2014, and started her fellowship at the Department of Vascular and Endovascular Surgery, Technische Universität München (TUM, Director Prof. H.-H. Eckstein) in 2015. Since 2012, she is a member of the Collaborative Research Center 127: "Biology of xenogeneic cell, tissue and organ transplantation --from bench to bedside." (Speaker Prof. B. Reichart). Her current research interests are in the field of experimental cardiac transplantation and xenotransplantation using small and large animal models at the Walter Brendel Centre of Experimental Medicine (Director Prof. U. Pohl), as well as clinical trials in human heart transplantation and aortic diseases.

Tanja Mayr is a veterinarian and works as an associate research fellow at the Walter Brendel Centre of Experimental Medicine, Ludwig-Maximilians-Universität München (LMU, Director Prof. U. Pohl). Her research interests are in the field of heart transplantation. She is a member of the Transregio Collaborative Research Centre 127: "Biology of xenogeneic cell, tissue and organ transplantation - from bench to bedside." (Speaker Prof. B. Reichart).

Stefan Buchholz is a resident at the Department of Cardiac Surgery, Ludwig-Maximilians-Universität München (LMU, Director Prof. C. Hagl). His research interest lies in xenogenic and allogenic rejection after heart and lung transplantation in rodents.

Jan-Michael Abicht is a consultant at the Department of Anaesthesiology, Ludwig-Maximilians-Universität München (LMU, Director Prof. B. Zwißler). He is also the Principal Investigator at the Transregio Collaborative Research Centre 127: "Biology of xenogeneic cell, tissue and organ transplantation—from bench to bedside" (Speaker Prof. B. Reichart). His current research interests are ex-vivo cardiac perfusions.

Alexander J. Kind is with the Chair of Livestock Biotechnology, School of Life Sciences Weihenstephan, Technische Universität München. Dr. Kind received his PhD from Cambridge University and has worked on diverse aspects of transgenic animal technology, including embryonic stem cells and the development of nuclear transfer to generate cloned and genetically modified large animals. His current research interests are in the development of large animals to model human disease and as xenotransplantation donors.

Paolo Brenner has been an assistant professor for cardiac surgery, Department of Cardiac Surgery, Ludwig-Maximilians-Universität München (LMU, Director Prof. C. Hagl) since 2011. He was previously a specialist for cardiac surgery, Dept. of Cardiac Surgery, at the LMU Munich under the supervision of Prof. Bruno Reichart. In 2004, Dr. Brenner completed his PhD fellowship at the Bavarian Research Foundation with the Xenotransplantation (XT) Project, which began in 1997. In addition, he has been a Principal Investigator in the DFG Transregio research group FOR 535 Xenotransplantation since 2004. Since 2012, he is the Head Principal Investigator of the cardiac xenotransplantation group at the Transregio Collaborative Research Centre 127 „Xenotransplantation" at the LMU. Additionally, he is a specialist for cardiac assist devices, as well as heart and lung transplantation.

Chapter 20
Xenotransplantation: The Last Best Hope? Ethical Aspects of a Third Way to Solve the Problem of Organ Shortage

Galia Assadi, Lara Pourabdolrahim and Georg Marckmann

20.1 Introduction

Regarding the constantly increasing number of people in desperate need of an organ worldwide, the gap between organ supply and demand can be called one of the major challenges in the area of modern medicine. Investigating the actual societal handling of the problem, two strategies can be identified. *First*, large-scale campaigns initiated and sponsored by Ministries of Health and conducted by health insurance companies and private institutions, e. g. the German Organ Transplantation Foundation, are undertaken in order to increase the public's willingness to donate. While this strategy can be called reactive, the *second* strategy focuses on the aspect of prevention. Therefore, biopolitical strategies are applied so as to enable the population to live a *healthier* life and to avoid pathogenic factors like smoking, obesity and hypertension. While the first policy aims at increasing the supply of organs, the second strategy targets reducing the demand. Even though it is not broadly recognized in the public sphere, transplantation medicine, from the start, has discussed and investigated a *third* policy: xenotransplantation. While the vision of providing an almost endless supply of organs by breeding animals for transplantation purposes nourishes the medical hope and intensifies research efforts, xenotransplantation still faces some severe problems, arising from e. g. the rejection of organs and cells

G. Assadi (✉)
Institute Technology -Theology-Science, Ludwig-Maximilians-University Munich, Munich, Germany
e-mail: galia.assadi@web.de

G. Marckmann
Institute for Ethics, History and Theory of Medicine, Ludwig-Maximilians-University Munich, Munich, Germany
e-mail: georg.marckmann@med.uni-muenchen.de

L. Pourabdolrahim
Graduate School of Systemic Neurosciences, Munich, Germany
e-mail: lara.pourabdolrahim@campus.lmu.de

R. J. Jox et al. (eds.), *Organ Transplantation in Times of Donor Shortage*,
International Library of Ethics, Law, and the New Medicine 59,
DOI 10.1007/978-3-319-16441-0_20

and the danger of cross-species infections. Nevertheless, remarkable progress has been made in the last decades, allowing xenotransplantation to be put back on the agenda of possible solutions for organ shortage.[1]

In order to assess the potential societal use of xenotransplantation, it is necessary to exceed the borders of medical science and undertake a systematic investigation of the ethical, political and conceptual issues raised by xenotransplantation. While some of the medical ethical aspects of xenotransplantation have already been well analyzed, the analysis of animal ethical issues proves to be less theoretically founded and consistent. In order to fill this gap and contribute to a broader discussion on the advantages and disadvantages of xenotransplantation, this article widens the perspective of the medical ethical analyses by pointing out some aspects regarding the principles of respect for patient's autonomy and justice and developing an order ethical perspective, which has not been reflected on in the literature so far (20.2). The final Sect. (20.3) provides a short summary of the central ideas of four of the most influential theoretical concepts and thereby contributes to a philosophical substantiation of the animal ethical analysis. Furthermore, some concluding reflections on the problem of guaranteeing an adequate consideration of animal welfare against the background of the pluralism of animal ethical theories and attitudes are presented.

20.2 The Medical Ethics of Animal-to-Human Transplant

In order to reach a substantiated decision about the ethical legitimacy and political feasibility of xenotransplantation, it is useful to take a widespread and – in the field of medical ethics – commonly accepted ethical approach, like principlism,[2] as a heuristic. In order to delimit the range of potential medical ethical problems, this chapter primarily poses the question, if and how the principles of respect for person's autonomy and justice are concerned.[3]

---

[1] For further information, see the contribution of Bruno Reichart et al. in this volume.

[2] The two bioethicists, Tom L. Beauchamp and James F. Childress, can be regarded as the theoretical founders of principlism. Published in 1977 for the first time and amended with every new edition, Principles of Biomedical Ethics, serves as an important point of reference for the international bioethical discourse. In order to construct an ethical theory fitting exactly to the special ethical and political needs in the bioethical context, Beauchamp and Childress combined two strategies of theory building. First, they investigated the common morality in a pluralistic society, in order to identify shared principles underlying the different moral standpoints. Second, they analyzed various and – at first glance – contradictory ethical theories, posing the question, if besides the differences regarding the question of ultimate justification, shared principles on a medium level can be found. This theoretical access allowed bioethicists to develop an ethical theory based on four principles (respect for autonomy, justice, beneficence, non-maleficence) shared by ethical theories and common morality. By returning to common morality, Beauchamp and Childress ensured the connectivity of their theoretical reflections to widespread public opinions and therefore reduced the gap between ethical reflections and political deliberations usually characteristic of ethical theories. Beauchamp and Childress (2008).

[3] As xenotransplantation has been ethically analyzed and evaluated since as late as the 1990s, a wide-ranging corpus of literature already exists. As the principlist approach is used in almost every

20.2.1 Informed Consent Versus Informed Contract

Based upon an individual ethical view of society as an ensemble of isolated, autonomous and sovereign individuals competing and cooperating within a societal framework, the first principle expresses the ethical norm that a patient must be able to decide autonomously about his/her body, potential therapies and limits of treatment. In order to call a decision an autonomous decision, Beauchamp and Childress point out that three criteria must be fulfilled. *First*, the patient has to understand the medical problem and the range of possible solutions, including all potential consequences regarding harms and benefits implied by these particular solutions. *Second*, based on the complete information provided by the physician, the patient's choice must be made consciously after a process of deliberation concerning the most suitable treatment. *Third*, this decision-making process must not be unduly influenced by external instances, e. g. physicians or relatives, in order to guarantee that the decision expresses the free will of the patient and is not influenced by persons whose expectations the patient is trying to meet.

Applied to the special context of xenotransplantation, several ethical issues regarding the feasibility of an autonomous patient's decision arise. Considering the special situation that the area of knowledge about the potential medical consequences and severe risks[4] of animal-to-human-transplantations is very limited due to a lack of experience, the process of informing the patient is extremely difficult and therefore the first criterion of providing extensive information can hardly be met.

Considering the interests of third parties and reflecting on the ethical obligations arising with regard to the principle of justice, the ignorance about the implications and consequences of this new technology furthermore poses the problem of justifying that public health and safety, as well as the health and safety of the affiliated and medical personnel, are put in jeopardy by technology that is only useful to a special part of the population. In order to solve the conflict between the obligations arising from the principles of respect for autonomy and justice and thereby minimizing the risk imposed on public safety and enabling an enormous growth in knowledge for research and development, lifelong post-operative monitoring has been demanded by the patient and his close next of kin in the medical as well as the ethical discourse and a prohibition to reproduce is being discussed. This solution, although compre-

publication, this article focuses on some blind spots of the existing discourse, in order to make an innovative contribution. For a complete analysis considering all ethical problems arising against the background of principlism, see e. g. Schicktanz. Interesting ethical contributions were also made in the anthologies edited by Helmut Grimm, Sheila McLean and Brigitte Jansen, to name but a few.

[4] In the scientific discourse, various severe risks are discussed. Consequences ranging from xenogeneic infections, treatable with a high dosage of immunosuppressants while bearing in the mind the risk of a decline of the physical condition of the patient, to the risk of death having been discussed controversially. The conflicting opinions within the field of medical science aggravate the process of informing the patient earnestly and therefore render grave obstacles with regard to the enabling of autonomous decision-making.

hensible, leads to serious restrictions of the autonomy of the patient, his next of kin and the medical personnel engaged in the post-operative treatment, which need a strong legitimization because they contradict the principle of respect for autonomy. Furthermore, as a legal framework regulating the practice of xenotransplantation is still missing, the problem of ensuring the cooperation of all concerned parties arises, heightening the fear of an uncontrolled spread of possibly dangerous xenogeneic infections.

In order to reconcile reasonable public claims for safety guaranteed by the state and the sensible demand of the patients affected, and thereby solving the conflict between the principles of respect for autonomy and justice, two different recommendations have been developed within ethical literature. *First*, answering primarily the problem of insufficient legal regulations and therefore answering claims arising from the consideration of the principle of justice, the juridical model of informed contract has been proposed. According to this recommendation, the individuals concerned sign a contract obligating themselves to regular post-operative monitoring and possible quarantine, if necessary, to protect the public by prohibiting a diffusion of xenogeneic pathogens. In the case of violations of the duties arising from this contract, the state should be given the right to restrict individual civil rights by forcing them to take part in monitoring procedures or quarantine measures. Assessing this proposition critically and reflecting on the political and juridical implications, it seems extremely unlikely that this solution will be implemented. Despite being intensively discussed within ethical literature, informed contract actually seems to be more of a theoretically interesting solution than a politically and juridical viable measure that is being undertaken within democratic societies that respect a citizen's autonomy. This position can be supported by reflecting on the comparable case of HIV, where no contrastable juridical measures were seized, thus rendering an extensive change of the existing legal framework to enable the execution of a cure like xenotransplantation almost impossible.

Second, reacting to the problem of restriction of autonomy, the already well-established model of informed consent has been suggested. As mentioned above, the criteria which must be met in order to call a decision autonomous and a consent informed are hardly to be met through the usual routines of patient-physician consultation, as xenotransplantation is being hallmarked by specific conditions. First, the range of available information concerning the benefits and the risks of this treatment strategy are constitutively limited, forcing the patient to decide under the conditions of risk. Second, the range of obligations, e. g. lifelong monitoring, quarantine and the prohibition of reproduction, exceed the normal scope of informed consent, making a decision extremely difficult. Third, the consequences of consent to a xenotransplantation affect not only the patient, but also his next of kin, possibly including children or other groups of persons not fulfilling the preconditions of informed consent.

20.2.2 Conditions of Consent

In order to develop practically useful solutions regarding the operationalization of the principles of respect for autonomy and justice, we want to propose focusing on the arrangement of conditions enabling the consent process, which must be specified for this situation. By recommending a set of conditions required in order to allow a durable, binding, informed consent by the affected persons, we intend to initiate a broader discussion within the ethical discourse.

The *first* condition to be considered in this context is the establishment of an objective, informational structure, enabling the patient, his next of kin and medical personnel to get access to all the relevant information. Therefore, detailed, comprehensible and specified information sheets must be produced in order to meet the different informational needs that patients, their next of kin and medical personnel have. Furthermore, this information needs to be presented and explained to the patients and their next of kin by a physician who is not involved in the xenotransplantation. He/She must have all available facts about possible benefits and dangers of xenotransplantation and alternative treatment, the expected success rates, and the limits of knowledge concerning the consequences available to them in order to ensure that the affected parties are able to make a medically informed – and therefore autonomous – decision. As the decision is very far-reaching and the patient and his/her next of kin are living with and under the threat and the strain of a terminal illness, it is extremely important to enable a sufficient amount of time for them to consider all relevant arguments. Therefore, *second*, the process of decision-making should be designed accordingly, providing the conditions for long-lasting reflections, discussions and consultations at intervals of several weeks. A *third* condition is that constant pre- and post-operative medical, psychological and ethical guidance should be provided. In order to facilitate the decision-making process for every party involved, a stable, professional structure of medical and psychological assistance is required prior to commencing treatment, allowing the patient and his/her relatives to express their concerns, fears and inner conflicts in a setting that is free from external and temporal pressure. Furthermore, from a perspective of justice, intensified attention should be given to the affiliates as they might experience conflicts of ethical liabilities. Feeling strongly bonded and ethically obliged to help and support their diseased partner in every way possible, they have to consider the consequences for them and their children as well, for whom they have to make a wide-ranging, representative decision under the condition of insecurity. Considering the case of an affiliate refusing to consent to the procedure, severe ethical and psychological problems will arise for all affected parties, due to the fact that a disagreement concerning the necessity and legitimacy of xenotransplantation between the patient and his/her next of kin either leads to the separation of the partners or to a complete refusal of the transplantation, leaving the life-threating situation of the patient unchanged.

Focusing on the reflection of the advantages and disadvantages of informed consent respectively informed contract, the existing ethical literature doesn't provide any practicable solutions for the case of conflict between a partner and his/her next of kin. In order to fill this gap within theory and practice, we want to propose the involvement of a professional ethics consultant, who is able to reflect the ethical aspects of the procedure, to structure the discussion, as well as to provide techniques of solving ethical conflicts by reconciling the different positions. Leaving the parties affected without any support structure to take care of and help solve the ethical problems, it can't be assured that the consent decisions are made autonomously in the sense Beauchamp and Childress proposed, meaning free of pressure and in consideration of all possible, known medical and social consequences.

In addition, considering arguments that are being proposed by virtue ethics, it is furthermore necessary to ethically support the attending physician to find an appropriate way of handling the conflict resulting from the double bind of obligations. As xenotransplantation – in the beginning[5] – has to be regarded as a technology that is still under development, the attending physician is on the one hand obliged to act in the patient's interest, but on the other hand he/she is bound to his/her role as a researcher and therefore obliged to achieve progress in the field of science. This situation makes it likely for the physician to experience serious ethical conflicts, which could be alleviated with the help of a professional ethics consultant. As xenotransplantation must be regarded as developing, experimental medical technology – at least in the beginning – professional ethics consultation proves to be a helpful necessity in order to guarantee the ethical justifiability of the process and therefore, the duration of consent.

20.2.3 A Third Way of Solving the Risk Ethical Challenges

Mainstream ethical literature focuses on the debate of the advantages and disadvantages of informed contract or informed consent. By posing the question this way, important aspects concerning the possibility of a third way of solving the problem are lost from sight. Changing the commonplace theoretical perspective and looking at xenotransplantation from an order ethical perspective, as it has been developed e. g. by Karl Homann (Homann and Suchanek 2000) and Ingo Pies (2009), might prove to be helpful in creating an innovative contribution to the discourse and a viable solution which could guide future political debates.[6] According to this theoretical approach, based on e. g. game theory reflections, a distinction is made between *moves in the game*, *rules of the game* and a *regulating framework of conditions*

[5] Due to the current limits of knowledge regarding the consequences of an animal-to-human-transplant, the question of whether xenotransplantation must be regarded as a method of healing or as human experimentation, is being discussed intensely. This distinction is not of academic interest alone, as the categorization of human experimentation changes the preconditions underlying the current ethical analyses. For an overview, presenting the most relevant arguments, see Schicktanz (2002).

[6] We want to thank Ingo Pies for his helpful and extensive comments on the order ethical aspects of xenotransplantation.

enabling rules and moves of the game. This distinction provides the theoretical and practical ground for escaping the narrow horizon of individual ethics. Thereby ethical claims towards and accusations of misbehavior or lacking sense of responsibility of individual actors (like e. g. company leaders) can be missed, as they prove to be ineffective, because they focus on *individual moves* instead of on the *framework enabling* only specific – and sometimes ethically illegitimate – moves.

Applied to the context of xenotransplantation, it is necessary to consider the fact that besides medical personnel, the state, the patient and his/her next of kin, companies providing transplantable cells and organs are an indispensable partner in the process of putting xenotransplantation into effect. As a legal regime regulating questions of liability in the case of an outbreak of xenogeneic infections is still missing, it proves to be most important to develop ideas for an ethically legitimate framework respecting and reconciling the interests of all parties (state, pharmaceutical companies, medical personnel and patients). Therefore, it is necessary to reflect on the different interests pursued by the different parties in order to recognize conflicts and convergences of interest and thereby develop frameworks that enable ethically legitimate moves.

The state simultaneously wants to achieve the aims of providing the best possible health care to sick citizens on the one hand, and to secure the safety of all its citizens on the other hand. The patient (as well as his affiliates) is most interested in getting the therapy that is the most beneficial and least harmful to him/her as well as to his/her loved ones. The medical personnel aim to provide the best possible and safest treatment for the patient without being exposed to the risk of acquiring a serious illness. The companies have the objective to sell safe products as profitably as possible. The absence of specific legal regulations clarifying the question of accountability in the case of an unexpected spread of xenogeneic diseases limits the available options by making it economically necessary for companies to establish disclaimers of warranties in order to avoid potentially ruining claims, e. g. by transferring the complete liability to the patient or medical personnel as consumers. This transfer of liability practically results in ethically problematic and unjustifiable restrictions of autonomy, like the prohibition of reproduction or the process of life-long monitoring. The ethical principle of respecting the patient's autonomy in the context of xenotransplantation must therefore lead to the development of a legal framework ensuring companies disclaimers of warranties by state guarantees, meaning that the state will take full accountability in the case of the outbreak of xenogeneic infections. In addition to the guarantees concerning disclaimer warranties, the state has to establish a legal framework of shared responsibilities in order to fulfill its constitutional duty to protect its citizens. According to this, each party (companies, state, medical personnel, patient and his/her next of kin) has a responsibility to avoid every practice known as potentially promoting a xenogeneic infection. Based on this system of shared responsibilities, the state takes responsibility in the case of an outbreak of a xenogeneic infection, while *regular* cases of liability will be treated according to the existing legal procedures regulating the use of pharmaceutical products by dividing the responsibility among pharmaceutical companies and medical personnel, respectively the medical institutions. If the framework of juridical conditions will be designed accordingly, neither the patients nor medical personnel nor the companies will have to bear the whole risk and restrictions of individual autonomy can be kept to a minimum.

As xenotransplantation does not only affect public, private and corporate interests, which can be illustrated within an order ethical framework, but also the wellbeing of animals needing specific reflection, this chapter concludes with a brief overview of the most important animal ethical positions in order to widen the theoretical perspective of the ethical discussion[7] on xenotransplantation.

20.3 Arguments Concerning Animal Welfare

Reflecting on the scope of rights being attributable to animals and, based on this, on human obligations towards animals, three different stances can be taken. These different positions result from different premises concerning the moral status of animals, which underlie the resulting ethical claims. As the choice of the fundamental argumentative position determines the range of ethical claims that are expressible, it is important to bring these positions to mind in order to ground the following presentation of the most influential ethical theories. *First*, the anthropocentric position is based on the assumption of an unalterable and qualitative difference between human and animal functioning as a basis of a hierarchy of rights. According to this position, humans are characterized through high-level properties like autonomy and rationality, while animals, being bound to their natural instinct, lack these capacities. This attribution of superiority, and the hierarchical system based upon it, results in the thesis that only humans can be considered ethically relevant subjects, while animals and nature as a whole possess only instrumental value depending on man's interest. While the anthropocentric position is based on the notion of asymmetry, the *second* viewpoint, the biocentric position, reverses this notion and is based on the premise of the symmetry of rights and liberties being attributable to all creatures because of their status as animated beings. Trying to combine insights from both precedent positions, the *third* viewpoint, the intermediary or pathocentric position, accepts the idea of human superiority, but connects it not only to fundamental rights of use, but also with responsibilities to protect. Therefore, it strengthens the rights of animals – and the resulting human duties – by arguing that animals possess sensitivity and the potential to experience pain, thereby including them in the field of ethically relevant objects. In order to assess the animal ethical implications of xenotransplantation and develop a solution to the problem of guaranteeing an adequate

[7] Important contributions to animal ethical aspects have been made e. g. by Edgar Dahl, Helmut Grimm and Silke Schicktanz. While Grimm presents an overview of considerable ethical questions and Dahl tries to prove the ethical legitimacy of xenotransplantation, Schicktanz follows up methodically on Beauchamp and Childress by identifying common, middle principles underlying all animal ethical theories. In contrast to this approach, it is the object of this chapter to present the differences between the theories in order to enrich the discourse and open up different perspectives of animal ethical thinking, resulting in different ethical claims.

consideration of animal welfare, the anthropocentric position can remain unconsidered. The anthropocentric position is built on the denial of animal rights and of the human responsibility to ensure animal welfare and, consequentially, no animal ethical problems arise against this theoretical background. Therefore, the following sections focus on the four prominent bio- and pathocentric arguments that are being developed by Peter Singer, Tom Regan, Bernard E. Rollin and David DeGrazia.

20.3.1 Utilitarian Ethics – Peter Singer

Based on the idea that creatures are characterized through their sensitivity and their potential to experience suffering and pain, in his book *Animal Liberation* Singer argues for the moral consideration of all sentient creatures by extending Bentham's utilitarian theory to all sentient creatures. By making sensitivity and the capacity to suffer preconditions[8] for having interests, Singer includes all creatures in the ethical calculation, regardless of their status within the field of nature. Thereby, Singer tries to surmount the so-called speciesism[9] through the abolishment of species-defined frontiers. Based on the attribution of symmetry of interest of avoiding pain, Singer points out that the decision on the ethical legitimacy of alternative options for action must be based on balancing all interests relevant in the specific context in order to make sure that the option maximizing happiness and minimizing pain for the greatest possible number of all parties affected will be chosen. This theoretical adjustment opens up the discourse of legitimization and allows new criteria to function as the argumentative basis for the differentiation of rights. Instead of transferring criteria used for categorization in the area of biology to the field of ethics, Singer establishes new heuristic categories enabling ethical differentiation, namely the capacity for suffering and enjoyment, self-awareness and the ability to plan for the future.[10] Based on this categorization, Singer enables a controversial ethical hierarchy within the field of life, arguing that neither the right to live nor the right

[8] "The capacity for suffering and enjoyment is a prerequisite for having interests at all, a condition that must be satisfied before we can speak of interests in a meaningful way. [...] The capacity for suffering and enjoyment is, however, not only necessary, but also sufficient for us to say that a being has interests – at an absolute minimum, an interest in not suffering" Singer (2009, pp. 7–8).

[9] "Speciesism – the word is not an attractive one, but I can think of no better term – is the prejudice or attitude of bias in favor of the interests of members of one's own species and against those of members of other species. [...] If possessing a higher degree of intelligence does not entitle one human to use another for his or her own ends, how can it entitle humans to exploit nonhumans for the same purpose?" Singer (2009, pp. 6).

[10] In *Practical ethics*, published in 1979, Singer deepens the discussion of criteria being able to differentiate between various spheres of value of lives, thereby initiating a controversial discussion on the ethical status of humans with consciousness disorders and infants. As this chapter aims to present only those theoretical arguments that are relevant in the context of xenotransplantation, the reconstruction of Singer's arguments and the following discussion exceed the limits of this contribution. For detailed information presenting Singer's arguments as well as the arguments brought forward by his critics, see Jamieson (1999).

to live free from pain are bound to membership within the human species, but are connected to self-awareness and the capacity of suffering and enjoyment. Applying these utilitarian arguments to the context of xenotransplantation, it would be ethically illegitimate to cause suffering to or even kill animals being self-aware and able to experience pain, like pigs and non-human primates. Following Singer, alternative treatments must thus be investigated, while any scientific and political efforts being undertaken to implement xenotransplantation must be stopped. Although Singer's theory proves to be the most influential and publicly recognized contribution to animal ethics in the twentieth century, several other models based on hierarchical rather than egalitarian premises circulate within the ethical discourse, legitimizing ethical thinking in a different way. To introduce an alternative approach, based on deontological reflections, the following paragraphs will present Tom Regan's and Bernard Rollin's theses.

20.3.2 Deontological Ethics – Tom Regan

Although Peter Singer and Tom Regan agree on many points, such as the need to avoid speciesism, animal ethicist Tom Regan has been criticizing Singer's utalitarian theory for not completely ruling out the permission to kill addressees of moral concern in order to prevent many individuals from comparatively smaller harm[11] and for additionally making the rightness of institutions like chattel slavery contingent on circumstances as to whether they promote overall better consequences.[12] Answering this problem, amongst others, he has developed the rights-based approach in animal ethics in *The Case for Animal Rights* (1983). As he is one of the first and most represented proponents of this view, we summarize Tom Regan's theses in the following paragraph. The aim is again to examine what can be derived for the assessment of xenotransplantation if we follow the theory.

Tom Regan attributes an equal amount of inherent value to all "subjects-of-a-life",[13] thus granting them the right to be treated with respect.[14] Criteria for being "subjects-of-a-life" are, according to Regan, having "beliefs and desires; perception, memory, and a sense of the future, including their own future; an emotional life together with feelings of pleasure and pain; preference- and welfare-interests; the ability to initiate action in pursuit of their desires and goals; a psychophysical identity over time; and an individual welfare [...]."[15] Because all "subjects-of-a-life's" inherent value is to be respected, they should not be treated "as if their value was reducible to their possible utility relative to our interests [...]. Animals are not to

[11] Regan (1985a).

[12] Regan (2004, p. 211).

[13] "Since inherent value is conceived to be a categorical value, admitting of no degrees, any supposed relevant similarity must itself be categorical"Regan (2004, p. 24).

[14] Regan (2004, p. XXVIII).

[15] Regan (2004, p. 243).

be treated as mere receptacles or as renewable resources."[16] As this value does not come in degrees[17] and is not reducible to a possible utility relative to others' interests, sacrificing "subjects-of-a-life" for the greater good is only allowed when there are equally great individual harms to be weighted against each other; harming one "subject-of-a-life" severely (or overriding one of his/her rights in a way that would make him/her severely worse-off) as an alternative to harming many individuals modestly is not allowed, no matter how big the latters' number is.[18] This prevents Regan from making judgments such as those he criticizes in utilitarian accounts.[19]

There are some exceptions to the prima facie right not to be harmed that every "subject-of-a-life" possesses. As mentioned above, in cases where the only choice is to either inflict severe harm on one subject or to inflict the same amount of harm on several, Regan holds that the right of the one individual is to be overridden as stated in the "miniride principle."[20] Additionally, the harm of death according to him is bigger in grown healthy humans than it is in animals like dogs.[21] In the case that being a vegetarian would severely threaten one's health (which he assumes to be wrong on empirical grounds), he would even consider it permissible to eat meat.[22]

Those exceptions taken together might be interpreted as allowing a grown-up human to use animals' organs to prevent themselves from dying due to organ failure: in that equal amounts of harm-per-subject can be weighed between individuals, and that in the case of xenotransplantation at least one receiver is threatened by death while at least one animal has to be killed to save him/her, might imply that it is permitted to kill one individual to take his/her organs to save several others from death. If the harm of death to grown healthy dogs, which could be seen as being

[16] Regan (2004, p. 384).

[17] Regan (2004, p. 244).

[18] This is the so-called "worse-off principle." Regan (2004, p. XXIX).

[19] "The rights view will not allow this. To suppose that we can justify harming an innocent individual merely by aggregating the consequences for all those affected by the outcome is to treat that individual as if he were a receptacle and thus is contrary to the respect to which, as a possessor of inherent value, he is due as a matter of strict justice. If his right not to be harmed is to be overridden, it cannot be overridden merely on the grounds that doing so is necessary to produce optimal outcomes for everyone" Regan (2004, p. 312).

[20] "Special considerations aside, when we must choose between overriding the rights of many who are innocent or the rights of few who are innocent, and when each affected individual will be harmed in a prima facie comparable way, then we ought to choose to override the rights of the few in preference to overriding the rights of the many" Regan (2004, p. 305).

[21] However, "[t]he loss death represents must be determined on a case-by-case basis. When it is, death represents a greater loss in the case of some animals than it does in the case of some humans." Regan (2004, p. XIII). "[T]he rights view's analysis implies that the value of a life, like the harm represented by death, increases as the number and variety of possible sources of satisfaction increase" Regan (2004, p. XXIV).

[22] "If we were certain to ruin our health by being vegetarians, or run a serious risk of doing so [...] and given that the deterioration of our health would deprive us of a greater variety and number of opportunities for satisfaction than those within the range of farm animals, then we would be making ourselves, not the animals, worse-off if we became vegetarians. Thus might we appeal to the liberty principle as a basis for eating meat, assuming the other provisos of that principle were satisfied" Regan (2004, p. 337).

similarly worse-off than pigs if they are killed, is smaller than the harm of death to grown healthy humans, then the amount of harm-per-subject would be greater for the humans than for the pigs if they die. Permission for humans to eat meat if their health is severely threatened otherwise could amount to a permission to kill animals for health reasons, which would then make killing animals to harvest their organs to prevent humans from serious health threats permissible.

On the other hand, Regan is very clear about the inherent wrongness of institutions that treat animals merely as a means to an end.[23] He also holds that no one has a right to have maladies treated by others who do not voluntarily assume a role within the medical profession and that those who do so are not morally permitted to "override the basic rights [as the one to be treated respectfully] of others in the process." Regan has stated repeatedly that animal testing of products needs to be abolished.[24] We assume, based on Regan's view on animal testing, that the exceptions mentioned above do not extend to the industrial use of animals as a means to an end. This view is suggested by the fact that the emphasis in his statements about the abolition of animal experimentation lies on the wrongness of using animals as resources and merely valuing them for their utility to others.[25]

What follows for xenotransplantation depends on whether the animals used for xenografts can be viewed as displaying the properties that Regan states as criteria for being "subject-of-a-life" and hence, an empirical question. To Regan, the answer to this question is that at least normal grown-up mammals should be treated as "subjects-of-a-life" and neither used for research nor in any other harmful way that does not benefit themselves.

[23] "That position cannot be any more adequate than the assumption that animals are things and, relatedly, that they have value 'merely as a means to an end,' that end being man. The assumption that animals are things is false at best" Regan (2004, p. 182). "An important part of Regan's theory is that all forms of institutionalized exploitation of animals violate the respect and harm principles because they fail to treat individuals as possessing equal inherent value, and rely on some form of utilitarian or perfectionist thought" Francione (1995, p. 87).

[24] "I regard myself as an advocate of animal rights – as part of the animal rights movement. The movement, as I conceive it, is committed to a number of goals, including: the total abolition of the use of animals in science [...]" Regan (1985b, p. 179). "The rights view abhors the harmful use of animals in research *and calls for its total elimination*" Regan (2004, p. 397); emphasis in the original. "Because these animals are treated routinely, systematically as if their value were reducible to their usefulness to others, they are routinely, systematically treated with a lack of respect, and thus are their rights routinely, systematically violated" Regan (2004, p. 531). "In the case of the harmful use of animals in science [...], animals are coercively placed at risk of harm, risks they would not otherwise run, so that others might benefit. This coercive transference of risks, from others to these animals, when the animals themselves would not otherwise be at risk of suffering the harms imposed on them, is, as I explain at length in *The Case*, an indefensible violation of their right to be treated with respect" Regan (1985b).

[25] Gary Francione interprets similarly: "For Regan, exceptional cases *exclude* the institutionalized treatment of rightholders solely as means to the ends of others" Francione (1995, p. 87).

20.3.3 Deontological Ethics Based on Teleological Considerations – Bernard E. Rollin

One branch of the rights view is held by Bernard E. Rollin. He considers those living beings that have interests as proper addressees of moral concern. Those interests need to be discerned from pure needs. Rollin would hold a car to have needs such as oil, petrol, anti-freeze admixture and the like. Those individuals that we would hold to be aware of whether their needs are fulfilled or not, have interests. Interests can consist of the mere urge to avoid pain.[26] If an animal experiences pain, that is a sufficient condition for the claim that it has interests.[27] However, according to Rollin, experiencing pain is a sufficient, but not a necessary condition for having interests. Living beings that are not able to perceive pain still have interests in different domains.[28] To Rollin, then, it is obvious that dogs and monkeys for example have interests.[29] Rollin goes so far as to state that "animals have a basic [...] right [...] namely, *the right to be dealt with or considered as moral objects by any person who has moral principles* [...]." This right is absolute, invariable, and inalienable.[30] He adopts the Kantian notion that we must not treat any objects of moral concern merely as a means to an end.[31] In addition, we must not keep any objects of moral concern from satisfying their respective *telos.*[32] A *telos,*[33] according to Rollin, is "the set of needs and interests which are genetically based, and environmentally expressed, and which collectively define the "form of life" or way of living exhibited by that animal and whose fulfillment or thwarting matter to the animal."[34] Rollin is not completely opposed to the use of animals. He states, in accordance with the above-

[26] Rollin (1981, p. 38).

[27] According to Rollin, in terms of evolutionary fitness, pain only makes sense if, "a creature can be aware of it and bothered by it", Rollin (1981, p. 42). His main argument to ascribe pain to (at least vertebrate) animals is their having similar bodily mechanisms to human pain mechanisms and a continuity in the evolution of such mechanisms. Rollin (1989, p. 154).

[28] Rollin (1981, p. 38).

[29] Rollin (1981, p. 42).

[30] Rollin (1981, p. 47); emphasis in the original.

[31] Rollin (1981, p. 51).

[32] Rollin (2008); Rollin (1981, p. 53); Rollin (2006a, p. 284).

[33] Quoted after Rollin on his notion of *telos*: "Major discussions of telos in Aristotle occur in Physics, Book II, Chaps. 2, 3, 5, 7, 8; Politics, Book I, Chap. 2; Metaphysics, Book I, Chap. 3; De Anima, Book II, Chap. 4; On the Heavens, Book I, Chap. 4; Posterior Analytics, Book II, Chap. 11. My view of telos has been most influenced by J. H. Randall (1960), and by his lectures at Columbia, 1965–1968" Rollin (2008, p. 156).

[34] He later goes on to elaborate: "Since, as many (but not all) *biologists* have argued, we tend to see animals in terms of categories roughly equivalent to species, the *telos* of an animal will tend to be a characterization of the basic nature of a species. On the other hand, increased attention to refining the needs and interests of animals may cause us to further refine the notion of *telos* so that it takes cognisance of differences in the needs and interests of animals at the level of subspecies or races, or breeds, as well as of unique variations found in individual animals, though, strictly speaking, as Aristotle points out, individuals do not have natures, even as proper names do not have meaning" Rollin (2008, p. 409).

mentioned Kantian notion, that "[i]f animals are going to be raised for food, they must live, in balance, happy lives, or at least lives free from pain and suffering. [...] It is, as I hope to have shown, ethically timely to use our science and technology for the benefit of the animals we use, not merely for their exploitation."[35]

In his assessment of xenotransplantation,[36] Rollin mainly refers to intuitions and attitudes of the public when he evaluates the ethical permissibility of the different aspects of xenotransplantation.[37] About the harms of transferring viruses, based on the state of knowledge in 2006, he writes that, "[t]his is a serious concern, and one cannot envision a future for xenotransplantation until it is resolved."[38] In his article on genetic engineering, he remarked on genetic modification[39] that, although the *telos* of the modified animals might be changed along with their genetic endowment, he does not categorically oppose such changes as long as this does not lead to harm towards the animal.[40] Concerning the use of pigs for harvesting organs, he concludes that people are more concerned with animal treatment than with animal deaths recently and that, "[i]t is difficult to believe that a society that accepts the killing of pigs for bacon will cavil at their more painless killing to save humans."[41]

As long as the animals are treated according to their nature and needs, e. g. are not kept from their *tele*, Rollin is a proponent of an animal rights account, which is not opposed to xenotransplantation on animal ethical grounds.

20.3.4 The Coherence Model – David DeGrazia

David DeGrazia wants to transcend the utility-vs.-rights-debate[42] by building up a web of principles that is informed by intuitions,[43] the best arguments from different theories[44] and empirical knowledge.[45] This is why he commits to the coherence model, which relies in great parts on John Rawls' *Theory of Justice*. Starting with considered judgments[46] and finding those principles that match them best,[47] those

---

35 Rollin (2004, p. 18).

36 Rollin (2006b).

37 This methodology reflects his conviction that the "demand that science pause to engage common sense, at least in those areas where failure to do so may have dangerous moral consequences" is legitimate and his hope "to demonstrate [...] that ordinary common sense and experience, philosophically shaped, still have something to say to science [...]" Rollin (1989, p. 21/22).

38 Rollin (2006b, p. 209).

39 A practice widely used in the field of xenotransplantation.

40 Rollin (2008).

41 Rollin (2006b, p. 209).

42 De Grazia (1996, p. 9).

43 De Grazia (1996, p. 16).

44 De Grazia (1996, p. 26).

45 De Grazia (1996, p. 25).

46 Rawls (1999, p. 42); De Grazia (1996, p. 19).

47 Rawls (1999, p. 17/18); De Grazia (1996, p. 20).

principles are then revised using induction and deduction considering judgments on every level of generalization from single cases to principles or even theories, until a reflective equilibrium is reached.[48] This equilibrium, however, is not final but remains open to revision whenever new information makes it necessary.[49]

This set of norms is justified if it matches coherence criteria such as logical consistence, argumentative support by good, generalizable reasons, simplicity, intuitive plausibility and compatibility with one's overall beliefs.[50] One of the basic principles he comes up with is impartiality, deducible from the fact that in moral practice, norms should be supported by reasons that "could be accepted from any point of view."[51] Animals "who have desires, preferences, or concerns, or who are capable of suffering and enjoyment", to DeGrazia have interests. This is a good reason for ethics to be concerned with animals. As addressees of ethical theories, in his book *Taking Animals Seriously* from 1996, DeGrazia holds that animals' interests should be considered equal to human interests and the burden of proof lies on theorists that do not agree because they are likely to be biased towards the human point of view.[52] "Equal consideration", according to DeGrazia, "means in some way giving equal moral weight to the relevantly similar interests in different individuals."[53] Considered judgments on this basis are that it is prima facie wrong to cause anyone, including animals, suffering. Additionally, DeGrazia agrees with Regan and Rollin that "equal consideration [...] is incompatible – if extended to animals – with all views that see animals as essentially resources for our use."[54]

In his later paper *On the Ethics of Animal Research* (2007) however, he takes a more agnostic stance on the issue of whether animals should be granted equal consideration of their interests.[55] In this article, he summarizes the common implications of theories that consider animals as proper addressees of moral treatment, but assigns their relevantly similar interests either less or equal consideration as compared to human beings. Those implications concern animal research issues, but given the similar conflict structure between animal suffering and human health benefits as in xenotransplantation, can be transferred to xenotransplantation.

He sums up that:

1. There should be a massive public investment in alternatives research. [...]
2. Animal experiments should not be permitted where viable replacement alternatives are known to exist. [...]

[48] Rawls (1999, p. 18); De Grazia (1996, p. 13/14).

[49] ibid.

[50] De Grazia (1996, p. 16/17).

[51] De Grazia (1996, p. 27/28).

[52] De Grazia (1996, p. 53).

[53] De Grazia (1996, p. 46).

[54] De Grazia (1996, p. 47).

[55] In this paper, DeGrazia expounds "Equal consideration"(EC) views as well as "unequal consideration"(UC) views and states that, "In this chapter, I assume that both EC and UC theories are fairly reasonable and will not attempt to adjudicate between them" DeGrazia (2007, p. 691).

3. Where animal research is permitted, housing conditions must meet the basic needs – physical, psychological and social – of animal subjects. [...]
4. Great apes should not be used in research unless their participation is voluntary and/or compatible with the best interests of individual research subjects.[56,57]

The necessary (but possibly not sufficient) preconditions for allowing xenotransplantation should then, according to DeGrazia, be that, despite great investments, an alternative for replacing it has not been found; the basic needs of the animals involved are met; and no great apes are used if not voluntarily or for their own benefit.[58]

20.4 Concluding Remarks

Reflecting on the animal ethical concepts presented in this section, some concluding reflections regarding the animal ethics of xenotransplantation and the safeguarding of animal welfare can be pronounced. A plurality of well-considered ethical theories can be asserted, making it difficult to determine the 'right' ethical position and action or even the best suitable criteria for distinguishing between right and wrong. As argued above, the plurality encompasses different concepts of the relationship between men and animals (anthropocentric, biocentric and pathocentric), as well as diverse types of rationales for a special concept. Furthermore, if the perspective is expanded from the ethical discourse to society as a whole, plurality of attitudes, values and fundamental positions (e. g. anthropocentric, biocentric or pathocentric) can be considered as a mark of democratic societies.

This situation of conflict and complexity can be resolved in two different ways. One way is to regard plurality and complexity as a problem, which can be solved only by reducing plurality by arguing for the superiority of a special position. A solution which confronts the proponent with the challenge of justifying the superiority of his/her position. The second way is to accept plurality as an irreducible fact in ethics and society and establish procedures guaranteeing that a transparent and fair sociopolitical process of social self-understanding in the respective community or society can take place. Only if different societal groups representing various positions can participate in the public discourse, can a democratic process of decision-making be ensured and can the resulting decision claim ethical legitimacy.

---

[56] He illustrates this by stating that, "[T]he cognitive, emotional and social complexity of great apes suggests that they are 'borderline persons' who deserve protections comparable with those afforded to humans of uncertain personhood [...]. (The same is true for dolphins. But as it appears impossible to meet their basic needs while they are held captive, I reject any research on dolphins that maintains them in captivity longer than necessary to benefit the dolphin subjects themselves.)", DeGrazia (2007, p. 694), based on DeGrazia (2005, p. 40–53).

[57] DeGrazia (2007, pp. 689–695; summary, p. 694).

[58] As the coherence model is dynamic, this view might change with time.

Transferring these reflections from a general level to the concrete level of xenotransplantation as a developing medical practice, it is important for the societies concerned to start a process of public debate about how to evaluate the use of animals for xenotransplantation and about what it means for humans to receive animal organs. From an ethical point of view, that various practices, using animals including e. g. industrial livestock farming, consumption of meat and animal experiments, are widely accepted in society is per se no sufficient justification for xenotransplantation, as the pure fact that these practices are performed doesn't establish their ethical legitimacy. Accordingly, the problem of plurality can't be solved by recurring to a dominant and therefore apparently legitimate position. In the context of democratic societies regarding freedom of opinion and public discourse as guiding ideals, an alternative way to deal with the plurality of animal ethical positions represented in society has to be found. It is therefore necessary to establish binding procedures to ensure that every position can be heard publicly, in that a well-considered societal judgment can only be reached on the basis of a public discourse respecting the plurality of opinions and enabling various forms of participation.

References

Beauchamp, T. L., and J. F. Childress 2008. *Principles of biomedical ethics*. Oxford: Oxford University Press.

Dahl, E. 2000. *Xenotransplantation. Tiere als Organspender für Menschen?* Stuttgart: Hitzel.

DeGrazia, D. 1996. *Taking animals seriously*. Cambridge: Cambridge University Press.

DeGrazia, D. 2005. On the question of personhood beyond Homo sapiens, In *In Defense of animals: The second wave*, ed. Peter Singer, 40–53. Oxford: Blackwell Publishing.

DeGrazia, D. 2007. On the ethics of animal research, In *Principles of health care ethics*, ed. Richard E. Ashcroft et al., 2nd ed., 689–695, Chichester: Wiley.

Francione, G. 1995. Comparable harm and equal inherent value: The problem of dog in the lifeboat, *Between the Species* 11 (3): 81–89.

Grimm H. (ed.) 2003. *Xenotransplantation. Grundlagen – Chancen – Risiken*. Stuttgart: Schattauer.

Homann, K., and A. Suchanek 2000. *Ökonomik. Eine Einführung*. Tübingen: Mohr Siebeck.

Jamieson, D. 1999. *Singer and his Critics*. Hoboken: Wiley-Blackwell.

Jansen, B. E. S., and J. W. Simon, eds. 2008. *Xenotransplantation. Ethical, legal, economic, social, cultural and scientific background.* 1 vol. Saarbrücken: VDM Verlag.

McLean, S. A. M., and L. Williamson, eds. 2005. *Xenotransplantation: Ethics and law*. Aldershot: Ashgate.

Pies, I. 2009. Können Unternehmen Verantwortung tragen? Ein ordonomisches Gesprächsangebot an die philosophische Ethik. In *Moral als Produktionsfaktor. Ordonomische Schriften zur Unternehmensethik*, ed. I. Pies. Berlin: Wissenschaftlicher Verlag Berlin.

Randall, J. H. 1960. Aristotle. New York: Columbia University Press.

Rawls, J. 1999. *A theory of justice*. Cambridge: Harvard University Press.

Regan, T. 1985a. Reply to Peter Singer, the dog in the lifeboat: An exchange. *The New York Review of Books 32(7). New York.*

Regan, T. 1985b. The case for animal rights. In *Ethics: The essential writings* (Reprinted), ed. G. Marino, 531–544. New York: Modern Library.

Regan, T. 2004. *The case for animal rights*. Berkeley: University of California Press.

Rollin, B. E. 1981. *Animal rights and human morality*. Buffalo: Prometheus Books.

Rollin, B. E. 1989. *The unheeded cry*. Oxford: Oxford University Press.

Rollin, B. E. 2004. The ethical imperative to control pain and suffering in farm animals. In *The well-being of farm animals: Challenges and solutions*, ed. J. J. Benson and B. E. Rollin, 1–19. Ames: Blackwell Publishing.
Rollin, B. E. 2006a. *An Introduction to veterinary medical ethics: Theory and cases*, Ames: Blackwell Publishing.
Rollin, B. E. 2006b. *Science and ethics*, Cambridge: Cambridge University Press.
Rollin, B. E. 2008. On telos and genetic engineering. In *The animal ethics reader*, eds. S. J. Armstrong and R. G. Botzler, 407–414, 2nd ed. London: Routledge.
Schicktanz, S. 2002. *Organlieferant Tier? Medizin- und tierethische Probleme der Xenotransplantation*. Frankfurt a. M.: Campus.
Singer, P. 2009. *Animal liberation: The definitive classic of the animal movement*. New York: Harper Perennial.

Galia Assadi She studied Social Work at the University of Applied Sciences Munich and mastered in Sociology at the LMU. Subsequently, she completed her PhD in Philosophy at the LMU. Her main research interests lie on the intersection of sociology, philosophy and politics. Her focus is on the critical reflection on normative orders of modern society and feminist theory. Following the works of Michel Foucault, she is currently investigating the connection between modern economical, philosophical, political and psychiatric thinking.1,*,

Lara Pourabdolrahim received her M.A. in Philosophy, Art History and English Literature at Ludwig-Maximilians-University Munich in 2011. She started her PhD studies in neurophilosophy at the Graduate School of Systemic Neurosciences in October 2011. Her research interests are theory of evolutionary psychology, trolley dilemmas, cognition in moral situations, modularity, ethics, and renaissance philosophy. She is currently working on her PhD project "Are Trolley Dilemma Judgment Mechanisms Evolutionary Adaptations?

Georg Marckmann studied medicine and philosophy at the University of Tübingen (Germany) and received a master's degree in Public Health from Harvard School of Public Health (Boston, MA). He was a scholar in the Postgraduate College "Ethics in the Sciences and Humanities" in Tübingen from 1992 to 1995. He received a doctoral degree in medicine in 1997. From 1998 to 2010, he was Assistant Professor at the Institute of Ethics and History of Medicine at the University of Tübingen and since 2003 served as vice director of the institute. Since 2010, he is full professor of medical ethics and director of the Institute of Ethics, History, and Theory of Medicine at the Ludwig-Maximilians-University of Munich. His main research interests include ethical issues of end-of-life care, distributive justice in health care, ethical issues in organ transplantation and public health ethics.

Chapter 21
Xenotransplantation and Tissue Engineering Technologies: Safeguarding Their Prospects sans Sacrificing our Future

Jan-Ole Reichardt

21.1 Introduction

The availability of comprehensive health care services is of paramount importance to all of us. Given this critical interest and our high willingness to pay for individual survival, large amounts of public and private resources are continuously invested into the advancement of our medical capabilities. Those investments bring technologies within our reach that may soon help us to overcome some major challenges of today's regenerative medicine. At the same time, new capabilities produce new responsibilities and revolutionary breakthroughs enforce new dimensions of awareness, thoughtfulness, self-control and institutional guidance. For this reason, our bioscientific research is closely accompanied by medical ethicists who try to ensure a smooth transition of ideas into practice and try to safeguard our progression into a more capable and yet sustainable future.

This is particularly true for *xenotransplantation research*, where high hopes have been raised that the fatal resource gap of today's transplant medicine might be bridged in the not too distant future. Regarding these hopes, most resources are currently *bet* on the genetical adaptation of swine to our human needs: sufficiently high performance levels with regard to the transplant recipients and sufficiently low risk levels with regard to those recipients and their respective environments. However, before translational success might be proclaimed here, some demanding challenges are to be met first:

J.-O. Reichardt (✉)
Institute for Ethics, History and Theory of Medicine, University Münster, Münster, Germany
e-mail: jan-ole.reichardt@uni-muenster.de

R. J. Jox et al. (eds.), *Organ Transplantation in Times of Donor Shortage*, International Library of Ethics, Law, and the New Medicine 59,
DOI 10.1007/978-3-319-16441-0_21

(i) *Bioscientific challenges*, related to the medical aspects of xenotransplantation,
(ii) *Economic challenges*, related to the funding of the translational efforts and the prospects of return for the investing bodies, and
(iii) *Political challenges*, related to the regulation of future xenotransplantation therapies and products.

The third set includes all legal, ethical, cultural and administrative aspects of the translational process. The present analysis is focused on the ethical challenges. It discusses a special form of externalities—some uncommon risks that are to be shouldered by uninvolved parties and the public. Its recommendations are given with the intent to eliminate unnecessary delays and to insure the protagonists' motivation to invest adequate amounts into quality control and risk mitigation.

21.2 Who Would Benefit and Who Would Suffer if Xenotransplants Became Available?

Technological developments described as *progress* usually have a positive cost-benefit ratio for its end-users, but can also come with net costs to others. The following part provides an overview about the stakeholders of xenotransplant medicine. The following cost and benefit prospects are neither exclusive, nor are most of them specific to the deployment of xenotransplant therapies. They are brought together to provide a more complete understanding of the translational scenario and its presumably supporting and objecting stakeholders and thereby ease our judgment of this development's legitimacy.

(A) It is undisputed that our medical system lacks the resources to treat all its patients with chronic organ failure and that we therefore are in need of additional organ substitutes with sufficient functional capabilities. The stem cell focused research in the field of regenerative medicine seems capable of closing these resource gaps over the next 20 years.[1] But until these presumably less invasive treatments become available, genetically engineered xenotransplants could offer some interim solutions, if their own bioscientific challenges were solved prior to this.[2] In that

[1] The potential of future stem cell based organ transplants has very recently been shown by Takebe et al. (2013), who provided a proof-of-concept demonstration of the generation of a vascularized and functional human liver from organ-buds that were transplanted into mice after their prior in vitro creation from human induced pluripotent stem cells (iPSCs). The potential of a more regenerative therapeutical approach has also been demonstrated—see for example the work of Yui et al. (2012).

[2] See Ekser et al. (2009, p. 87): "Xenotransplantation is a potential answer to the current organ shortage. Its future depends on: (1) further genetic modification of pigs, (2) the introduction of novel immunosuppressive agents that target the innate immune system and plasma cells, and (3) the development of clinically-applicable methods to induce donor-specific tolerance." Others think that these challenges might be overcome in the not too distant future and that our arrival at that point would be a plain question of money expenditures, for example Petersen et al. (2009, p. 101): "The techniques for introducing beneficial genes or removing undesired genes are avail-

case, *all patients with chronic organ failure* (waiting for a respective transplant) would benefit: either directly, via xenotransplantation, or indirectly, via a reduced waiting time for the ordinary allograft.

(B) At the same time, not only current patients, but *all those with financial access to the transplant system* would statistically benefit from the availability of an additional transplant source, because it would raise their own prospects of survival should they suffer from chronic organ failure in the future.

(C) higher availability of transplants and a more controllable provision of those transplants would allow the *organizations that provide the transplant services* (hospitals, transportation and logistics) to maximise their efficiency by a reduction of idle time and a volume boost of scheduled transplantations. This would reduce their costs per patient and thereby allow them to bill less per case, cross-finance less profitable activities or distribute higher earnings to their *shareholders* if run on a for-profit basis.

(D) An increasing number of transplants would also benefit those individuals who are actively involved in the provision of transplant services: the so-called *transplant community*. It would increase the demand for their expertise, thereby enhancing job security, increasing their bargaining position in salary negotiations and their bonus payments in case of revenue-related salaries.

(E) Those who would produce the yet to become bedside-ready xenotransplants would also profit: *the emergingbiotech industry* that developed over the past 30 years in the field of regenerative medicine and that has to be differentiated from the medical device industry and the pharmaceutical industry (although not necessarily with regard to ownership and control).[3]

(F) As long as xenotransplants would require a complex regime of pharmaceutical immunosuppression, *the pharmaceutical industry* would also benefit from an increasing demand of new long-term customers. And as some insiders—on condition of anonymity—suggested in personal conversation, this group would financially profit the most from the availability of new xenotransplant therapies.

(G) The last group of beneficiaries would only benefit under very special circumstances: *the for-profit health care insurance industry*. They would profit from new therapies if they were cheaper than their current equivalents (like a kidney transplantation in comparison to a continuous dialysis treatment), but would suffer losses from medically preferable but more expensive therapies (like a heart or liver transplant in comparison to the patient's sad but financially inexpensive death). Non-profit oriented health insurance funds would neither benefit nor lose, but their two important tasks to keep health care services top-notch and as affordable as possible, could mislead their administrations to deploy *rationing* principles in addition to their actual task of *rationalisation*. Although the decisions about rationing in health care are tasks that are exclusive to the political representatives of the insured, the administrative body could be misled to weigh the potential benefits of some

able, but genetic modification of pigs and testing of these modifications in nonhuman primates is a very expensive and time- and labour-consuming interdisciplinary endeavour."

[3] For further information on the industry's development, see Nerem (2010).

against the potential costs to the whole community of the insured and to judge the cost-benefit ratio of xenotransplants as *imbalanced* or *economically unfavourable* without any legitimization to do so. Neither would respective cost savings qualify as *benefits*, nor would respective payments qualify as *losses*.

(H) The first group of loss sufferers would consist of *those animals that would function as transplant sources* and from which the tissue parts, cells and organs would be harvested for transplantation purposes. This analysis doesn't support an attitude of ignorance towards animals and their human-induced suffering. Instead, it argues that as long as a large majority accepts animal consumption not only for scientific experiments (and for *the greater good*), but also for culinary delights and the sheer joy of wearing leather clothes, as long as that doesn't change, the legitimacy of animal consumption for the rescue of human lives should not be questioned. For that reason, the potential suffering of animals due to new techniques of xenotransplantation will not be taken into account in the following parts.

(I) The second group of net losers would consist of *the large fraction of the community ofpeople who are insured who*—from an ex-post perspective—*will never need an organ transplant* but will nevertheless have to pay for the costs of those who do. They might not qualify as loss sufferers in the proper sense, since this situation is exactly what insurance funds are invented for: to protect the insured against the financial fiasco of an improbable but expensive event's actual occurrence. Some of the insured might nevertheless suffer *statistical losses* if an expensive treatment gets covered, but their individual risk level to develop a condition where they would finally profit from the availability of expensive treatments is much lower than those of other community members, and the associated savings are not deducted from their personal contribution to the insurance fund. On the other hand, a deliberate omission of risk-based cost adjustments can also be interpreted as a genuine act of solidarity—and to one-sidedly call these a *personal loss* or *bad deal* seems to imply a rejection of solidarity. However, some very healthy people could nevertheless regard the availability of (expensive) xenotransplant therapies as annoying.

(K) Then, there might be those who are insured, who will develop symptoms of chronic organ failure in the future, will get a xenotransplant in time but would have gotten an even better allotransplant, if xenotransplants were still unavailable then. But, since becoming worse off in that specific way would require a lot of genuine bad luck, this allocation issue is almost irrelevant. And bad luck in a fair lottery, where nobody knows one's outcome in advance, provides no justification for those who become worse off later on to complain about specific measures that actually increase everyone's expected utility prior to the draw. So *the unlucky few, who would end up with a worse transplant in an era of xenotransplantation than they would today*, aren't an ethical hurdle to the progress of transplant medicine. And in most cases, they will not even know that they would be better off under counterfactual conditions.

(L) Those *commercially involved in the provision of transplant services that become obsolete* by the introduction of medical innovations also lose—namely the profitability of their existing investments (in expertise and technology): for example, those who deliver artificial heart assist or replacement devices, those who deliver or deploy haemodialysis devices, the pharmaceutical producers of insulin analogues and so on. But investments into treatment capabilities do not come with moral claim rights to an omission of progress beyond the status quo, while other people's suffering might well impose some prima facie duties to allow and support relief promising changes. For that reason, economic losses of medical progress are in themselves morally irrelevant.

(M) The last group of negatively affected stakeholders suffers an increase in exposure-related risks. Although this group includes every human on this planet, some would be more exposed and some would be more vulnerable to the threat. These risks accrue to us from the possible existence, evolution and spread of xenozoonotic pathogens—a possible side effect, specific to the transplantation of animal cells, tissue parts and organs into human bodies. These side effects threaten the transplanted as well as their *innocent bystanders* (who have nothing to do with this particular transplantation and have not consented to any risk exposures in advance). For that reason, a patient's informed consent to her xenotransplant therapy is not enough to justify her bystander's risk increase and special attention to this problem is required to reach both: translational success and the moral legitimacy of this translation. The following parts of this analysis focus on these third person risks, which represent the by far most important (if not only relevant) *ethical* challenge to xenotransplantation's translational success.

21.3 Third Person Risks—What do we Know?

To debate the acceptability of third person risks and the adequacy of risk-mitigating measures, a profound analysis of these risks is paramount. So what makes these risks so special? What do we know about such unintended side effects? As we will soon see, truthful answers to these questions might illuminate the topic at hand, but without a satisfactory disclosure of the facts we're after. The reason for this dissatisfaction is that the risks at hand are of unknown probability and severity.[4] On the other hand, we *do* know some aspects of those risks involved: The perceived dangers consist of the possibility that immunosuppressed patients with porcine organ transplants could function as bioreactors, breeding new cross-species pathogens, thus causing outbreaks of zoonotic diseases. This idea is based on the fact that xenotransplanted patients lose the repellent effects of two bodily barriers between their human tissue and the transplanted animal graft. Furthermore, the presumably necessary pharmaceutical suppression of their bodies' graft rejection will simultaneously suppress their immune response capabilities, transforming a body's hos-

[4] Compare Bruine de Bruin et al. (2009, p. 1…9): "As with other novel technologies, if xenotransplantation is to be judged fairly, proponents must explain its complex, uncertain, and unfamiliar risks and benefits. Xenotransplantation's risks include the possibility of a recombinant virus infecting human transplant recipients, potentially causing an epidemic of an unfamiliar disease. […] However, because the actual probability of these events is unknown, the accuracy of [our evaluational] judgments cannot be evaluated."

tile environment for infectious agents into *fertile soil* for hazards. This is a rough sketch of the threats we might face, if the transplantation of xenografts becomes a widely used standard therapy in the not too distant future. But at the moment, this basic idea is just a hypothetical scenario without empirical plausibility and bears no moral weight when actual lives are at stake. To demonstrate that this idea is not an *empty challenge*, some evidence has to be given to support its plausibility and thereby its ethical relevance claim. And indeed, the perception of these dangers is neither rooted in mere paranoia, nor in technophobes' apocalyptic fantasies. On the contrary: there is a well-documented history of species-crossing pathogens and their causation of *zoonotic diseases*. As Taylor et al. (2001, p. 983) demonstrated, a sometimes one- sometimes multidirectional pathogen transmission between humans and one or more animal species is quite common, since more than 60 % of all human diseases currently known to us are caused by species-crossing pathogens.[5] And as Karesh et al. (2012) highlighted, their negative impact on human well-being can hardly be overestimated:

> The greatest burden on human health and livelihoods, amounting to about 1 billion cases of illness and millions of deaths every year, is caused by endemic zoonosis that are persistent regional health problems around the world. Many of these infections are enzootic (i.e., stably established) in animal populations, and transmit from animals to people with little or no subsequent person-to-person transmission [.] Other zoonotic pathogens can spread efficiently between people once introduced from an animal reservoir, leading to localized outbreaks (e.g., Ebola virus) or global spread (e.g., pandemic influenza) (Karesh et al. 2012, p. 1936 f).

Although only a few of these (and some yet unknown) pathogens might be of relevance in xenotransplant cases, current research on the emergence of new diseases emphasizes the close connection between new infectious agents and changes in the relationship between humans and wildlife, mediated by livestock animals. As Pearce-Duvet (2006) puts it:

> Agriculture may have changed the transmission ecology of pre-existing human pathogens, increased the success of pre-existing pathogen vectors, resulted in novel interactions between humans and wildlife, and, through the domestication of animals, provided a stable conduit for human infection by wildlife diseases (Pearce-Duvet 2006, p. 369).

The surveys of Jones et al. (2013) confirm this observation. They found several examples in which an increase in the intensity of our interaction with livestock and wildlife was associated with an increasing risk of zoonotic disease emergence. For this reason, they regard these intensifications as major factors with regard to the development of new diseases:

> Expansion of agriculture promotes encroachment into wildlife habitats, leading to ecosystem changes and bringing humans and livestock into closer proximity to wildlife and vectors, and the sylvatic cycles of potential zoonotic pathogens. This greater intensity of interaction creates opportunities for spillover of previously unknown pathogens into livestock or humans and establishment of new transmission cycles (Jones et al. 2013, p. 8399).

[5] Taylor et al. (2001, p. 983): "A comprehensive literature review identifies 1415 species of infectious organisms known to be pathogenic to humans [.] Out of these, 868 (61 %) are zoonotic, that is, they can be transmitted between humans and animals [.]"

Swine can be regarded as an archetypical livestock animal and the transplantation of porcine cells, tissue parts and organs into human bodies does indeed qualify as an intensification of our relationship with this species. Furthermore, swine—or swine cells, tissue parts and organs—are, with regard to some zoonotic pathogens, less resistant to an infection than humans. At the same time, infected swine are a known source of pathogen recombination, regularly giving rise to new breeds of influenza. For this reason, Ma et al. (2009) recommend a thorough prevention strategy regarding possible contact of swine with infectious agents:

> Although HPAIV H5N1 viruses have been transmitted directly to man, it may be that some species of carnivores could act as an intermediate host as they are quite susceptible to infection with this subtype [.] In the case of swine, empirical and experimental evidence demonstrates swine can generate novel influenza A viruses that have the potential to infect humans and some avian species. At present, it is difficult to predict which virus, if any, might induce a human pandemic. History would suggest that the likelihood of such an event is low; however, it seems prudent to minimize the risk of transmission of swine viruses to people as well as minimize the risk of transmission of novel viruses to swine (Ma et al. 2009, p. 332).

This seems plausible, but the minimization of a xenotransplant's pathogen exposure is easier planned than done. Moreover, as Millard and Mueller (2010) put it, infections of the human body are almost inevitable during a xenograft's operating life and some infections of the xenograft as well:

> Reactivation of latent human viruses or new infection will inevitably occur in prospective recipients of xenografts. Emerging data challenge the concept of species-specificity for human viruses considered strictly adapted to their host. These pathogens may have the potential to infect a porcine xenograft resulting in tissue alterations and damage (Millard and Mueller 2010, p. 9).

So the history of the emergence of new zoonotic diseases does indeed provide some reasons to worry about unintended side effects of porcine xenotransplants. On the other hand, a lot of research was done to identify the yet unknown and to eliminate the already suspected risk factors of zoonotic infections. As Millard and Mueller emphasize, these endeavors were quite successful:

> With the exception of endogenous retroviruses and porcine lymphotropic herpesvirus, exclusion of known pathogens was successful and has eliminated a majority of donor pathogens [.] (Millard and Mueller 2010, p. 6).

A lot of effort has been put into the sustainable deactivation of porcine endogenous retroviruses (PERV), but since some PERVs are part of every pig genome and at least for now too difficult to remove, there is no once-and-for-all solution available yet.[6] Anyhow, as Scobie et al. (2013) reported, not a single incident of PERV infection could be found in patients, which have already been treated with porcine xenografts for at least some weeks:

> [Our] results provided no evidence of PERV transmission or presence of specific anti-PERV [antibodies] in [burn patients who had received living pig-skin dressings for up to 8 weeks], consistent with previous studies [.] (Scobie et al. 2013, p. 2909).

---

[6] See Denner et al. (2009, p. 239) and Denner and Tönjes (2012).

While these risks of PERV infection might be a lesser hurdle than previously assumed, another one remains: the risk of unknown pathogens which could succeed in hiding their infectiousness throughout any reasonable period of quarantine, as Denner and Tönjes (2012) point out:

> At present, it is possible that a still unknown microorganism is transmitted from pigs to human xenotransplant recipients or from other animals via pigs to humans. Nevertheless, the probability is extremely low, assuming that such transmission would have been observed much earlier due to the close contact between pigs and humans over a long time. Thanks to improvements in virus diagnostics, new, previously unknown viruses have been described for pigs, but most of them are nonpathogenic. Some examples are new paramyxoviruses, tiomanviruses, and kobuviruses. It is almost impossible to develop systematic strategies to detect such unknown viruses and other microorganisms, e.g., by coculture of human and pig cells and screening for cytotoxic effects (Denner and Tönjes 2012, p. 334).

So for all we know, it is still possible that some widely unsuspicious microorganisms unveil their negative impact on our health only after it's too late to prevent a nightmare scenario. Of course, the relationship between humans and their livestock has been a close one for a long time, although not as close as it will become in an era of xenotransplantation. In the end, only time (and respective experiments) will tell, if those 'extremely low probabilities' are indeed as low as they seem to some of us now—as Denner and Tönjes acknowledge:

> The efficacy and safety of xenotransplantation will be shown—according to the proverb "the proof of the pudding is in the eating"—in the first clinical trials. The ongoing study of pig islet transplantation to diabetic individuals in New Zealand, the first clinical study officially approved by a governmental regulatory authority, in 2009, will be one of the first steps on the way to the clinical application of xenotransplantation [.] Pig heart and kidney transplantation may follow, using the experience obtained during the first islet cell trials. Immunological, microbiological, and physiological hurdles may be overcome step by step (Denner and Tönjes 2012, p. 335).

Knowing that every xenotransplant would increase the probability of an emerging new infectious agent—be it by viral cross-over, be it by graft-induced exposure to the patient—only their clinical usage will tell us if the suspected improbability of large scale pandemics and other dystopian scenarios is indeed sufficiently small enough to justify this technology's deployment. In that we can neither quantify nor qualify the occurring risks as cogently as we would have to in order to truly understand what we are dealing with exacerbates our assessment of the technology at hand. But this kind of uncertainty is a well-known one in the area of technology assessment, where it impedes our understanding of the circumstances at hand and becomes—as Gethmann (2000, p. VII) puts it—"a real dilemma for those moral philosophers who strive for a rational evaluation of new technologies not *ex post*, but *ex ante*." Sadly, this lack of information doesn't legitimize a blunt prima facie ignorance of the yet unknown, because—as Hüsing et al. (2001) stated correctly, to rashly regard the hypothetical as basically irrelevant is a pragmatic fallacy:

> The lack of knowledge regarding some individual factors or causal relationships is part of the risk itself, and it would be wrong to conclude from its hypothetical nature or not given quantifiability alone that it's probably improbable (Hüsing et al. 2001, p. 209).

At the same time, we aren't totally blind. We can at least base our policy decisions on our experts' *informed uncertainty* and their *gut feelings* regarding the possible outcomes. But unfortunately, their expertise comes at a price: their deep involvement in the development of xenografts means that even if they try to be impartial in their counseling and filter their intuitions accordingly, their involvement might lead to an overly optimistic attitude. At least this is one of the lessons learned from nuclear energy research, asbestos usage in construction, the planning of military *humanitarian interventions* and so on. Where big money is involved and big profits are to be earned and where people are betting their future on a project's success, an optimistic attitude regarding the long-term harmlessness of their 'baby' shouldn't surprise us. Therefore, the translation of xenotransplants—like the deployment of any other potentially hazardous technology—asks for a well-designed regulatory framework to protect the public from an optimism bias and the additional delusiveness of an almost omnipresent strategy of "Positive Thinking" that Ehrenreich (2009) described so tellingly in her diagnosis of the American Society. And that framework has to be put into life soon, since in 2009, the biotech company *Living Cell Technologies* (LCT) already started its first clinical xenotransplantation trials in New Zealand. Focusing on the safety and efficacy of their commercial product DIABECELL®, they transplanted encapsulated islet cells of porcine origin to fourteen human patients with type 1 diabetes mellitus. And as the LCT scientists around Garkavenko et al. (2012) report, although pig cellular material was found in several patients' blood, no virus transmission (including PERV) could be found. Beyond these satisfying results, the mere conduct of the study highlights a point already made by Bach et al. (1998), namely the fact that we seem unable to refrain from gambling if great individual rewards are at stake and the involved risks are too abstract and of only hypothetical nature:

> The history of medical innovation has shown us unwilling to resist tangible individual benefit even in the face of unknown risks. It is incumbent upon us now to prepare for the moment when the decision to begin organ xenotransplantation will be well-nigh irresistible (Bach et al. 1998, p. 144).

By 2014, LCT's translation of cell-based xenografts had reached Phase IIb, with plans to release a finalized product in 2016.[7] While LCT's reports on the avoidability of xenozoonosis are indeed optimistic, a potentially less optimism biased counsel on the recent developments in xenotransplantation research is difficult to obtain, since the information providing institutions fell victim to the cuts (or changed focus again) after they provided a status report at the peak of xenotransplant medicine's hype cycle more than 10 years ago. Those institutions were (among others and each with its most recent publication on xenotransplantation) the German Federal Parliament Committee 19 (2000), the German Medical Association's Scientific Advisory Board on Xenotransplantation (1999), the Nuffield Council on Bioethics' Working Party on Xenografts (1996), and the U.S. Food and Drug Administration's Xenotransplantation Guidance (2003). At the same time, the WHO (2004) "urged"

[7] See www.lctglobal.com.

its member states to collaborate and coordinate their efforts for "the prevention and surveillance of infections resulting from xenogeneic transplantation," but better funding of national and international health institutions (like the German Robert Koch Institute (RKI)) to provide the respective surveillance services has not kept pace with the funding of xenotransplantation research itself. Priority has been given to the product and not to its risk management, so far. So it seems as if a *business as usual* approach and a passive attitude towards the recent developments in xenotransplantation research are widespread, although an industry driven by financial expectations and a *pragmatic* optimism bias with regard to its caused externalities should not be left alone to proceed at will and as desired. Instead of *waiting it out* it seems more reasonable to develop a protective strategy that keeps both our aims in focus and balance: the health of those who are in need of organ substitutes and our very own health that we should protect from excessive risks. Since being too strict or too careless could both cost too much, the next part asks for the right balance of optimism and pessimism with regard to new and potentially hazardous technologies with great benefit prospects, like xenotransplantation medicine.

21.4 Benefit Optimism and Disaster Pessimism—is There a Right Balance?

To act reasonably when doomsday scenarios are involved requires *the right* amount of precaution: one that lets us refrain from irresponsibly reckless ventures but allows and motivates the realization of those benefits that are within reach of responsible interventions. But where those lines between reasonable and unreasonable or responsible and irresponsible actions are to be drawn is far from obvious. The heading under which these questions of judgement have recently been discussed is called *theprecautionary principle* and some bioethicists base very cautious recommendations on this principle.[8] The following part explores this principle's potential to provide sound advice with regard to the question at hand. So what is meant with this notion of a precautionary principle? As Rath (2012) demonstrates, caution is advised whenever this *principle* is mentioned, because it has different possible interpretations and comes with different duties attached:

> While the weak version suggests that scientific uncertainty should not be a ground for refusing counteractive measures, the strong one obliges the decision maker to implement a risk reaction, even if no clear evidence is available as to how such a reaction would influence the risk situation (or other situations). [...] In the course of events, when further information on the risk situation in question is gained, the implemented reactions have to be evaluated and possibly adjusted. Hence, the precautionary principle [...] implies a duty to [...] continuously reconsider the decision made at an earlier stage. This is the reason why the precautionary principle is best understood as a dynamic decision process rather than a fixed principle (Rath 2012, p. 22 f).

[8] Extensively discussed in Paslack et al. (2012).

What the weak version claims is almost self-evident, but it requires too little to reach a sound regulation of xenotransplantation. The strong version seems to come in two flavors—*strong* and *ultra*:

> The first type allows continuing the course of action but the agent is obliged to implement accompanying risk reducing measures. The second type prohibits the risky course of action until the scientific uncertainty disappears and it is secured that the socially chosen level of security is met [.] (Rath 2012, p. 17).

In the case of xenotransplantation, there is no non-risky option, because to refrain from a therapy isn't *safe* for those in need, who could be saved with the help of that therapy. Here, the risk-averse scenario of *ultra precautiousness* asks for a consequentialist sacrifice of the needy for the sake of a supposedly larger group of xenozoonosis victims. For letting that *supposedly* larger group exceed and outweigh those *actually* in need, a good dosage of pessimism regarding the probability of such a dystopic scenario is needed. At this point, it might be difficult to convince others of one's ultra-pessimistic expectations, and it seems much easier to argue for a less pessimistic precautionary approach that asks only for an implementation of accompanying risk-reducing measures (the *strong* flavour of the precautionary principle). Taking that path, it no longer becomes necessary to justify the actual sacrifice of real patients for the sake of an only hypothetically larger group of only hypothetical victims. One wouldn't have to give up on pessimism either and there would be much room left for one's personal expectations with regard to xenotransplantation. One could easily ask for the amount of risk-reducing security measures that would actually correspond to one's level of pessimism. But how much pessimism would be a compelling level not only to us but to others as well? How much pessimism gets us the most plausible position? Are there any meta-arguments to judge what can't be judged from within? While some arguments were given to put a potentially optimism-biased counselling back into perspective, it's also paramount to avoid a pessimism-biased position that we might feel attracted to. Since disastrous worst-case scenarios have their own narrative beauty, they tend to be (story-wise) more compelling versions of their more moderate alternatives. But the better novel is not to be conflated with the more reasonable approach regarding the regulation of risky technologies. So while we should stay aware of an optimism bias of those involved in the development of xenografts, we shouldn't be less attentive with regard to a bumbledom tendency to exaggerate this topic's importance by opting for the highly dramatic scenario. Of course it's still possible to follow one's optimistic or pessimistic expectations to the extreme, but before we do so, we should check first that we haven't fallen victim to one of the two manipulative mechanisms.

21.5 Putting the Risks of Xenotransplantation into Perspective

After having done that, and for as long as neither chronic pessimists nor strong optimists can be proven plainly right or wrong, it might be helpful to put our xenotransplant stories into perspective by highlighting other real-life risk factors that we and our health are already exposed to. This is in itself a somehow manipulative approach, and although the disclosure of an already existing leak in a lifeboat does not justify the drilling of another albeit smaller hole, it helps to redirect our attention to some more urgent threats to public health if we are interested in safeguarding our future. One of these problems is the continuous emergence and facilitated spread of antimicrobial resistance that "demands concerted efforts from multiple health and industry sectors in both developed and developing countries, as well as the strengthening of multinational/international partnerships and regulations" as DiazGranados and McGowan (2009, p. 1274) put it. This problem is facilitated by a widespread usage of antibiotics for animals and crops, as Shlaes (2010, p. 16) reports:

> At least half of all the antibiotic use in the United States is for animals and crops. This has been a controversial topic for over 30 years. [...] Nobody knows to this day why low doses of antibiotics make animals grow faster, but it's true. They grow about 4–8% faster than animals not fed on low dose antibiotics.

And while our current antibiotics are overcome by an increasing number of pathogens, our market-driven system of pharmaceutical research fails to provide the necessary incentives for large pharmaceutical companies to invest in the research of replacement substances.[9] At the same time, a global coordination of regulatory measures to prevent the worst is lacking behind:

> One area of obvious restriction in the distribution of antibiotics is their use for growth promotion in animal husbandry. This was suggested with great foresight in 1969 by a report presented to the British government by a committee chaired by M. M. Swann. It took almost 40 years, however, for these ideas to be translated into legislation in Europe. In the United States, rules in this area are still awaiting realization (Sköld 2011, p. 192 f).

Gastmeier et al. (2010) estimate that 400,000–600,000 hospital-acquired infections occur in Germany every year, but Walger et al. (2013, p. 335) argue convincingly that these numbers are far too low and closer to 1,000,000, with an average lethality rate of 2–7% (USA 100,000 of 1.7 million = 5.9%, UK 6.7%), resulting in 20,000–70,000 deaths by nosocomial infection per year in Germany. A lot of these infections should (and could) be avoided in the first place, but it would also help to protect our capabilities to fight these infections whenever they occur. But while thousands of lives are lost every year, regulatory activities to curb the most significant sources of pathogen resistance proceed at snail speed. Under these circumstances of unnecessary deaths and unprevented dying, it becomes pointless to fear a dystopian scenario with regard to xenotransplantation, since there are less hypothetical man-made disasters in the works already. Knowing that there are indeed more imminent threats to public health than xenotransplants makes it more difficult to lightheartedly sacrifice the survival of thousands for better protection against zoonotic diseases of a hypothetical nature. And it can make it easier to proceed with the respective research as long as we know that xenotransplants might pose a threat to public health, but a relatively unimportant one if compared to the other apocalyptic riders mentioned above. At the same time, this should not lead to flip-

[9] See Shlaes and Projan (2009, p. 49).

pancy, since a careful translation of risky technologies is still advisable. What such a careful approach could look like is the leading question of the next and final part.

21.6 Discussion—Shaping our Institutions in Accordance to our Needs

As the strong precautionary principle demands, the risks of questionable technologies and our respective options to handle them should constantly be re-evaluated. At least in this regard, a precautionary principle seems plausible and acceptable. In the case of xenotransplant medicine, the option to long-term quarantine xenotransplanted patients has already been rejected on the basis of a sound reasoning by Beckmann et al. (2000), since such measures would fail to respect the dignity of the transplanted by impairing their self-determination and would—beyond that—also be so overly expensive that comprehensive quarantine scenarios are unrealistic options. At the same time, Beckmann's recommendation to refrain from xenotransplant therapies, if these quarantine measures were regarded as unbearably cruel,[10] would be heartless towards the needy and unrealistic with regard to the probability of such reservations as Bach et al. (1998, p. 144) suggested when they stated that "The history of medical innovation has shown us unwilling to resist tangible individual benefit even in the face of unknown risks." Therefore, a strategy is needed that accepts the translation of xenotransplant medicine into clinics while constraining its hazardous potential as much as possible. Such a strategy should also provide the necessary means for the risk-reducing measures it recommends, because without the necessary funding, nothing will ever happen.

My recommendations aim at a continuous assessment of xenotransplant technologies as recommended by the favoured interpretation of the precautionary principle and a minimally invasive surveillance of xenotransplant patients to protect them and the public against a sudden lack of funding and the following disruption of postoperative monitoring. If every transplant would come with a fee attached that could be interpreted as a contribution to something like a liability insurance fund (in the broadest sense), the necessary funding for an international network of biosecurity experts would seem within reach. Such a network could be established by already existing national institutions (like the German *Robert Koch Institute*) and already existing transnational institutions (like the *World Health Organization*) and opened up—in addition to xenotransplantation medicine—to agriculture and farming as well as all the other players whose potentially negative contributions to public health should be targeted and taxed (as Rothblatt 2004 recommends) or liability insured. Since the idea behind such an obligatory *Biosecurity Fund* is not that

[10] See Beckmann et al. (2000, p. 259): "If [the quarantine related restrictions of our social life and our personal freedom] would exceed the limits of acceptability, it does not follow that the protection of other people's lives should be suspended, but that a transition to the clinic would be unjustifiable given these conditions." [Translation by the author.]

of an indulgence fee, but of a flexible amount that corresponds to recommendable safeguarding actions, which become necessary given the respective action, the fee could increase or shrink with regard to the agent's transparency level and his other contributions to our biosecurity. The fund should provide emergency prophylaxis and support the already existing national bodies. Its most important aim should be the identification of potential outbreaks, the communication of anything that might be related to such an outbreak and the initiation of an adequate reaction to such outbreaks in a very timely manner. To reach those aims, national and international infrastructures have to be closely intertwined and have to be well equipped with qualified manpower—thus generating costs that have to be dealt with by the insurance fees of all xenotransplantations and otherwise risky actions. Given the desirability of such a system, the next step should elaborate on its pragmatic hurdles and sketch, in more detail, what this kind of *Biosecurity Fund* could look like and how it should be structured to reach the aim of a sustainable translation of even those technologies that could otherwise come at a prize that would be too steep for all of us.

References

Bach, Fritz H., et al. 1998. Uncertainty in Xenotransplantation: Individual benefit versus collective risk. *Nature Medicine* 4 (2): 141–144. doi:10.1038/nm0298-1418.

Beckmann, Jan P., et al. 2000. *Xenotransplantation of cells, tissues or organs. Scientific developments and ethico-legal implications. Xenotransplantation von Zellen, Geweben oder Organen. Wissenschaftliche Entwicklungen und ethisch-rechtliche Implikationen.* Berlin: Springer.

Bruine de Bruin, Wändi, et al. 2009. Communicating about xenotransplantation: Models and scenarios. *Risk Analysis* 29 (8): 1–11. doi:10.1111/j.1539-6924.2009.01241.x.

Denner, Joachim, and Ralf R. Tönjes. 2012. Infection barriers to successful xenotransplantation focusing on porcine endogenous retroviruses. In: *Clinical Microbiology Reviews* 25 (2): 318–343. doi:10.1128/CMR.05011-11.

Denner, Joachim, et al. 2009. Strategies to prevent transmission of porcine endogenous retroviruses. (The International Xenotransplantation Association consensus statement on conditions for undertaking clinical trials of porcine islet products in type 1 diabetes—Chap. 5). *Xenotransplantation* 16 (4): 239–248. doi:10.1111/j.1399-3089.2009.00544.x.

DiazGranados, Carlos A., and John E. McGowan Jr. 2009. Antimicrobial resistance: An international public health problem. In *Antimicrobial drug resistance. Clinical and epidemiological aspects*, ed. Douglas L. Mayers, 1267–1276. Totowa: Humana Press. doi:10.1007/978-1-60327-595-841.

Ehrenreich, Barbara. 2009. *Bright-Sided. How the relentless promotion of positive thinking has underminded America.* New York: Metropolitan Books.

Ekser, Burcin, et al. 2009. Xenotransplantation of solid organs in the pig-to-primate model. *Transplant Immunology* 21 (2): 87–92. doi:10.1016/j.trim.2008.10.005.

Garkavenko, Olga, et al. 2012. The first clinical xenotransplantation trial in New Zealand: Efficacy and safety. *Xenotransplantation* 19 (1): 6–7. doi:10.1111/j.1399-3089.2011.00680_3.x.

Gastmeier, P., et al. 2010. How many nosocomial infections are avoidable? [Wie viele nosokomiale Infektionen sind vermeidbar?]. *Deutsche medizinische Wochenschrift* 135 (03): 91–93. doi:10.1055/s-0029-1244823.

German Bundestag—Committee 19. 2000. Printed Matter 14/3144. Report of the Committee on Education, Research and Technology Assessment (Committee 19) in accordance with § 56a of the Rules of Procedure. Technology Assessment, here: Monitoring "Xenotransplantation"

[Bericht des Ausschusses für Bildung, Forschung und Technikfolgenabschätzung (19. Ausschuss) gemäß § 56a der Geschäftsordnung. Technikfolgenabschätzung, hier: Monitoring „Xenotransplantation“]. http://dip21.bundestag.de/dip21/btd/14/031/1403144.pdf. Accessed 23 April 2015.

German Medical Association—Scientific Advisory Board on Xenotransplantation. 1999. Advisory Opinion of the Scientific Advisory Board of the German Medical Association on Xenotransplantation [Stellungnahme des Wissenschaftlichen Beirates der Bundesärztekammer zur Xenotransplantation]. http://www.aerzteblatt.de/pdf/97/6/a320-5.pdf. Accessed 23 April 2015.

Gethmann, Carl Friedrich. 2000. Editor's Preface to Volume 8 of his series "Ethics of Science and Technology Assessment": Beckmann et al. 2000. [Geleitwort zu Band 8 der von ihm herausgegebenen Reihe "Wissenschaftsethik und Technikfolgenbeurteilung"], p. VII–VIII.

Hüsing, Bärbel, et al. 2001. *Technology assessment of cellular xenotransplantation. Final report for the swiss science and technology council by the center for technology assessment of the fraunhofer institute for systems and innovation research (ISI)* [Technologiefolgen-Abschätzung Zelluläre Xenotransplantation. Abschlussbericht für den Schweizerischen Wissenschafts- und Technologierat, Zentrum für Technologiefolgen-Abschätzung]. Karlsruhe: Fraunhofer ISI.

Jones, Bryony A., et al. 2013. Zoonosis emergence linked to agricultural intensification and environmental change. *Proceedings of the National Academy of Sciences of the United States of America* 110 (21): 8399–8404. doi:10.1073/pnas.1208059110.

Karesh, William B., et al. 2012. Ecology of zoonoses: Natural and unnatural histories. *Lancet* 380 (9857): 1936–1945. doi:10.1016/S0140-6736(12)61678-X.

Ma, W., et al. 2009. The role of swine in the generation of novel influenza viruses. *Zoonoses and Public Health* 56 (6–7): 326–337. doi:10.1111/j.1863-2378.2008.01217.x.

Millard, Anne Laure, and Nicolas J. Mueller. 2010. Can human viruses infect porcine xenografts? *Xenotransplantation* 17 (1): 6–10. doi:10.1111/j.1399-3089.2009.00566.x.

Nerem, Robert M. 2010. Regenerative medicine: The emergence of an industry. *Journal of The Royal Society Interface* 7 (Suppl 6): 771–775. doi:10.1098/rsif.2010.0348.focus.

Nuffield Council on Bioethics—Working Party on Xenografts. 1996. Animal-to-Human Transplants: the ethics of xenotransplantation. London: Nuffield Council. http://nuffieldbioethics.org/wp-content/uploads/xenotransplantation.pdf. Accessed 23 April 2015.

Paslack, Rainer, et al. ed. 2012. *Proceed with caution? Concept and application of the precautionary principle in nanobiotechnolgogy*. Münster: LIT.

Pearce-Duvet, Jessica, M. C. 2006. The origin of human pathogens: evaluating the role of agriculture and domestic animals in the evolution of human disease. *Biological reviews of the Cambridge Philosophical Society* 81 (3): 369–382. doi:10.1017/S1464793106007020.

Petersen, Björn, et al. 2009. The perspectives for porcine-to-human xenografts. *Comparative Immunology, Microbiology and Infectious Diseases* 32 (2): 91–105.

Rath, Benjamin. 2012. Political and philosophical foundations and practical applications of the precautionary principle. In *Proceed with caution? Concept and application of the precautionary principle in nanobiotechnolgogy*, ed. Rainer Paslack et al., 5–25. Münster: LIT.

Rothblatt, Martine. 2004. *Your life or mine. How geoethics can resolve the conflict between public and private interests in xenotransplantation.* Aldershot/Burlington: Ashgate Publishing.

Scobie, Linda, et al. 2013. Long-Term IgG response to porcine Neu5Gc antigens without transmission of PERV in burn patients treated with porcine skin xenografts. *Journal of Immunology* 191 (6): 2907–2915. doi:10.4049/jimmunol.1301195.

Shlaes, David M. 2010. *Antibiotics. The perfect storm.* Dordrecht: Springer Netherlands. doi:10.1007/978-90-481-9057-7.

Shlaes, David M., and Steven J. Projan. 2009. Antimicrobial resistance versus the discovery and development of new antimicrobials. In *Antimicrobial drug resistance. Mechanisms of drug resistance*, ed. Douglas L. Mayers, 43–50 Totowa: Humana Press. doi:10.1007/978-1-59745-180-24.

Sköld, Ola. 2011. *Antibiotics and antibiotic resistance*. Hoboken, NJ: Wiley-Interscience.

Takebe, Takanori, et al. 2013. Vascularized and functional human liver from an iPSC-derived organ bud transplant. *Nature* 499 (7459): 481–484. doi:10.1038/nature12271.

Taylor, Louise H., et al. 2001. Risk factors for human disease emergence. *Philosophical Transactions of the Royal Society of London. Series B, Biological sciences. The Royal Society* 356 (1411): 983–989. doi:10.1098/rstb.2001.0888.

U.S. Food and Drug Administration of the U.S Department of Health and Human Services—Center for Biologics Evaluation and Research (CBER). 2003. Guidance for Industry. Source Animal, Product, Preclinical, and Clinical Issues Concerning the Use of Xenotransplantation Products in Humans. Final Guidance. http://www.fda.gov/downloads/BiologicsBloodVaccines/GuidanceComplianceRegulatoryInformation/Guidances/Xenotransplantation/ucm092707.pdf. Accessed 23 April 2015.

Walger, Peter, et al. 2013. Report of the German Society for Hospital Hygiene (DGKH) on prevalence, mortality and the potential for prevention of nosocomial infections in Germany 2013 [Stellungnahme der DGKH zu Prävalenz, Letalität und Präventionspotenzial nosokomialer Infektionen in Deutschland 2013]. *Hygiene & Medizin* 38 (7/8): 329–338.

WHO [57th World Health Assembly]. 2004. WHA57.18 – Human organ and tissue transplantation. http://www.who.int/ethics/en/A57_R18-en.pdf. Accessed 23 April 2015.

Yui, Shiro et al. 2012. Functional engraftment of colon epithelium expanded in vitro from a single adult Lgr5 + stem cell. *Nature Medicine* 18 (4): 618–623. doi:10.1038/nm.2695.

Jan-Ole Reichardt is a lecturer and research associate in Ethics at the Institute for Medical Ethics, History and Philosophy of Medicine at the University of Münster and an associate member of its Centre for Advanced Study in Bioethics. Dr. Reichardt has degrees in philosophy, formal logics and theory of sciences from the University of Leipzig. His research interests lie at the intersection of ethics, moral and political theory, with a particular interest in topics related to normative concepts of living well, notions of human dignity, autonomy and institutional justice.

Part IV
Crossing Borders: International and Intercultural Perspectives

After the discussion of the medical and ethical challenges and implications of crossing the species border in Part III, Part IV crosses national and cultural borders by opening up the perspective for remedies being practiced in countries other than Germany or Austria, whose situation was discussed primarily in Sect. I through III.

In the opening chapter of this section, *Kristof Thys*, *Fabienne Dobbels*, *Paul Schotsmans* and *Pascal Borry* compare the underlying rationales for living kidney donation from an international perspective. While in most countries minors are legally prohibited from acting as living kidney donors, in some countries, like Sweden, the United Kingdom and the United States, living kidney donation by minors may be lawful under well-defined conditions and circumstances. Based on the results from a previous study investigating guidelines and position papers on the topic, they argue that these guidelines express conflicting views concerning the ethical and legal legitimacy of donation by minors. In order to critically re-evaluate the appropriateness of living kidney donation by minors and to take a more unified approach towards this phenomenon, they undertake a close analysis of the arguments in favor of and against an absolute prohibition of living kidney donation by minors. The arguments are presented in three thematic categories, representing the main ethical aspects that have been identified in the previously discussed review. These aspects concern the ability of minors to make an informed and deliberate decision about living kidney donation, the assessment of whether acting as a living kidney donor could be in accordance with the best interest of the minor, and the appropriateness of parental consent and independent authorization.

Karen de Looze's article looks at some of the difficulties that arise in the process of implementing national policies that deal with organ donation and transplantation. It particularly focuses on the pressures that emerge from the international discourse on organ transplantation and limit the capacity of national governments to think and act outside the box to address their specific circumstances. As a case in point, she discusses the situation in India, based on 18 months of fieldwork conducted in the country. In 1994, India implemented the Transplantation of Human Organs Act (THOA) in order to alleviate organ shortage. De Looze explains that this Act has its roots in universalist ethics based on Euro-American preferences that have sought to discourage organ sale and encourage cadaveric organ donation. She argues that medical policy is tightly interwoven with an economic perspective that works through a discourse of scarcity. Against this background, she looks at the double significance of India's "kidney belt", a region in Southern India (more specifically Tamil Nadu) that is renowned for both medical tourism and organ sale. She concludes by discussing the tension between a culture-sensitive directive to render medical policy effective in the field and certain restraints that arise from international pressures tightly interwoven with universalist ethics and a strictly neoliberal discourse that focuses on modernization through economic (and technological) development.

Kiarash Aramesh provides an overview of the ethical and legal history of one of the most noteworthy renal transplantation programs in the developing world, the Iranian model. With an annual rate of around 24 transplantations per million population the Iranian model of paid and regulated living-unrelated kidney transplantation (IMKT) was the subject of extensive ethical reviews, discussions, and controversies in the past two decades. Opponents and proponents of this model explained their arguments, ideas and concerns in many articles and books. Sometimes, the authors' political viewpoints influenced their judgments and ethical conclusions. Aramesh recapitulates the most important facts and events, arguing that it is a noteworthy experience of health-related problem solving in critical situations. In addition to sketching the ethical battleground of opponents and proponents (describing their main theoretical and factual arguments and inferences), the text includes a description of the Brain Death Act (intended to facilitate post-mortem organ donation) and the religious grounds and challenges behind ratifying this Act and explaining why this model of organ donation has not gained popularity in Iran. He finishes by recommending the promotion of organ donation from brain-dead persons as an innovative way to solve the problem of organ shortage in Iran, particularly as the prevalence of accidents resulting in brain death in Iran is high and the public attitude towards brain-dead organ donation is positive.

The article contributed by *Per Pfeffer* expatiates upon the organization of the Norwegian program of renal transplantation which was officially started in 1967. Pfeffer argues that some crucial decisions had to be made right from the start, like the assessment of the superiority of transplantation to dialysis and the aim to offer transplantation to all patients who will benefit from it. Furthermore, family members are given the opportunity to donate a kidney to bridge the gap between need and supply of organs. This argument is strengthened by the fact that after more than 40 years, these conditions still constitute Norway's national guidelines for end-stage renal decease. Pfeffer explicates the special characteristics of the Norwegian model of combining living and post-mortem donor donation, yet emphasizing the advantages of live donation. According to him, a cost-benefit analysis of live donation shows that many advantages face few costs. Some of the benefits of live donation are better graft and recipient survival and a shorter waiting time after a suitable donor has been found. Following that line of argumentation, Pfeffer concludes that

Norway's active policy towards live donation has taken the pressure off the transplantation waiting list.

Rafael Matesanz' and *Beatriz Domínguez-Gil's* contribution is dedicated to the regulatory framework and the ethical and organizational preconditions of the successful Spanish model of organ transplantation. They argue that the increase in postmortem donation, and consequently in the number of solid organ transplants, has been the result of the implementation of a set of measures, mainly of an organizational nature. Their article reviews the elements of this system, a global reference in the pursuit of the self-sufficiency paradigm. They illustrate that the measures composing the Spanish Model were adopted after the *Spanish National Transplant Organization* (Organización Nacional de Transplantes – ONT) was created in 1989. The specific organization of the process of donation was the result of the cooperation of organizations on three different but interrelated levels: national, regional and hospital. The authors argue that even though the Spanish success is often attributed to the legal system of presumed consent (opt-out regulation), this policy is not strictly applied in practice as relatives are always approached and have the final veto. In contrast, improvements in the system through the development of a properly trained and devoted network of transplant coordination teams, led by intensive care physicians and supported by regional authorities and the ONT, have been the key features of the Spanish success. Social acceptance of donation by the Spanish population may also be seen as a component of this success, which results from the close cooperation with the mass media, but also from the response of society to the creation of a solid system of organ donation and transplantation, which has been sustainable over time.

The article contributed by *Thomas Mone* demonstrates models of organization and operation that transcend political and cultural variances and can help to improve donation and transplantation in Germany and elsewhere by presenting the principles and interventions employed to dramatically improve donation in Southern California. In order to reach this goal, Mone names eight principles that are followed by successful programs, e.g. an ethics-based regulation and oversight for public trust, the separation of donation and transplantation, the communication of the value of donation to the public, the existence of transparent allocation rules to ensure fairness, and the innovation in the science of donation – to name only a few. But Mone does not stop at naming abstract principles, he also illustrates how these principles can be operationalized in a systematic process of delineating the tasks, recruiting and training specialists and developing programs, policies and procedures to accomplish donation. In this context, he points at the importance of donation development to educate and inspire the general and healthcare professional communities, family support and authorization for donation and aftercare. In conclusion, he advises that only by ensuring that the identified principles and processes of organ donation are implemented and continually monitored for adherence and improvement, the goal of ending deaths on the waiting lists can be reached.

Sohaila Bastami centers on the ethical challenges raised by the reimplementation of controlled donation after cardiac death in Switzerland in 2011. As brain death is becoming an increasingly rare phenomenon due to better road safety and neurological interventions in this area of the world, controlled donation after cardiac death (cDCD) permits physicians to continue post-mortem organ donation, with the advantage of not harming the living. The aim of Bastami's chapter is twofold: First, to present the six challenges that result from a narrative literature review on the ethics of cDCD. Second, to demonstrate the relationship between these challenges and several research questions that her research team plans to ask in a study on next-of-kin's experiences with cDCD. As ethical challenges she names the appropriate consent to cDCD, potential conflicts of interest, choosing the ideal location of death, implementing pre-mortem organ-protective measures for the recipient, impact of cDCD on medical care at the end of life and, finally, challenges to the dead donor rule. Furthermore, she demonstrates the relationship between four of the six ethical challenges set forth in the review and several of the research questions that the study aims to answer. She concludes by arguing that in order to advance the organ donation in a responsible way accompanying research on the impact on families is necessary, especially pertaining to DCD, as very little research exists on family members' experiences.

In order to investigate and discuss the strengths and ethical challenges of uncontrolled donation after cardiac death (uDCD), *Iván Ortega-Deballon, David Rodríguez-Arias* and *Maxwell J. Smith* compare the uDCD protocol introduced in New York City to the current Spanish and French protocols. They expose that, since their inception, uDCD programs have generated both promise and concern. On the one hand, these protocols potentially increase organ donation rates by harvesting organs from individuals who suffer out-of-hospital cardiac arrests (OHCA). On the other hand, they raise a number of ethical concerns regarding the truthfulness of the information provided to donor relatives and the possibility that organ donation could compromise treatment of patients. By elucidating ethical concerns with existing uDCD protocols, it is their goal to effect positive policy change in those protocols and others that will likely be developed worldwide. They argue that uDCD protocols and non-conventional resuscitation procedures (NCRP) programs can and should coexist, although the former should be subjected to the failure of the latter. Thus, they point out that only after every medically useful and ethically justifiable effort to save a patient's life has been tried without success should an OHCA victim be considered a potential organ donor, as agreed upon and published by international consensus on DCD. They stress that the NYC uDCD protocol has proven to be a laudable effort in this direction, but also remind about the importance to identify the aspects of uDCD protocols that need improvement as a result of the cumulative scientific evidence in the management of cardiac arrest before giving up resuscitative attempts. Both European protocols and the NYC uDCD protocol should be evaluated with this in mind.

Chapter 22
Is an Absolute Prohibition of Living Kidney Donation by Minors Appropriate? A Discussion of the Arguments in Favor and Against

Kristof Thys, Fabienne Dobbels, Paul Schotsmans and Pascal Borry

22.1 Introduction

Kidney transplantation is the treatment of choice for many patients suffering from end-stage renal disease and is associated with a lower incidence of morbidity,[1] a higher quality of life[2] and favorable cost effectiveness[3] as compared to chronic renal dialysis therapy. As a consequence of organ shortage, however, the average waiting time for a deceased donor kidney has steadily increased over the last decade and currently exceeds 1.5 years for children and 3.5 years for adults in the Eurotransplant region.[4] In order to reduce long waiting times on the deceased donor list, living donor kidney transplantation has become a well-established practice in many countries.[5] Living donor kidney transplantation not only reduces the risk of future

[1] Wolfe et al. (1999).

[2] Sayin et al. (2007).

[3] Winkelmayer et al. (2002).

[4] Rahmel (2013).

[5] Horvat et al. (2009).

K. Thys (✉) · P. Schotsmans · P. Borry
Centre for Biomedical Ethics and Law, University of Leuven, Leuven, Belgium
e-mail: kristof.thys@med.kuleuven.be

P. Schotsmans
e-mail: paul.schotsmans@med.kuleuven.be

P. Borry
e-mail: pascal.borry@med.kuleuven.be

F. Dobbels
Centre for Nursing Studies and Health Care Research,
University of Leuven, Leuven, Belgium
e-mail: fabienne.dobbels@med.kuleuven.be

R. J. Jox et al. (eds.), *Organ Transplantation in Times of Donor Shortage*,
International Library of Ethics, Law, and the New Medicine 59,
DOI 10.1007/978-3-319-16441-0_22

morbidity as a consequence of long-term dialysis, but also confers better graft and patient outcomes as compared to deceased donor transplantation. A thorough donor screening process ensures optimal quality of the donor kidney and semi-elective timing of the donation allows for a minimal cold ischemia time. Indeed, increasing the duration of pre-transplant dialysis treatment has been associated with an increased risk of patient death and graft failure.[6] Specifically, one study found that patients undergoing pre-emptive kidney transplantation, defined as kidney transplant procedures without preceding dialysis treatment, had a 37 % lower risk of death-censored graft loss compared to kidney transplant patients that received a 6–12 months dialysis treatment prior to transplantation.[7]

Living donor kidney transplantation, however, is only possible when a suitable living kidney donor is available. Even though for young recipients, parents or other family members often step forward to donate a kidney, it remains unclear whether, and under what conditions, minors should qualify to become a living kidney donor as well. In most countries, minors are legally prohibited from acting as living kidney donors in order to "provide legal certainty and maximize the legal protection of minors"(Lopp 2013). In other countries, such as Sweden, the United Kingdom and the United States, living kidney donation by minors may be legal under well-defined conditions and circumstances. In the United States, for example, 49 minors under the age of 18 donated a kidney between 1988 and 2013 (U.S. Organ Procurement and Transplantation Network 2013). Also in Europe and Canada, cases of living kidney donation by minors were reported.[8]

In a previous study,[9] we found that guidelines and position papers adopt different approaches, and under what conditions, living kidney donation by minors could be appropriate. Most guidelines advocate an absolute prohibition on living kidney donation by minors. These guidelines express concerns about minors' lack of cognitive and psychosocial maturity to make a decision about the donation; the conflict of interest that parents might experience when making a decision about living kidney donation by one of their children for the benefit of another child; and the medical and psychological harm a minor might be exposed to as a consequence of donation. Finally, the concern exists that minors might be considered as potential living kidney donors, "without there being a desperate medical need or reasonable chance of success"(Thys et al. 2013), given that other treatment options are available, including kidney grafts from deceased donors or living donors that are over 18 as well as dialysis treatment.

Other guidelines, however, would occasionally allow living kidney donation by minors under the provision of adequate safeguards. Four different safeguards were identified in our systematic review. First, the donation should be authorized by a qualified independent body, such as a court or an ethics committee. Second, the minor's decision-making capacity and autonomy should be independently assessed. Third, the procedure should be deemed consistent with the minor's best interest.

[6] Meier-Kriesche et al. (2005); Papalois et al. (2000).

[7] Meier-Kriesche et al. (2005).

[8] Webb and Fortune (2006).

[9] Thys et al. (2013).

Fourth, living kidney donation by minors should only be allowed as an *ultima ratio*, when all other opportunities for donation or treatment alternatives have been exhausted.

In the light of these conflicting views, a more scrutinized analysis of the arguments in favor of and against an absolute prohibition of living kidney donation by minors may help us to critically re-evaluate the appropriateness of living kidney donation by minors and to take a more unified approach towards this phenomenon. Therefore, in this chapter, we aim to present the main arguments in favor of and against an absolute prohibition of living kidney donation. These arguments will be presented in three thematic categories, representing the main ethical aspects that have been identified in the previously discussed review.[10] These aspects concern the ability of minors to make an informed and deliberate decision about living kidney donation, the assessment of whether acting as a living kidney donor could be in accordance with the best interest of the minor and the appropriateness of parental consent and independent authorization.

22.2 The Decision-making Capacity of Minors

The first aspect concerns the ability of minors to provide informed and free consent to living kidney donation. Opponents of an absolute prohibition of living kidney donation by minors argued that the ability to make an informed and deliberate decision about living kidney donation does not primarily depend on one's chronological age, but rather on one's level of maturity and understanding.[11] It was argued that decision-making capacity does not suddenly appear at the age of 18, but gradually develops during childhood and adolescence. Therefore, minors may already possess sufficient maturity to understand the nature of the procedure, to weigh the risks and benefits of the procedure, and to make and communicate an autonomous decision. Referring to the Piagetian theory of cognitive development, one study suggested that minors age 13 and older, that are in the formal operations stage of cognitive development, may have similar capacities as adults to provide informed consent.[12] Moreover, some commentators remarked that in many countries, minors who can demonstrate sufficient maturity are legally allowed to make their own decisions in many health-related areas, including consent to treatment and participation in research.[13] Indeed, a study by Stultiëns et al. concluded that minors are allowed to make legal decisions concerning the provision of their own health care in many European countries, either from a fixed minimal age onwards or based on an *ad hoc* evaluation of their age and level of maturity.[14] Correspondingly, one commentator contended, that "allowing mentally sophisticated minors to consent to organ dona-

[10] Thys et al. (2013).

[11] Webb and Fortune (2006); Broeckx (2013); Brierley and Larcher (2011).

[12] Zinner (2004).

[13] Brierley and Larcher (2011).

[14] Stultiëns et al. (2007).

tion appears to be a logical step" (Zinner 2004). Another commentator stated, that "if the minor is found sufficiently competent, then he should be treated no differently from a competent adult donor"(Broeckx 2013).

However, the idea that minors may be competent enough to consent to living kidney donation was criticized. Critics held that the former position focuses too strongly on minors' cognitive capacities, disregarding the psychosocial factors that may prevent minors from making a sufficiently deliberate and autonomous decision. A study about the ethical aspects of living liver donation by minors emphasized that the transition period from childhood to adulthood is characterized by several psychosocial developmental challenges that may impact their decision-making capacity.[15] These psychosocial factors are at least partly associated with biological developments and brain maturation processes that may continue until one's mid-twenties.[16] They include an increased susceptibility to peer pressure, higher perceptions of invulnerability and a lack of sensitivity to long-term consequences of one's actions.[17] Moreover, it was argued that minors are largely dependent on their parents for financial, emotional and psychosocial support, and therefore might be prone to conscious or unconscious family pressure or coercion.[18]

22.3 The Best Interest of the Minor

The second aspect concerns whether living kidney donation by minors could still be considered appropriate, if the procedure is deemed compatbile with the minor's best interests . In this regard, Crouch and Elliott (1999) made a distinction between two types of interests. First, minors have interests in their own physical and psychosocial wellbeing that are referred to as self-regarding interests. Second, minors also have other-regarding interests, which are defined as interests in the wellbeing of other people, "at least partly as an end in itself"(Crouch and Elliott 1999). In the following paragraphs, we will discuss each of these types in turn.

22.3.1 Minors' Self-Regarding Interests

Opponents of an absolute prohibition have argued that living kidney donation may be in the minor's best interest provided that there is a beneficial cost-benefit analysis for the potential donor.[19] The anticipated benefits that a minor might experience from acting as a living kidney donor are psychosocial in nature and include

---

[15] Capitaine et al. (2013).

[16] Giedd (2008).

[17] Capitaine et al. (2013).

[18] Webb and Fortune (2006); Kallich and Merz (1995); Shartle (2001).

[19] Cheyette (1999).

benefits as a consequence of altruistic behavior, such as increased self-esteem and self-worth, as well as psychosocial benefits because of the improved health status of their sibling and the improved relationship with the recipient.[20] The anticipated risks may be both medical and psychosocial. Irrespective of the age of the donor, the medical risks of living donor nephrectomy involve a 0.03 % mortality risk, approximately a 10 % risk of perioperative complications and the possibility of long-term complications of living with a solitary kidney.[21] Moreover, minors may also suffer psychosocial harm as a consequence of living kidney donation, mainly because the donor's psychosocial wellbeing is often closely attached to the medical and psychosocial outcomes of the recipient.[22] If the anticipated psychosocial benefits that the minor may experience are likely to outweigh the medical and psychosocial risks, the donation could be considered in the minor's best interest.

By contrast, critics argued that living kidney donation by minors could not be justified by referring to the minor's self-regarding best interest. First, it was argued that the long-term medical outcomes of living donor nephrectomy in minors have not been adequately observed and studied so far. One study found that the long-term effects of unilateral nephrectomy are not to be neglected, as several patients suffered a decline of renal function 20 years after the procedure.[23] Moreover, little is known about the minor donor's risk of developing a hereditary form of diabetes, in the case that the recipient is diagnosed with diabetes mellitus.[24] Second, the long-term psychosocial effects of living kidney donation in minors are currently unknown, as well. It is therefore uncertain whether minors would be able to experience the same type of psychosocial benefits as adults, as they are still in the process of emotional development.[25] Moreover, one scholar remarked that the amount of benefits a minor may experience by acting as a living kidney donor has often been overestimated in law cases, while the potential for psychosocial risk has been largely neglected.[26]

22.3.2 Minors' Other-Regarding Interests

Some opponents of an absolute ban contended that living kidney donation by minors may also be appropriate if the minor has an intrinsic interest in the wellbeing of the recipient, especially if the recipient is an intimate family member.[27] These commentators held that the interests of minors "are intimately bound up with the interests of their families"(Crouch and Elliott 1999), implying that the wellbeing of the donor

---

[20] Schover et al. (1997); Johnson et al. (1999).

[21] Matas et al. (2003).

[22] Cheyette (1999).

[23] Davis (2004).

[24] Salvatierra (2002).

[25] Crouch and Elliott (1999).

[26] Cheyette (1999).

[27] Crouch and Elliott (1999); Jansen (2004).

is intrinsically related to that of the recipient. From this perspective, it was strongly emphasized that members of intimate families should not primarily be considered as isolated individuals, but as relational agents that "incorporate each other and each other's goals as part of themselves"(Friedman 1994) and whose interests are often intertwined. Dwyer and Vig argued that family relations carry moral significance and therefore import special obligations towards each other. They emphasized that "siblings also have some obligations to each other and to the family unit"(Dwyer and Vig 1995) that might justify them taking several risks for the benefit of each other. Some commentators even argued that the recipient should not necessarily be a close family member of the minor, but could also be a non-relative with whom the donor has a close emotional bond, like a close friend.[28]

This approach received several criticisms, however. First, the idea of family obligations to sacrifice the wellbeing of one family member for the benefit of another family member was opposed in the literature. Critics held that the mere fact of belonging to a family is not a sufficient argument for justifying living kidney donation by a minor and "doesn't imply an exemption from moral scrutiny"(Steinberg 2004). The mere existence of such obligations themselves was even doubted, as "parents choose to have children and thus take on the duties associated with parenthood. Children do not choose to be born, do not contract with their parents, and so incur no debt towards them"(Lyons 2011). Moreover, it was argued that family relationships are inherently characterized by a natural imbalance of power between parents and their children. If confronted with the possibility of living kidney donation by a healthy child for the benefit of an ill sibling, parents may likely attribute more weight to the interests of the prospective recipient as compared to those of the potential donor.[29] Therefore, these critics held the view that, although family relationships may be a relevant factor to include in the ethical decision-making, "an idealized vision of the family shouldn't blind us to the fact that families are also home to child abuse, other forms of domestic violence, divorce, and sometimes even murder"(Steinberg 2004).

Second, it was emphasized that the decision-making would be even more burdensome for proxy decision-makers if the donation is intended for a recipient outside the immediate family, especially when there is no close emotional bond between the donor's parents and the recipient or the recipient's family. Moreover, critics argued that it would be difficult to decide on the degree of emotional attachment between donor and recipient that would be required in order to justify such donations.[30]

Third, it was emphasized that family attachments, and the moral significance that is attached to them, are not fixed but change over time. It was argued that these changes are often predictable by an impartial observer, but are often unexpected for the potential donors themselves.[31] As persons can only donate a kidney once in a lifetime, minor donors will not be able to make the same choice again for their

---

[28] Jansen (2004).

[29] Lyons (2011).

[30] Fleck (2004).

[31] Holm (2004).

own children, with whom they are likely to have a more intimate bond than with the prospective recipient. In the light of this consideration, the Danish Council of Ethics recommended that living kidney donors should preferably be older than 35 years of age, as most people of that age "know whether they are going to have children, and they know how their adult relationship with their parents is going to be" (Holm 2004).

22.4 The Appropriateness of Parental Consent and Independent Authorization

The third aspect concerns the appropriateness of parental consent and independent authorization of the donation. Commentators who argued against an absolute ban on living kidney donation by an incompetent minor emphasized that parents or legal guardians could act as substitute decision-makers for their children in case they are not able to consent to living kidney donation themselves. It was argued, that "due to the nature of the family and the general relationship between guardians and those for whom they are responsible, it might be assumed that decisions made by parent-guardians are in the best interests of their children" (Morley 2002).

Critics expressed the concern that parents or guardians are likely not able to make these decisions in the best interest of the child. First, parents may not be able to adequately understand and appreciate the long-term medical and psychosocial risks and benefits of the donation.[32] Second, parents may experience a conflict of interest in making this decision, as they are supposed to further the interests of all their children, both the donor and the recipient.[33]

Commentators that would occasionally allow living kidney donation by minors formulated diverging responses in reaction to these criticisms. A first response is that the requirement for parents to decide in their children's best interest may be considered too strict. In her model of constrained parental autonomy, Friedman Ross held that parents should not be expected to always promote the best interests of their children, as the best interest standard "is incompatible with the family as an intimate group with goals that do not maximize the best of each child member"(Friedman 1994). Instead, she argued that parents have the autonomy to raise their children according to their own perception of a good life. This implies that parents sometimes have to make trade-offs between the interests of their children in order to support the wellbeing and functioning of the family as a unit. In making these trade-offs, however, parents are constrained by the principle of respect for persons. This principle implies that a decision that involves more than minimal harm for the child, as in the case of kidney donation, requires both the informed and voluntary consent from the competent minor and his parents. On the one hand, this model does not support living kidney donation by minors who are not competent enough to consent,

[32] Broeckx (2013).

[33] Broeckx (2013); Lyons (2011).

as parents do not have the right to sacrifice or abuse one child to benefit the greater good of the family. On the other hand, competent minors are not considered capable of consenting to living kidney donation without the accompanying consent of their parents, as parents remain responsible for the "financial and physical harms accrued by their child" (Friedman 1994).

A second response to these criticisms is that minors should only be allowed to become a living kidney donor provided that the donation is approved by an independent body. In a position paper that was published in 2008, the American Academy of Pediatrics recommended that this approval preferably should be given by a donor advocacy team with sufficient expertise in pediatric psychology, communication skills and transplantation medicine. This donor advocacy team should be responsible for assessing the minor's level of maturity and understanding of the risks and benefits of the procedure, as well as the voluntariness of the minor's decision.[34] Other commentators, however, argue that approval by an independent committee is insufficient to protect the minor's interests and the donation should preferably be authorized by a hospital ethics committee, a national pluridisciplinary committee or a court.

However, the ability of courts to approve living kidney donation by minors was also questioned. First, some critics held that court interventions intrude on the autonomy of families to develop their own conception of a good life. These critics argued that "judges may not superimpose their own arbitrary values and preferences over those of the parent-guardians"(Morley 2002) and courts should only intervene when parents "are grossly unfit, unable or unwilling to adequately care for their child"(Friedman 1994). Second, it was argued that courts are just as poorly equipped to adequately consider all the potential risks and benefits that are involved as the parents are, and therefore cannot substitute the medical judgment of the transplant professionals, who are responsible for guaranteeing that all potential medical risks are adequately considered.[35] Third, it was claimed that the involvement of courts in the decision-making process may be emotionally burdensome for the potential donors, recipients and parents and may withhold parents from providing adequate emotional support to their child during the process.[36]

22.5 Discussion and Conclusion

In this chapter, we aimed to present the arguments in favor of and against an absolute prohibition of living kidney donation by minors. These arguments focused on three ethical aspects that are central to the decision-making process on living kidney donation by minors. These aspects include the minor's competence to provide informed consent to the donation, the best interest of the minor and the appropriate-

[34] Friedman et al. (2008).

[35] Broeckx (2013); Friedman (1994).

[36] Broeckx (2013).

ness of parental consent and court approval. In general, advocates of an absolute prohibition held that living kidney donation by minors could neither be justified by referring to the minor's capacity to consent to the donation by himself, nor the ability of parents or a court of law to make a decision in the minor's self-regarding or other-regarding interests. By contrast, critics of an absolute prohibition held that living kidney donation by minors may be appropriate, provided that the minor has sufficient decision-making capacity to consent to the donation himself or, if the minor is considered unable to provide informed consent himself, the donation is considered to be in the minor's interest.

Until now, the debate concerning the appropriateness of living kidney donation by minors has mainly focused on the decision-making capacity and best interest of the potential donor. The interests of the recipient have received far less attention in this debate. Although living donor kidney transplant recipients generally report positive medical and psychosocial outcomes, these transplantations may also have far-reaching negative psychosocial consequences for the recipients. If the recipient displays feelings of ambivalence towards the donation, for example, or experiences feelings of indebtedness towards the donor, this may adversely impact the long-term psychosocial outcomes of the recipient and his ability for self-management. To date, these phenomena have not been adequately researched, especially in cases where the intended recipient is a child.[37] It is therefore uncertain whether the young age of the donor might increase the recipient's risk for adverse psychosocial outcomes. Further research on the attitudes of transplant recipients towards receiving a kidney from a minor donor may shed more light on the recipient's perspectives.

Moreover, the perspectives and attitudes of transplant professionals warrant further exploration. To our knowledge, only one study addressed the willingness of these professionals to allow living kidney donation by a minor. The study concluded that approximately one third of U.S. physicians would be willing to allow living kidney donation by a 15-year old.[38] However, this study did not explore in-depth the motivations and reasons for or against allowing living kidney donation by minors. An in-depth exploration of the attitudes of these important stakeholders may help us to better understand the norms and values that are implicitly present in practice. Insight in these implicit norms and values may challenge us to critically re-evaluate normative arguments and theories concerning the appropriateness of living kidney donation by minors.

Finally, to our knowledge, no studies have addressed the specific challenges that occur when young adults (18–25 years old) donate a kidney. Although young adults are considered legally competent to consent to living kidney donation, many of the above-mentioned challenges might also be applicable to the young adult age group. First, any of the psychosocial aspects that characterize the transition from childhood to adulthood—including increased susceptibility to peer pressure, perceptions of invulnerability and impulsivity, may continue until the mid-twenties and therefore challenge young adults' capacity to provide informed consent. Second, similarly as

[37] Aujoulat et al. (2012).

[38] Joseph et al. (2008).

minors, young adults may still be very socially and financially dependent upon their families and have not accomplished their own family planning yet. Third, just as in minors, the long-term medical and psychosocial outcomes of young adult donors and their recipients are currently unknown. More research on the decision-making process and outcomes of these young adult donors may therefore provide valuable insights for the debate concerning the appropriateness of living kidney donation by minors.

References

Aujoulat, I., K. L. Schwering, and R. Reding. 2012. Living-related donation: A challenge to adolescent transplant recipients who transit from parental care to self-managed care. *Child Care Health Development* 38:146–148.

Brierley, J., and V. Larcher. 2011. Organ donation from children: Time for legal, ethical and cultural change. *Acta Paediatrica* 100:1175–1179.

Broeckx, N. 2013. Living organ donation and minors: A major dilemma. *European Journal of Health Law* 20:41–62.

Capitaine, L., K. Thys, K. Van Assche, et al. 2013. Should minors be considered as potential living liver donors? *Liver Transplantation* 19:649–655. doi:10.1002/lt.23633.

Cheyette, C. 1999. Organ harvests from the legally incompetents: An argument against compelled altruism. *Boston College Law Review* 41:465–515.

Crouch, R. A., and C. Elliott. 1999. Moral agency and the family: The case of living related organ transplantation. *Cambridge Quarterly of Healthcare Ethics* 8:275–287.

Davis, C. L. 2004. Evaluation of the living kidney donor: Current perspectives. *American Journal of Kidney Disease* 43:508–530.

Dwyer, J., and E. Vig. 1995. Rethinking transplantation between siblings. *The Hastings Center Report* 25:7–12.

Fleck, L. M. 2004. Children and organ donation: Some cautionary remarks. *Cambridge Quarterly of Healthcare Ethics* 13:161–166.

Friedman, L. R. 1994. Justice for children: The child as organ donor. *Bioethics* 8:105–126.

Friedman, L. R., J.R. Jr. Thistlethwaite, and The Committee on Bioethics. 2008. Minors as living solid-organ donors. Pediatrics 122 (2): 454–461.

Giedd, J. N. 2008. The teen brain: Insights from neuroimaging. *Journal of Adolescent Health* 42:335–343.

Holm, S. 2004. The child as organ and tissue donor: Discussions in the Danish Council of Ethics. *Cambridge Quarterly of Healthcare Ethics* 13:156–160.

Horvat, L. D., S. Z. Shariff, A. X. Garg, et al. 2009. Global trends in the rates of living kidney donation. *Kidney International* 75:1088–1098.

Jansen, L. A. 2004. Child organ donation, family autonomy, and intimate attachments. *Cambridge Quarterly of Healthcare Ethics* 13:133–142.

Johnson, E. M., J. K. Anderson, C. Jacobs, et al. 1999. Long-term follow-up of living kidney donors: Quality of life after donation. *Transplantation* 67:717–721.

Joseph, J. W., J.R. Jr. Thistlethwaite, M. A. Josephson, et al. 2008. An empirical investigation of physicians' attitudes toward intrasibling kidney donation by minor twins. *Transplantation* 85:1235–1239.

Kallich, J. D., and J. F. Merz. 1995. The transplant imperative: Protecting living donors from the pressure to donate. *The Journal of Corporation Law* 20:139–154.

Lopp, L. 2013. Best practice proposal: Legal safeguards for living organ donation in Europe in consideration of the current national regulations. In The EULOD project living organ dona-

tion in Europe. results and recommendations, eds. F. Ambagtsheer and W. Weimar. Lengerich: Pabst Science Publishers.
Lyons, B. 2011. Obliging children. *Medical Law Review* 19:55–85.
Matas, A. J., Bartlett, S. T., A. B. Leichtman, et al. 2003. Morbidity and mortality after living kidney donation. *American Journal Of Transplantation* 3:830–834.
Meier-Kriesche, H. U., F. K. Port, A. O. Ojo, et al. 2005. Effect of waiting time on renal transplant outcome. *Kidney International* 58:1311–1317.
Morley, T. M. 2002. Proxy consent to organ donation by incompetents. *The Yale Law Journal* 111:1215–1249.
Papalois, V. E., A. Moss, K. J. Gillingham, et al. 2000. Pre-emptive transplants for patients with renal failure, an argument against waiting until dialysis. *Transplantation* 70:625–631.
Rahmel, A. 2013. Eurotransplant International Foundation. Annual Report 2012. Leiden, The Netherlands.
Salvatierra, O. 2002. Transplant physicians bear full responsibility for the consequences of kidney donation by a minor. *American Journal of Transplantation* 2:297–298.
Sayin, A., R. Mutluay, and S. Sindel. 2007. Quality of life in hemodialysis, peritoneal dialysis, and transplantation patients. *Transplantation Proceedings* 39:3047–3053.
Schover, L. R., S. B. Streem, N. Boparai, et al. 1997. The psychosocial impact of donating a kidney: Long-term follow-up from a urology based center. *Journal of Urology* 157:1596–1601.
Shartle, B. 2001. Proposed legislation for safely regulating the increasing number of living organ and tissue donations by minors. *Louisiana Law Review* 61:431–471.
Steinberg, D. 2004. Kidney transplants from young children and the mentally retarded. *Theoretical Medicine* 25:229–241.
Stultiëns, L., T. Goffin, and P. Borry. 2007. Minors and informed consent: A comparative approach. *European Journal of Health Law* 14:21–46.
Thys, K., K. Van Assche, H. Nobile, et al. 2013. Could minors be living kidney donors? A systematic review of guidelines, position papers and reports. *Transplant International* 26 (10): 949–960.
U.S. Organ Procurement and Transplantation Network. Living donors recovered in the U.S. by donor age. http://optn.transplant.hrsa.gov/latestData/rptData.asp. Accessed 26 June 2013.
Webb, N. J. A., and P. M. Fortune. 2006. Should children ever be living kidney donors? *Pediatric Transplantation* 10:851–855.
Winkelmayer, W. C., M. C. Weinstein, M. A. Mittleman, et al. 2002. Health economic evaluations: The special case of end-stage renal disease treatment. *Medical Decision Making* 22:417–430.
Wolfe, R. A., V. B. Ashby, E. L. Milford, et al. 1999. Comparison of mortality in all patients on dialysis, patients on dialysis awaiting transplantation, and recipients of a first cadaveric transplant. *New England Journal of Medicine* 34:1725–1730.
Zinner, S. 2004. Cognitive development and pediatric consent to organ donation. *Cambridge Quarterly of Healthcare Ethics* 13:125–132.

Kristof Thys holds a master's degree in Theology and Religious Studies (KU Leuven; 2010) and an Erasmus Mundus master's degree in Bioethics (KU Leuven, RU Nijmegen, Università degli Studi di Padova; 2011). He is currently enrolled as a PhD candidate at the Centre for Biomedical Ethics and Law of the KU Leuven (Belgium). His research focuses on the ethical aspects of living kidney donation by minors and young adults.

Fabienne Dobbels is professor at the Centre for Nursing Studies and Health Care Research of the KU Leuven (Belgium), conducting research on adherence, self-management and patient-reported outcomes in the field of both adult and pediatric organ transplantation. She is a former Director of the International Society for Heart and Lung Transplantation and International Pediatric Transplant Association. She is currently the co-chair of the working group on Psychological Care for Living Donors and Recipients of the European platform on the ethical, legal and psychosocial aspects of transplantation (ELPAT) and a founding member of the European Transplant allied health professionals (ETAHP) working group of the European Society of Organ Transplantation. Being trained as a psychologist, she had more than 15 years of clinical experience in the field of heart transplantation. Her research resulted in more than 130 papers and book chapters on psychosocial issues related to transplantation and numerous lectures at national and international conferences.

Paul Schotsmans is professor of biomedical ethics at the Centre for Biomedical Ethics and Law (KU Leuven, Belgium). He is honorary president of the European Association of Centres of Medical Ethics (EACME), where he served consecutively as treasurer, secretary-general and president. He is also a board member of the Belgian Advisory Committee on Bioethics. He was board member of the International Association of Bioethics. He is a member of the ethics committee of Eurotransplant. He is also member of several local and international ethics committees. He is also the co-chair of the working group on Pediatric Organ Donation and Transplantation of the European platform on the ethical, legal and psychosocial aspects of transplantation (ELPAT). His research interest is mainly the application of 'personalism' as an ethical model for the integration of reproductive technologies, pre-implantation and prenatal diagnosis, clinical genetics, stem cell research, organ transplantation and end-of-life decision-making. He is the author and co-editor of several books in bioethics and papers in leading journals.

Pascal Borry is assistant professor of bioethics at the Centre for Biomedical Ethics and Law (University of Leuven, Belgium). His main research activities are concentrated on the ethical, legal and social implications of genetic and genomics. Pascal Borry is involved in various national and international research projects. He was awarded the prize for biomedical ethics 'Professor Roger Borghgraef' (2006), the Innovation Prize of the Dutch Association for Community Genetics and Public Health Genomics (2014) and the Prize of the Dutch Association for Bioethics (2015) He was a visiting scholar at the Case Western Reserve University, the Université de Montréal and McGill University, and the VU Medical Center Amsterdam. He is programme coordinator of the Erasmus Mundus Master of Bioethics. Moreover, he is member of various policy committees such as the Flemish Commission on neonatal screening (2012–2017), the Belgian Consultative Committee on Bioethics (2014–2018) and the Superior Health Council (2014–2020). Within the European Society of Human Genetics he is member of the Public and Professional Policy Committee (2008–2014) and elected member of the Board (2012–2017).

Chapter 23
India's Kidney Belt and Medical Tourism: A Double-edged Sword

Karen De Looze

23.1 Introduction

This chapter looks at some of the difficulties that arise in the process of implementing national policies that deal with organ donation and organ transplantation in local contexts. It particularly focuses on the pressures that emerge from international discourse on organ transplantation that limit the capacity of local governments to think and act *outside of the box* to address local circumstances. As a case in point I discuss the situation in India. This article is based on 18 months of fieldwork which I conducted in the country. The Transplantation of Human Organs Act (THOA) was implemented in India in 1994 with the aim to alleviate organ shortage. This Act has its roots in Universalist ethics based on Euro-American preferences that have sought to discourage organ sale and encourage cadaveric organ donation.[1]

Medical policy is tightly interwoven with an economic perspective that works through a discourse of scarcity. The logic of supply and demand, applied to matters of organ transfer, oversimplifies the context in which the THOA struggles to be implemented. Medical discourse and in particular the discourse on medical tourism connects organ transfer to profitability. Bearing this in mind, I will look at the double significance of India's kidney belt, a region in South India and more specifically Tamil Nadu that is renowned for both medical tourism and organ sale.

Glossing over the complexities presented in this chapter, I will then discuss the tension between a culture-sensitive directive to render medical policy effective in the field, and certain restraints that arise from international pressures that are tightly interwoven with Universalist ethics and a strictly neoliberal discourse that focuses on modernization through economic (and technological) development.

[1] The definition of brain death, on which cadaveric organ donation rests, is questioned (Evans 2007), and with it the practice of organ donation at the end of life can altogether be expected to undergo some significant changes in the years to come.

R. J. Jox et al. (eds.), *Organ Transplantation in Times of Donor Shortage*,
International Library of Ethics, Law, and the New Medicine 59,
DOI 10.1007/978-3-319-16441-0_23

23.2 Organ Shortage as a Central Marker

The issue of organ shortage arose at a particular moment in history, following the growing practice of organ transplantation from the 1960s onwards.[2] To augment the number of available organs, advancements in organ transplant technology are eagerly sought: printing organs in 3D,[3] growing kidneys, nanotechnology, and so on. In such a neoliberal account, *organ shortage* and the ethical dilemma of finding *good solutions* is seen as a temporary problem that will cease to exist once a limitless amount of organs can steadily be produced. It downplays the cost of implementing such technologies, as well as foreseeable problems that can be expected with their implementation and distribution. In the meantime, in Euro-American countries, the introduction of a new definition of death—brain death—and the harvesting of organs from brain dead patients contributed to countering the shortage of organs.[4] India, a country that shares the concern of organ shortages, introduced the Transplantation of Human Organ Act in 1994 in order to set up a cadaver donor program. Yet, there are some major disparities in such programs that seem to be accepted worldwide.[5] A report from the World Health Organization presents the following deceased donor numbers: 20.7 per million in the USA, 15.9 in Europe, 2.6 in South America and 1.1 in Asia in 2000.[6]

23.3 The Transplantation of Human Organs Act

Bioethics is cast in Universalist terms, looking for principles that hold true everywhere. These ethical principles favor the values of a particular Euro-American white middle-class.[7] Following the example of Europe and America, the Transplantation of Human Organs Act (THOA) aimed to implement a definition of brain death and a practice of cadaveric organ harvesting in Indian society in order to increase organ supply. Indirectly, it sought to eradicate organ sale. The logic of the THOA was that by increasing the supply of organs by harvesting organs from the brain dead, the demand for organs would be met, and hence the prices that render illegal organ sale so attractive would drop.[8] I will consider how this logic has worked in practice.

[2] Gervais (1986); Lock (2002).

[3] Atala (2011).

[4] Gervais (1986); Youngner (2007).

[5] Lock (2002).

[6] WHO (2003).

[7] Ohnuki-Tierney et al. (1994).

[8] Legislative Department (1994).

23.3.1 The Supply Side

The success of the THOA discouraging organ sale significantly depends on an actual rise in cadaveric organ procurement. It is striking that 18 years after the implementation of the THOA, there have been relatively few cadaver donations. In India, a mere 0.05 per million of the population are brain dead donors.[9] Among cadaveric organ transplantations done over a period from 1995 to 1999, 141 transplants took place in Chennai, the capital of Tamil Nadu, as compared to 60 in Delhi, and 21 in Mumbai. In other cities, Varanasi for example, there are no cadaveric organ retrievals happening at all; only living donations are allowed. While, in terms of size and magnitude of the city, it might be more honest to compare numbers in Chennai with numbers in Lucknow, the capital of Uttar Pradesh, it became apparent that even in Lucknow only four cadaver organ retrievals took place while I was doing my research (P.C. 05/03/ 2011). Given its cadaver donation numbers, Tamil Nadu is said to be "at the forefront in India" (Shroff et al. 2007).

The pronounced interregional differences have a complex set of related causes, of which I will mention two. First, Chennai immediately moved on to include multi-organ harvesting. Second, Tamil Nadu has more infrastructural and administrative support available to medical care as compared to other regions. Yet, during my fieldwork I found that cultural attitudes regarding death and the ritualized handling of decaying bodies help explain why a widespread acceptance of cadaveric organ harvesting and transfer in India is problematic and why regional differences are as blatant as they are.[10] In the context of this chapter I can only touch on a few of these cultural attitudes.

In India, a gift is seen as potentially poisonous and harmful,[11] especially when gifts are given anonymously as prescribed by universalistic bioethics. Indian gifts can be considered a context for a transmission of "spirit" to occur (Laidlaw in Copeman 2011). Food, clothing, and body parts are especially powerful media for the transmission of bio-moral qualities.[12] Considering that certain castes are considered to be more "polluting" than others, gifts are not easily given across caste boundaries. The risk of pollution is annihilated when a payment is made in exchange for the gift: payment cancels out the wings of indebtedness on which pollution travels. From this perspective, organ sale offers a comparative cultural benefit over organ donation.[13] A similar risk is present for an organ donor. He or she becomes responsible for the *karma* of actions performed by the recipient whose life was saved. Secondly, obtaining organs from the bodies of the dead interferes with a cultural attachment to full-body cremation.[14] A death ritual is enacted according to a blueprint

[9] Mudur (2008).

[10] De Looze (2011); De Looze (2013).

[11] Raheja (1998).

[12] Parry (1994).

[13] De Looze (2013).

[14] De Looze (2013); Copeman and Reddy (2012).

of a regenerative ritual that operates in adherence to a sacrifice of the self to the cremation fire.[15] Many informants fear that when organs are donated before the full body has been cremated, they will not have these organs in their next life. The *use* of organs from the dead is not without conflict either, since it mixes up categories of the pure and impure: the dead live on in the bodies of the living, which resembles the feared affliction of spirit possession.[16] Furthermore, regional differences coincide with leanings towards Vaishnavite, Shaivaite or Shaktist streams of Hinduism, the latter being prevalent in the region of Tamil Nadu. All have different ways of looking at the body-mind-soul complex and prescribe different procedures to untie it. Tamil Nadu is a region where Christianity is more present, which influences the acceptance of practices of cadaveric organ donation in and of itself.

I elaborate on cultural aspects in more detail elsewhere.[17] What is important is that cultural reasons help explain the unpopularity of the practice of cadaveric organ donation in India,[18] regardless of the universalistic pretenses of the practice. As a result, the first important *crack* in the success of the THOA has been that the rise in organs available from brain dead patients has been minimal. This has consequences for the second aim of the Transplantation of Human Organs Act, namely, the goal to eradicate illegal kidney trafficking. It is estimated that an average of 2000 people sell their kidney annually,[19] whereas there are only 50 cadaver donors per year.[20]

23.3.2 The Demand Side

With the THOA, by better meeting the high demand for organs, policy makers aimed to reduce the possibility of making lucrative financial gains on illegal organ markets and thus nip sales in the bud. The THOA thus rests on the assumption that cadaveric organ donation is suitable in an Indian context and, that organ shortage can be met, at least enough to bring about a significant drop in (mostly) kidney prices. Yet, as I pointed out, the increase in supply from cadaver organ donations has been minimal in India. Is there a ceiling to the need for organs? In this section, to get a better perspective on the gap between supply and demand, I scrutinize how the demand for organs has evolved.

If around 200,000 kidneys and 100,000 livers are needed every year in India, only 2–3 % will become available.[21] The *claimed demand* can thus be expected to continue to grow with the availability of organs and the increasing acceptance of organ transfer as a procedure. Researchers have indeed argued that a higher avail-

15 Parry (1994).

16 De Looze (2011).

17 De Looze (2011); De Looze (2013).

18 Shroff (2008).

19 Shimazono (2007).

20 Shroff (2012).

21 Dutta (2012).

ability of organs often coincides with an increase of referrals to waiting lists.[22] The rising incidence of diabetes and hypertension further increases the rate of organ failures. Even in countries that have had successful cadaver donation programs, organs from this source have failed to meet an ever-increasing demand, which led to a resurgence of transplant programs that focus on living donors to complement the former.[23] On top of an increasing national demand, the rise of medical tourists traveling to India to obtain a kidney further enhances the gap between supply and demand.

23.4 Systemic Difficulties with the THOA

Looking at the evolution on both the supply and the demand side, it becomes clear that the gap between both is increasing as opposed to decreasing. Yet the THOA is based on the reasoning that scarcity can be dealt with *enough*. Scheper-Hughes (2000, p. 198) urges us to reconsider what *scarcity* and *need* mean exactly, and how these terms and policies, by chasing their fulfillment, blind us in our capacity to see alternative ways to deal with issues of importance in the field of organ transplantation. The question is to what extent policies become ever more permissive to meet the insatiable demand.

Secondly, with the THOA, a market mechanism is applied to solve the issue of organ sale. Paradoxically, this reinforces the perspective of organs as commodified goods[24] that are potentially *fungible*, i.e. subjective to buying and selling.[25] The THOA, using a market logic to de-economize organ exchange, then paradoxically reinforces the *economization* of bioethics and biosociality.[26]

Lastly, policy discussions in India not only suffer from the pressure of a national organ shortage. The shortage of indigenous supplies is closely intertwined with international shortage. Networks of medical tourism, whereby recipients travel abroad to obtain organs through commercial transactions, bear witness to this.[27] I will now look at how medical tourism is connected to economic development in the international discourse, and discuss how this influences the situation in India.

---

22 Abadie and Gay (2006).

23 Shimazono (2007); De Looze and Shroff (2012).

24 Sharp (2000).

25 Radin (1996).

26 Rabinow (1999).

27 Shimazono (2007).

23.5 The International Context

Earlier we saw that India has about 0.05 cadaver donors per million.[28] Tharakan (2012) sees in this number, which is a mere fraction of the 25 cadaver donors per million in the United States, a sign that India "lags well behind other nations in organ donation rates." The statement that a country "lags behind" reveals the pressure to be *competitive* in international rankings. In the first instance, competition rests on the number of organs harvested, and secondly, the extent to which these organs become available through the application of Universalist policy, in this case cadaveric organ donation. Competition among medical establishments and governments is even more obvious when it concerns efforts to attract medical tourists. Medical tourism is not only seen as an opportunity for development[29] but also as a signpost thereof. It is considered a prime example of a market-driven, commercialized medical service and encouraged as a vehicle for economic development in *lagging* economies, such as India.[30] In the international discourse as well then, a discourse of economic competitiveness penetrates medical discourse.

23.6 The Situation in India

The practice of medical tourism in India is proof for the national and international medical community that the nation has become a player on the international scene;[31] that it has the infrastructure and know-how available to attract medical tourists from the *developed world*. The number of foreigners obtaining medical services in India has risen from 10,000 7 years ago to 450,000 a year today, while it is speculated that revenues have increased from US $ 350 million annually to US $ two billion in 2012.[32]

The slogan "First World Treatment at Third World Prices" (Smith 2012) illustrates that there is a *split*. Whereas medical tourism is seen as an opportunity to spur economic development, its success rests on its low prices and the minimal purchase power of a big part of the local population. India is a player in medical tourism, which reveals medical expertise and cutting-edge technology, yet these are available only to a select group of people, often foreigners. "The flow of organs follows the modern routes of capital: from South to North, from Third to First World, from poor to rich, from black and brown to white, and from female to male" (Scheper-Hughes 2000, p. 193). The split is between two *developmental perspectives*: one being development in the form of techno-scientific advancement, the other being

[28] Mudur (2008).

[29] Bookman and Bookman (2007); WHO (2007); Smith (2012); Gautam (2008).

[30] Smith (2012).

[31] Smith (2012).

[32] Smith (2012).

development in the form of the democratization of human rights and a widespread access to medical services. Economic development through the former only makes a fickle trickle-down promise to the latter. India, while being home to the most innovative medical practices, is getting "bad credits" in the area of equity considerations (Smith 2012). As an example, I will discuss India's kidney belt.

23.7 India's Kidney Belt

The Tamil Nadu region in India is also called the *kidney belt*, in that it is renowned as an area of kidney trade. Villivakkam, a slum in Chennai (the capital of Tamil Nadu), obtained the nickname *kidneyvakkam*. So many of its inhabitants have sold a kidney that Cohen (1999) wonders what it would be like *not* to have done so. Communities such as Villivakkam are also called "one kidney communities" (The Hindu Publishers 1997).

Regions in India where medical tourism is most successful are those where the infrastructure for intensive transplantation practices is available, and where transplantation is more widely known among the public. These regions, because of their familiarity with practices of organ donation, are also areas where organ markets are mostly located. These markets often supply organs to medical tourism networks. This is not surprising, since the international discourse on medical tourism establishes the link between medical services and business thus inserting a factor of economic profitability into medical discourse, which compromises simultaneous attempts to discourage organ sale.

23.8 A Double-Edged Sword

While transplant technology and medical tourism in India are perceived as a route to collective development and Tamil Nadu is considered exemplary of the *way ahead*, India's kidney belt, located in the same region, points out the limits of this strategy. It has been realized that many development programs implemented in the past have been unable to bridge the gap between the rich and the poor, regardless of the trickle-down promise.[33]

Thus, medical tourism offers a means for India to be a player in a globalized world, whereby Tamil Nadu is proof of India's ability to offer cutting-edge medical applications. Yet, the organ trade in Tamil Nadu also shines light on human rights that are sometimes compromised in this process. India is then considered to be *lagging behind*, since the access to infrastructure and know-how has not spread nationwide. Moreover, it is considered to be lagging behind since few of the organs that

[33] Smith (2012).

provide India's supply are harvested from brain dead bodies, as Universalist global ethics would want to see being done.

The result of this tension has been a dynamic of shame. As I read in a newspaper article during my fieldwork, sellers in *one kidney communities* have been harassed for damaging the name and fame of the village and of India as a nation. In academic articles, India is portrayed as a notorious agent in organ sale and since the early 1990s has been referred to as the "organs bazaar of the world" (Scheper-Hughes 2000), much to the despair of the country. In individual situations, organ sellers have frequently been harassed. Cohen gives the example of children that are shouted at: "your mother is a kidney seller" (Cohen 1999, p. 140). To come to a better understanding of this collective double edge, I will draw the parallel of how the kidney scar has received a double meaning for individuals, based on research done by Cohen (1999) in India.

23.9 The Kidney Scar: A Parallel

Cohen goes beyond doctors' perception of kidney scars as medical post-operative signs that can and do heal and uncovers the *real wound* of the kidney scar: poverty. The scar that marks the post-operative condition of living kidney sellers, he says, has two moments. On the one hand, it signifies a successful effort to get out of debt, on the other hand it signals the limits of such success in the long run.[34] Soon after a kidney is sold, a condition of debt often readily re-emerges[35] and this *resource* can no longer be called on.

Aside from seeing the kidney scar as a wound that signals a successful albeit temporary attempt to get out of a situation of poverty, Cohen also sees in the kidney scar an attempt to participate in civil society (Cohen 1999, p. 140). "The operation here is a central modality of citizenship, by which I mean the performance of agency in relation to the state. (…) In other words, having an operation (…) has become a dominant and pervasive means of attempting to secure a certain kind of future, to the extent that means and ends collapse: to be someone with choices is to be operated upon, to be operated upon is to be someone with choices."

Analogously, whereas medical tourism allows India to partake in the global civil society, and medical tourism signals a successful effort towards the economic development of the nation, it also exemplifies the limits of this system in that the sacrifices made along the way are huge. In a sense, India's biocapital is *explanted* in a way that reminds one of a nation's resources being confiscated in colonial times.

---

[34] Cohen (1999).

[35] 96 % of the 305 participants who sold a kidney about 6 years before they were interviewed in 2001, sold their kidney in order to pay off debts. Six years after having sold their kidney, 75 % of the participants were still in debt and the number of participants living below the poverty line had increased. Goyal et al. (2002).

23.10 Primary and Secondary Transactions

In the meantime, the debate on the legalization of organ sale in India is still going on. Proponents argue that the THOA has not succeeded in banning the market[36] or even in providing the organs needed. Publicity for organ sale rests on the argument that there is a *win-win* situation: a donor gains money and a recipient a life-saving kidney.[37] In this type of publicity, only "primary transactions" (Cohen 1999) are taken into account, while "secondary phenomena", such as the socio-economic systems that are structurally disadvantageous to sellers, are left out of the equation.

In the same way, the Transplantation of Human Organs Act only takes into account primary transactions. It has its foundation in the logic of supply and demand, while it loses sight of secondary phenomena such as the difficulty to inscribe cadaveric organ donation in a specific local cultural context. At the same time, it tends to neglect the intricacies that come with the larger international context of medical practices in India as part of, and in particular, the outflow of organs to medical tourists. Promotion campaigns for medical tourism overlook how India might be structurally disadvantaged as part of international socio-economic configurations. They too proclaim a win-win in that India gains economic development, while the lives of first world buyers are saved. Discourses that highlight the opportunities for economic development risk simplifying the rhetoric of development through neglect of a long tradition of hegemonic and counter-hegemonic struggle, which is visible in India's attempts to be considered a *modern* player in the global arena. It also ignores the structural disadvantage brought to India's own citizens.

23.11 The Tradeoff

Counselors in the area of organ transplant policy in India are, on the one hand, pressured to localize their regulations and make them more sensitive to the meaningful structures that are prevalent in civil society.[38] It is important that local circumstances and cultural factors are integrated at the basis of and all throughout policy development and are more than just an appendix to Universalist ethics. The rise in cadaver donations has been insufficient in significantly altering the landscape of organ sale in India. Part of this has to do with the way a polished and often textual cultural discourse is applied in slogans of publicity, whereas this cultural discourse does not address concerns of the people as they arise in cultural action logics.[39] References to the Bhagavad Gita, for example, are commonplace. In these examples of publicity it is said that upon death the body is separated from the soul, similar

[36] Cohen (2010).

[37] Cohen (1999).

[38] De Looze (2011); De Looze (2013).

[39] De Looze (2013).

to a person disposing of garments before going to sleep; that we are imperishable souls living in perishable bodies. Therefore, it is said, organs can be used freely upon death. However, this is a cultural ideal that only speaks to the experience of an accomplished *sannyasin* or renouncer. For lay people, such disassociations of soul and body for the common man only happen during cremation. Such top-down approaches of culture sensitivity to seek ways to connect culture to the technology of organ transplantation a posteriori have proven ineffective.[40]

On the other hand, policy makers are compromised by a situation of international interdependence, the global exchange of organs, and a competitive international discourse. In contrast to the need to render policies sensitive to cultural context and thus *go local*, effective national policies also require awareness of global interaction patterns. "In the age of globalization, having local regulation is almost equal to no regulation at all, because people can easily travel to those places where there is no regulation" (Bunzl 2011). While strictly Universalist ethics are not advisable, simultaneous policy changes in several countries are required, considering the difficulty that nations face to make real policy changes in the context of inter-nation competition.[41]

Lastly, the above-mentioned makes the interdependence of different rights clear. As long as bioethics are not handled together with the securing of other fundamental needs, such as the right of a basic income for all, the exploitation of certain groups of the population will continue.

23.12 Tentative Solutions

I argue to include systems of awareness that acknowledge cultural values and challenges as well as the impact of international discourses and practices when tailoring as well as seeking to implement policies. Pressures arise from international discourse that may be counterproductive to constructive local experimentation. Another obstruction to the search for long-term solutions that are firmly embedded in local contexts may be the pressure to conform to a strategy of *the fast lane* when aiming to increase numbers of organs available. While policies are often tendentious today, following the proclamations of Universalist ethics, global bioethics may instead benefit from a true conversation based on *good local examples* as well as from pragmatic international policy agreements that emerge from such conversations. At the same time, international medical discourse would want to make sure to address development, not only from a techno-economic and neoliberal point of view, but also include its humanitarian side while integrating lessons from the post-modern and post-colonial age. Moreover, it would challenge the paradoxes that are interwoven in its discourse: on the one hand, promoting economic, collective

[40] De Looze (2013).

[41] Bunzl (2011).

profitability through organ transfer, while on the other hand, seeking to relinquish the connection between medical practice and individual profitability through organ sale.

23.13 Conclusion

The central concern of medical policies on organ transplantation today is to alleviate organ shortage. This concern also underpins the Transplantation of Human Organs Act (THOA) that has played a decisive role in transplantation policy in India since 1994. Yet, India faces some empirical difficulties in implementing the THOA. All too easily, these difficulties are considered a sign that organ sale ought to be legalized. In this chapter, I have undertaken an analysis of the complexities of the situation in the hope that these complexities may be taken into account in future discussions.

The THOA is built on the argument that a rise in the supply of organs as a result of implementing a cadaveric organ donation program nationwide would indirectly help put an end to illegal organ sale. Yet, cadaver organ donation has shown a limited and region-specific increase. One of the major causes for this is that this practice may not be sensitive to local culture. When practices are implemented in India, it would be good for advocacy movements to address the fact that a gift in India could potentially be considered a polluting agent, as well as to interact with concerns that arise when using body parts from the (brain) dead. Perhaps even more creative policies can be considered that respond to local concerns in their makeup. On the other hand, I have wondered whether the demand for organs can indeed be expected to diminish if there is a rise in the availability of donor organs. I conclude that this is not the case: the demand for organs tends to increase with an increase in supply. Moreover, medical tourism puts a strain on the national supply of organs. International inequities in economic buying power cause the gap between supply and demand in India to be extended rather than bridged.

While the THOA wishes to de-economize organ exchanges, it relies on an economic rationale of supply and demand to do so. All the while, international discourse on organ transfer has a heavy economic component, as well. This is especially visible in promotion campaigns for medical tourism that publicize it as a major opportunity for the development of *lagging economies*. India's kidney belt reflects the pride India has in being an international player in the medical field, on the one hand. Its well-established centers for medical tourism show that it possesses *first-world* infrastructure and expertise. On the other hand, kidney sales in these regions, as well as the selectivity with which this first-world infrastructure benefits local communities, hampers the image of India as a developed nation, in that it is unsuccessful in providing its citizens with basic human rights. India's kidney belt as such has two sides to it: it is a region that exemplifies India's participation in global dynamics, yet along the way, many sacrifices have to be made. This reminds us of Cohen's analysis of the double meaning of the kidney scar, which on the one hand signifies a successful attempt by individuals in getting out of a situation of debt and be a citizen with access to modern choices, while on the other hand it shows the limits hereof: a kidney can only be sold once.

Looking at the supply side of the THOA it becomes clear that measures more sensitive to local culture contexts are needed; at the same time, there is very little room for such adaptations, considering international competition, the pressure to follow Universalist ethics, and global problems, such as medical tourism. Medical policies often involve a reduction of complexity of the medical situation to primary transactions, while they leave out a consideration of secondary phenomena or the context that is vital to estimate their success. These include socio-economic inequities within India, but also counter-hegemonic struggles on an international scale. Combined care for the localization of policy development and simultaneous international policy implementation is needed, and I have suggested that both are to be founded on conversational ethics. Conversational and interactive bioethics contextualizes global interdependence[42] exacerbated by organ trafficking and medical tourism,[43] such conversations must start by paying attention to how ensuing tensions are handled in practice[44] and the *good examples* that emerge from this.[45] Through conversation, we may arrive at what I call *shared ethics*: an ethics that is able to deal with the tension of universalism and particularism without denying one or the other; an ethics that is not imposed but agreed on; that does not rest on moral a priori but is discovered through practice and through intimacy between different stakeholders as well as system-awareness.

References

Abadie, A., and S. Gay. 2006. The impact of presumed consent legislation on cadaveric organ donation: a cross-country study. *Journal of Health Economics* 25:599–620.

Atala, A. 2011. Printing a human kidney. http://www.ted.com/talks/anthony_atala_printing_a_human_kidney.html. Accessed 28 April 2011.

Bookman, M. Z., and K. R. Bookman. 2007. *Medical tourism in developing countries*. New York: Palgrave Macmillan.

Bunzl, J. 2011. *The simultaneous policy*. London: New European Publications.

Cohen, L. 1999. Where it hurts: Indian material for an ethics of organ transplantation. *Daedalus* 128 (4): 135–166.

Cohen, L. 2010. Ethical publicity: On transplant victims, wounded communities, and the moral demands of dreaming. In *Ethical life in South Asia*, ed. A. Pandian and D. Ali, 253–274. Bloomington: Indiana University press.

Copeman, J. 2011. The gift and its forms of life in contemporary India. *Modern Asian Studies* 45 (5): 1051–1094.

[42] McConnell (1999); Turner (2005).

[43] Turner (2008).

[44] Cf. e.g. Morioka (2001); Souter (2010).

[45] The idea of conversational ethics arose in cooperation with Annemarie Mol and Priya Satalkar.

Copeman, J., and D. Reddy. 2012. The didactic death. *HAU Journal of Ethnographic Theory* 2 (2): 59–83.
De Looze, K. 2011. My heart will go on: The cybernetics of organ harvesting donor (im)mortality and the politics of the non-self. In *Worldviews, science and us: Bridging knowledge and its implications for our perspective of the world*, ed. Aerts Diederik, Bart D'Hooghe, and Nicole Note. Singapore: World Scientific.
De Looze, K. 2013. Interweaving fragments of ethical publicity and ethical resistance: The quest for cadaver organs in India. *Contemporary South Asia* 21 (3): 304–317.
De Looze, K., and S. Shroff. 2012. Can presumed consent overcome organ shortage in India? Lessons from the Belgian experience. *National Medical Journal of India* 25 (3): 168–171.
Dutta, N. 2012. Organ donation—all your queries answered. Health.India.com. http://health.india.com/diseases-conditions/organ-donation-all-your-queries-answered/. Accessed 4 May 2013.
Evans, D. 2007. Seeking an ethical and legal way of procuring transplantable organs from the dying without further attempts to redefine human death. *Philosophy, Ethics, and Humanities in Medicine* 2 (1): 11.
Gautam, V. 2008. Healthcare tourism opportunities for India. www.eximbankindia.com/ht/prelime.pdf. Accessed 14 Jan 2013.
Gervais, K. 1986. *Redefining death*. New Haven: Yale University Press.
Goyal, M., R. L. Mehta, L. J. Schneiderman, and A. R. Sehgal. 2002. Economic and health consequences of selling a kidney in India. *The Journal of the American Medical Association* 288 (13): 1589–1593.
Legislative Department India, Ministry of Law, and Justice and Company Affairs. 1994. The transplantation of human organs act. india.gov.in/allimpfrms/allacts/2606.pdf. Accessed 28 April 2011.
Lock, M. 2002. *Twice dead: Organ transplants and the reinvention of death*. Berkeley: University of California Press.
McConnell, J. 1999. The ambiguity about death in Japan. *Journal of Medical Ethics* 25:322–324.
Morioka, M. 2001. Reconsidering brain death: A lesson from Japan's fifteen years of experience. Hastings Center Report: 41–46.
Mudur, G. 2008. Indian doctors hope kidney scandal will spur cadaver donation programme. *British Medical Journal* 336 (7641): 413.
Ohnuki-Tierney, E., M. Angrosino, et al. 1994. Brain death and organ transplantation: Cultural bases of medical technology. *Current Anthropology* 35 (5): 233–254.
Parry, J. 1994. *Death in Benares*. Cambridge: Cambridge University Press.
Rabinow, P. 1999. Artificiality and enlightenment: From sociobiology to biosociality. In *The Science Studies Reader*, ed. M. Biagioli, 407–416. New York: Routledge.
Radin, M. J. 1996. *Contested commodities*. Cambridge: Harvard University Press.
Raheja, G. G. 1998. *The poison in the gift: Ritual prestation and the dominant caste in a North Indian village*. Chicago: University Press.
Scheper-Hughes, N. 2000. The global traffic in human organs. *Current Anthropology* 41 (2): 191–224.
Sharp, L. 2000. The commodification of the body and its parts. *Annual Review of Anthropology* 29:287–328.
Shimazono, Y. 2007. The state of the international organ trade: A provisional picture based on integration of available information. *Bulletin of the World Health Organization* 85 (12): 901–980.
Shroff, S. 2008. Cadaver organ donation and transplantation: An Indian perspective. http://www.mohanfoundation.org/SlidesSection.asp. Accessed 15 Jan 2008.
Shroff, S. 2012. Organ donation and transplantation—tribulations and triumphs—an Indian perspective. http://www.mohanfoundation.org/organ-donation-transplant-resources/tribulations-triumphs-indian-perspective.asp. Accessed 20 Sept 2012.
Shroff, S., and Pushpa Singh. Personal communication on 05/03/2011.
Shroff, S., S. Rao, G. Kurian, and S. Suresh. 2007. Organ donation and transplantation—Chennai experience in India. *Transplantation Proceedings* 39 (3): 714–718.

Smith, K. 2012. The problematization of medical tourism: A critique of neoliberalism. *Developing World Bioethics* 12 (1): 1–8.

Souter, M. 2010. Ethical controversies at end-of-life after traumatic brain injury. *Critical Care Medicine* 38:502–509.

Tharakan, A. 2012. India moves to contain organ donation havoc. *Canadian Medical Association Journal* 184 (8): E387–E388.

The Hindu Publishers. 1997. One-kidney communities. Frontline 15 (25). http://www.frontlineonnet.com/fl1425/14250730.htm. Accessed 14 Jan 2013.

Turner, L. 2005. From the local to the global: Bioethics and the concept of culture. *Journal of Medicine and Philosophy* 30:305–320.

Turner, L. 2008. 'Medical tourism' initiatives should exclude commercial organ transplantation. *Journal of the Royal Society of Medicine* 101: 391–394.

World Health Organization. 2003. Ethics, access and safety in tissue and organ transplantation: Issues of global concern. Report of the conference in Madrid, Spain, 6–9 October 2003. http://www.who.int/transplantation/en/Madrid_Report.pdf. Accessed 5 May 2013.

World Health Organization. 2007. Medical visas mark growth of Indian medical tourism. *Bulletin of the World Health Organization* 85 (3): 164–165.

Youngner, S. 2007. The definition of death. In *The oxford handbook of bioethics*, ed. B. Steinbock. New York: Oxford University Press.

Karen De Looze is an affiliate researcher at the Interdisciplinary Center Leo Apostel, Brussels Free University. She obtained her PhD in interdisciplinary studies with a study on post-mortem organ donation.

Her research investigated complexities surrounding post-mortem organ donation in India and drew lessons from local cases that are relevant globally. This research study included 19 months of fieldwork in India, and more specifically in Chennai, Varanasi and Vrindavan. Karen's background is in social and cultural anthropology, cultural and developmental studies, and educational sciences. Her research interests include intercultural and comparative philosophy, bioethics, and end-of-life research.

Chapter 24
Iran's Experience on Living and Brain-Dead Organ Donation: A Critical Review

Kiarash Aramesh

24.1 Introduction

Located in the Middle East region, Iran is a large country with an area covering about 1.65 million km^2 and a population of some 75 million. The prevalence of End Stage Renal Disease (ESRD) in Iran is increasing, e.g. the prevalence and incidence rates of ESRD in Iran increased from 238 per million people (pmp) and 49.9 pmp in 2000 to 357 pmp and 63.8 pmp in 2006, respectively.[1] Accordingly, each year an increasing number of patients in Iran find themselves in desperate need of kidney replacement therapy in the form of dialysis or transplantation; the latter being the permanent treatment.

Being one of the most noteworthy renal transplantation programs in the developing world, with an annual rate of around 24 transplantations per 1 million population, the Iranian model of paid and regulated living-unrelated kidney transplantation (IMKT) was the subject of extensive ethical reviews, discussions, and controversies among scholars in the past 2 decades.

Opponents and proponents of this model explained their arguments, ideas and concerns in many articles and books. Sometimes, the authors' political viewpoints influenced their judgments and ethical conclusions. This chapter provides an overview of what has happened in this area, in that it is a noteworthy experience of health-related problem solving in critical situations. In addition to sketching the ethical battleground of opponents and proponents (describing their main theoretical and factual arguments and inferences), the text includes a description of the *brain*

[1] Hosseinpanah et al. (2009); Mahdavi-Mazdeh (2012).

K. Aramesh (✉)
Medical Ethics and History of Medicine Research Center, Tehran University of Medical Sciences, Tehran, Iran
Center for Healthcare Ethics, Duquesne University, USA
e-mail: kiarasharamesh@tums.ac.ir; arameshk@duq.edu

R. J. Jox et al. (eds.), *Organ Transplantation in Times of Donor Shortage*,
International Library of Ethics, Law, and the New Medicine 59,
DOI 10.1007/978-3-319-16441-0_24

death act aimed to facilitate brain-dead organ donation and the religious grounds and challenges behind ratifying this act and explaining why this model of organ donation has not gained popularity in Iran.

24.2 A Brief History

In Iran, the first hemodialysis facility was established in 1974[2] and the first renal transplantation was carried out in 1967 in Shiraz, a city in the southern part of Iran.[3] Between that time and 1978, when the Islamic revolution occurred, a total of around 100 renal transplantations had been performed in Iran. In many cases, kidneys used for transplantation were obtained from the European Transplantation Network.[4]

After the revolution, renal transplantation programs were temporarily stopped. In the early 1980s, patients who needed renal transplant had to seek this treatment abroad, most of them travelling to the UK. However, because of the high costs, many patients could not do so. At the same time, because of the shortage of facilities needed for hemodialysis (mainly due to the Iraq-Iran war) a large number of these patients died.[5] During the last half of the 1980s, renal transplantation teams gradually formed in Iran. From 1985 to 1987, 274 renal transplantations were performed using living organ donors.[6]Collaborations among physicians and religious authorities paved the way in 1988 for the formal development of the Iranian organ transplantation program.[7] In that year, a large number of patients with end stage renal disease needed renal transplants and established a long waiting list to travel abroad using government support for kidney transplantations. The financial burden, along with the deficiency of dialysis facilities, which resulted in some patients dying during the war (1980–1988), urged health authorities to find a way out. The decrees (*Fatwas*)of the religious authorities prepared for the establishment of a compensated, living-unrelated donor renal transplantation program, which was named the Iranian model of kidney transplantation (IMKT). Even though most Shiite authorities do not regard selling organs a right for Muslims,[8] it seems that compensation is accepted. After the establishment of this model, the number of renal transplantations that were performed in Iran increased rapidly and by 1999, the renal transplant waiting list was eliminated.[9]

---

[2] Aghighi et al. (2008).

[3] Larijani (2010).

[4] Larijani (2010); Mahdavi-Mazdeh (2012).

[5] Larijani (2010).

[6] Larijani (2010); Mahdavi-Mazdeh (2012).

[7] Larijani et al. (2004); Aramesh (2009a).

[8] Aramesh (2009b).

[9] Larijani et al. (2004); Ghods and Savaj (2006).

Reportedly, Iran has the largest program of unrelated live donor kidney transplantation in the region.[10]

24.3 How the IMKT Works

According to the formal formulation of the IMKT, the first step is that every person who is a candidate for receiving an unrelated live kidney transplant and every person who wants to donate (or basically, sell) his or her kidney should be referred to the Iranian Patients' Kidney Foundation for registration, which is free of charge. After primary evaluations and obtaining consent from the intended recipient and donor, the Foundation introduces each matched couple (recipient and donor) to each other, so they can negotiate the amount of money the recipient should pay.[11]

After the transplantation is complete, a non-governmental organization (NGO) named the Charity Foundation for Special Diseases is responsible for providing monetary compensation (namely, the gift for altruism, which is provided by the government) and 1-year of medical insurance coverage for the donor. However, as mentioned above, in reality, since the donor and the recipient already know each other a sort of informal payment occurs, which makes it more like buying an organ from the free market. Consequentially, this model has given rise to numerous ethical controversies and debates.

All the transplantation centers in the country are located at university hospitals and are responsible to the Ministry of Health and Medical Education. The medical team does not receive any part of the share of money paid to the donor by the recipient.[12]

24.3.1 Advantages of IMKT

Elimination of Waiting List The elimination of the waiting list for kidney transplantation is the most important claimed advantage of the IMKT.[13] Although some writers have called this claim into question,[14] it is evident that kidney transplantation candidates get the required organ shortly after their registration in the related organization, provided they can pay enough money to find an organ donor. As a matter of fact, given the relatively low price of such organs, buying the one that is needed is affordable for most people.[15] Indeed, the effectiveness of the paid model

[10] Einollahi (2010); Simforoosh (2007).

[11] Mahdavi-Mazdeh (2012).

[12] Mahdavi-Mazdeh (2012).

[13] Ghods and Savaj (2006).

[14] Griffin (2007).

[15] Malakoutian (2007).

with regards to the elimination of the waiting list has inspired some famous western ethicists to propose a modified version of it as a solution to the problem of organ shortage.[16]

Elimination of Organ Trafficking Because of the role played by the Iranian Patients' Kidney Foundation in introducing the potential recipients and donors to each other for a face-to-face negotiation (see above) there is no room for brokers within this system. Also, according to an act ratified by the Iranian Parliament, if anyforeign person wants to get a kidney transplant in Iran, his or her donor must be of the same nationality.[17] Accordingly, it is impossible to transplant a kidney from an Iranian donor to a foreign recipient. It has been claimed that this provision has eliminated organ trafficking and the possibility of exploiting impoverished Iranians as organ donors for rich foreigners.

The Better Quality of Organs Organs donated by living donors are of better quality when compared to organs harvested from brain dead individuals or cadavers.

24.3.2 Weaknesses of IMKT

Commercialization of Human Organs The existence of direct financial relations between kidney donors and recipients is the major ethical Achilles' heel of the IMKT.[18] Direct monetary exchanges between donor and recipient leads to the commercialization and commodification of human organs, which is a violation of human dignity. Although it is argued by the authorities of the Ministry of Health that the IMKT includes formal compensation in the form of charity, there is, in reality, a sort of regulated market for organ transplantation.

Some authors mention the similarities of socioeconomic standing of donor and recipient populations in Iran as an argument for justifying the paid unrelated donation.[19] They argue that such similarities show that in this model the exploitation of the poor by the wealthier part of society does not occur.[20] Ethically speaking, however, this similarity does not justify the model; it just keeps the price of organs low! Around the hospitals where kidney transplantations are performed, you can see several hand-written announcements on the walls written by somebody who is willing to sell a kidney (see Fig. 24.1).

Exploitation of Poor People Given the choice, nobody wants to sell his or her organs. Therefore, the burden of commercialization of human organs is placed on underprivileged social groups and the poor. It has been reported that many donors are addicts seeking money to buy drugs or sometimes, women forced by their husbands to sell their kidneys. In some cases, in families encountering financial prob-

[16] Friedman (2006); Erin and Harris (2003); Delmonico et al. (2003).

[17] Mahdavi-Mazdeh (2012).

[18] Griffin (2007).

[19] Malakoutian et al. (2007).

[20] Mahdavi-Mazdeh (2012).

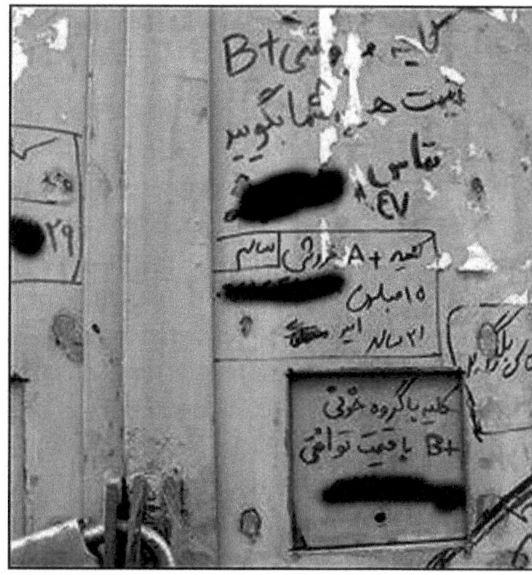

Fig. 24.1 Hand-written announcements for kidney sale

lems, they expect the husband or father to sell his kidney to solve or alleviate the problem.[21]

Although the informed consent is obtained from all donors, nobody can ignore the fact that the main drive behind kidney donation in IMKT is financial. In an attempt to make the donation a consensus within the family, and as a unique feature of the IMKT, informed consent is necessary from both the donor and his or her next of kin (husband or wife in the case of married donors),[22] which obviously does not solve the problem of financial coercion.

Stigmatization of Donors Organ donors are considered organ sellers with no honor, therefore, they tend not to disclose their true identity and address to the hospital's administration, which makes their medical follow-ups very difficult and often impossible.[23] The resulting absence of an effective registration system for donors and the long-term follow-up of donors have been named as significant disadvantages of the IMKT.[24]

Suppression of Altruistic Donation Since organs for transplant are available in the market for a relatively low price, family members of patients who need organs prefer to buy an organ for their loved ones instead of donating their own organs. Also, the stigmatization surrounding organ donors lowers the rate of altruistic donation in society.[25]

21 Zargooshi (2001).

22 Mahvadi-Mazdeh (2012).

23 Zargooshi (2001).

24 Mahdavi-Mazdeh (2012).

25 Zargooshi (2001).

24.4 Organ Transplantation and Brain Death Act

As an attempt to use organs harvested from brain-dead persons, the *Organ Transplantation and Brain Death Act*, previously rejected in 1995, was approved by Iran's parliament in 2000, permitting organ transplantation using brain-dead donors.[26] According to this Act, brain-dead persons' organs, with the consent of their close relatives, can be transplanted to persons in need provided that doing so is necessary in order to save their lives. Accordingly, only heart transplantation can be considered a legitimate reason for terminating a brain-dead person's life. Harvesting other organs, like kidneys, pancreas, liver or cornea is permitted only after harvesting the heart, which turns a brain-dead person into a dead person.

Considering that in Iran, legislation is based on Islamic (*Shiite*) jurisprudence (*Fiqh*), this Act is based on religious decrees allowing such practice. In Shiite jurisprudence, a brain-dead person is not considered dead but, rather, as being in a stage of life (namely: *Hayat-e-Gheyr-e Mustagherreh*, which means unstable life) where she or he could only be sacrificed for the sake of saving a stable human life.[27]

In contrast with living donation, organ donation from brain-dead persons are completely altruistic without any monetary incentive for donors. A virtual network, covering the entire country (encompassing 13 procurement units and 18 brain death identification units), facilitates this sort of organ donation. The declaration of brain death is based on the diagnosis of five physicians (consisting of an internist, a neurologist, a neurosurgeon, an anesthesiologist, and a forensic medicine specialist) and according to neurological tests and after obtaining a confirmatory electroencephalogram.[28] The consent for donation should be obtained from the first-degree relative of the donor. Before transplantation, recipients and donors are anonymous to each other. These organs are being allocated based on a first come, first serve policy.

However, because of the availability of better quality organs obtained from live donors, most recipients prefer to receive their organs from a live donor rather than a deceased one. Consequently, in contrast to developed countries, 76 % of kidneys come from living unrelated donors and only 12 % of kidneys are from deceased donors.[29] In comparison, consider for example that in the US in 2006, 65 % of transplanted kidneys were from deceased donors and less than 1 % of them were from anonymous living donors. Consequently, the health authorities do not feel any urge to improve the quality of organs obtained from deceased donors or adopt any essential policy aimed at increasing the number of organs obtained in this way.

26 IR Iran Parliament (2000).

27 Larijani (2010).

28 Mahdavi-Mazdeh (2012).

29 Larijani (2010).

24.5 Conclusions

In light of the substantial advantages as well as weaknesses of the IMKT, its ethical flaws cannot be ignored. Arguably, despite some notable practical successes and advantages of this model, it should be substituted with another model that is mainly based on altruistic donation. Of course, given long waiting lists and the large number of people who die before getting their transplant in developed countries, one should not fail to appreciate the value of the elimination of these deadly waiting lists. One the other hand, without the act of paying enough money, it is impossible to achieve a sufficient number of unrelated donors to eliminate the waiting list. Thus, while compensatory payment by an NGO could be considered an acceptable incentive for donors, such processes would, quite clearly, not eliminate the waiting list. Accordingly, a model of indirect and regulated payment from recipients to donors can be considered as a possible solution for the future.

Considering the high prevalence of accidents resulting in brain death in Iran, and the positive public attitude towards brain dead organ donation,[30] the problem of a shortage of organs could be solved by promoting organ donation from brain-dead persons. Consequently, adopting the opt-out approach rather than the opt-in one would be a great step forward.

Acknowledgement The abstract of this article was first presented at the International Bioethics Workshop for Young Scholars, titled *Organ Transplantation in Times of Donor Shortage: Interdisciplinary Challenges and Solutions*, held by the Ludwig-Maximilians-University (LMU) Munich, Germany, February 25-March 2, 2012. I would like to express my gratitude to the leaders and organizers of that workshop, especially Prof Dr. Georg Marckmann and PD Dr. Ralf J. Jox for that great and fruitful event. Also, I would like to extend my many thanks to Dr. Galia Assadi for all her assistance and cooperation through the workshop and the process of writing and finalizing this article. Last but not least, I would like to appreciate the helpful and informative comments provided by Dr. Barbro Fröding, the reviewer of this article.

References

Aghighi, M., A. Heidary Rouchi, M. Zamyadi, et al. 2008. Dialysis in Iran. *Iranian Journal of KidneyDisease* 2:11–15.

Aramesh, K. 2009a. Iran's experience on religious bioethics: An Overview. *Asian Bioethics Review* 1 (4): 318–328.

Aramesh, K. 2009b. The ownership of human body: An Islamic perspective. *Journal of Medical Ethics and History of Medicine* 2:4. http://journals.tums.ac.ir/upload_files/pdf/13449.pdf. Accessed 8 June 2013.

Boroumand, M., A. Parsapour, and F. Asghari. 2012. Public opinion of organ donation: A survey in Iran. *Clinical Transplantation* 26:E500–E504. doi:10.1111/ctr.12001.

Delmonico, F. L., R. Arnold, N. Scheper-Hughes, et al. 2003. Ethical incentives—not payment—for organ donation. *The New England Journal of Medicine* 346 (25): 2002–2005.

[30] Boroumand et al. (2012).

Einollahi, B. 2010. Kidney transplantation in Iran. *Iranian Journal of Medical Sciences* 35 (1): 1–8.
Erin, C. A., and J. Harris. 2003. An ethical market in human organs. *Journal of Medical Ethics* 29:137–138.
Friedman, A. L. 2006. Payment for living organ donation should be legalized. *British Medical Journal* 333:746–748.
Ghods, A. J., and S. Savaj. 2006. Iranian model of paid and regulated living-unrelated kidney donation. *Clinical Journal of the American Society of Nephrology* 1:1136–1145.
Griffin, A. 2007. Kidney on demand. *British Medical Journal* 334:502–505.
Hosseinpanah, F., F. Kasraei, A. A. Nassiri, et al. 2009. High prevalence of chronic kidney disease in Iran: A large population-based study. *BMC Public Health* 9:44. doi:10.1186/1471-2458-9-44.
IR Iran Parliament. 2000. Deceased or brain dead patients organ transplantation act. H/24804-T/9929, 6-4-2000.
Larijani, B. 2010. *Bioethics in organ transplantation, an Islamic perspective*. Tehran: Medical Ethics and History of Medicine Research Center.
Larijani, B., F. Zahedi, and E. Taheri. 2004. Ethical and legal aspects of organ transplantation in Iran. *Transplantation Proceedings* 36:1241–1244.
Mahdavi-Mazdeh, M. 2012. The Iranian model of living renal transplantation. *Kidney International* 82:627–634.
Malakoutian, T., M. S. Hakemi, A. A. Nassiri, et al. 2007. Socioeconomic status of Iranian living unrelated kidney donors: A multicenter study. *Transplantation Proceedings* 39:824–825.
Simforoosh, N. 2007. Kidney donation and rewarded gifting: an Iranian model. *Nature Clinical Practice Urology* 4 (6): 292–293.
Zargooshi, J. 2001. Iranian kidney donors: Motivations and relations with recipients. *The Journal of Urology* 165:386–92.

Kiarash Aramesh is a medical doctor who was born and raised in Iran. His specialty is in Community Medicine. He is Associate Professor and Vice-President for Research at the Medical Ethics and History of Medicine Research Center at Tehran University of Medical Sciences. In addition, he is a member of the National Committee of Bioethics of the Iranian National Commission for UNESCO. From August 2013 until July 2014 he worked as a visiting scholar at the Department of Bioethics at the National Institutes of Health (NIH) in the United States of America. Subsequently, he joined the Healthcare Ethics Center at the Duquesne University in Pittsburgh, USA, as a PhD candidate. His research interests are Biomedical Research Ethics, Religious Ethics, Human Dignity, Beginning and End-of-Life Issues, and Public Health Ethics.

Chapter 25
The Norwegian Model Full Utilisation of Both Living and Deceased Donors to Meet the Need for Organs

Per Pfeffer

25.1 Introduction: The Right Set of Rules from the Beginning

The Norwegian national renal transplant program was officially started in 1967 (Pfeffer and Albrechtsen 2011). Dialysis at that time was rudimentary and deceased donor (DD) transplantations had significantly worse outcomes than transplantations with organs from living donors (LD). The access to organs from DDs was also very limited. Some crucial decisions had to be made right from the start, which, after more than 40 years, still constitute Norway's national guidelines for end-stage renal decease:

- Transplantation is superior to dialysis.
- Transplantation should be offered to all patients who may benefit from it.
- Family members should be given the opportunity to donate a kidney to bridge the gap between need and supply of organs.
- Pre-dialytic transplantation is preferable.

This type of activity required the establishment of a new law for the transplantation and donation of organs.[1] A particularity of the Norwegian Transplantation Law of 1973 was the provision made in 1977 requiring cerebral angiography and later alternatively arcography to visualise the cessation of intracranial circulation. This is, of course, the absolute proof of brain death and has led to great confidence in the population and among health care workers in Norway.

[1] Lovdata (1973).

P. Pfeffer (✉)
Oslo University Hospital, Oslo, Norway
e-mail: per.pfeffer@gmail.com

R. J. Jox et al. (eds.), *Organ Transplantation in Times of Donor Shortage*,
International Library of Ethics, Law, and the New Medicine 59,
DOI 10.1007/978-3-319-16441-0_25

The transplantation law includes presumed consent, even though this has, as is the case in most other countries as well, not been practised. Relatives will be consulted, however the emphasis is placed on the deceased donor's wish or attitude towards organ donation. The transplantation law also includes a paragraph on live donation, which, among other things, states that live donors can be used if there is no obvious risk or danger for the donor's life or health.

25.2 An Active Approach to Live Donation

The Norwegian Model of renal transplantation has been associated most commonly with its long-term emphasis on LDs. This was often criticised as unethical activity by many other transplantation centres, but has, over time, proven to be both sound and necessary in that in over 2700 LDs there has been no operative mortality. In 1983, use of LD was widened by the introduction of cyclosporine. The improved immunosuppression made it possible to put less emphasis on HLA compatibility while still achieving good graft survival. Non-genetically related donors, such as spouses and distant relatives, were introduced and later also long-term, close friends. Even with these organsources and even with full HLA-mismatch, the long-term graft survival has been better than with organs taken from deceased donors (Fig. 25.1).

A further peculiarity of the Norwegian living donor program is that no patient with end-stage renal disease is put on the DD wait list before the possibility of a LD has been thoroughly evaluated. In other words, the DD wait list should be reserved

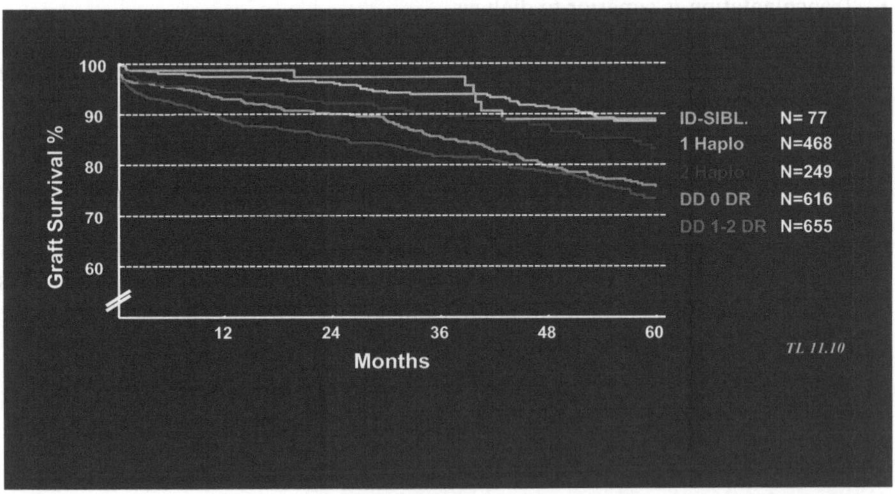

Fig. 25.1 Survival of first renal grafts by donor source and HLA-match. Data from 2000–2009. *ID-SIBL* HLA-identical sibling, *1 Haplo* 1 HLA haplo-identical living donor, *2 Haplo* 2 HLA haplotype-mismatched living donor, *DD 0 DR* deceased donor, no HLA DR mismatch, *DD 1–2 DR* deceased donor, 1–2 HLA DR mismatches. (Data taken from: Norwegian Renal Registry 2010)

for those patients who do not have the opportunity of receiving a LD graft. The availability of a sufficient amount of organs in Norway can only be made possible by the extensive use of LDs over time. Countries that traditionally do not use LDs will typically only be able to supply an organ to one third of those on the wait list. The Norwegian Ministry of Health has concluded that neither the Oviedo directive of the Council of Europe nor the organ directive of the European Union are legally in conflict with the Norwegian practise.[2]

After more than 7300 renal transplantations, of which over 2700 were with a kidney from a living donor, 72% of the Norwegian uremic population is successfully transplanted at any given time. This is the highest coverage compared to other countries. In 2011, the total transplantation rate per million was 60.4, including all kidney sources (Fig. 25.2).

This is made possible by the high rate of LDs, averaging 37% over the years of the program. There is no age limit for transplantation or dialysis in Norway. Patients that are deemed unsuitable for transplantation at primary evaluation will, among other things, be offered heart-, aortic-, or carotid artery surgery where indicated, in order to make them eligible. Norway has a universal health care system. Dialysis

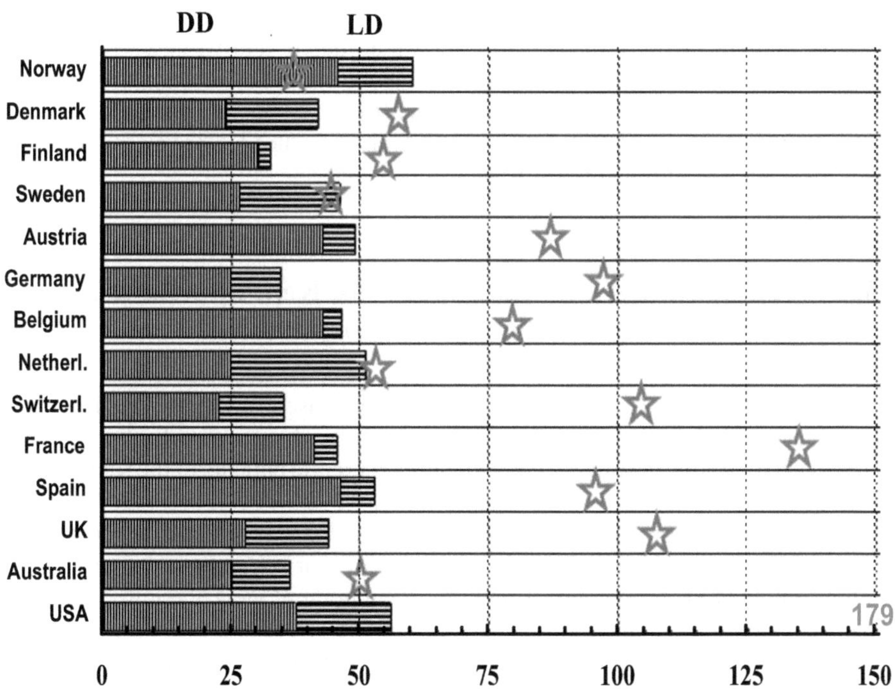

Fig. 25.2 Renal transplantation and wait lists in 2011. Graft sources: *DD* deceased donor, *LD* living donor. *Stars* DD wait list. All data per million. (Newsletter Transplant 2012)

[2] Council of Europe (1997), Directive 2010/53/EU (2010).

also belongs to this public system and there are no private dialysis units in Norway. Recipients and potential LDs are processed at the 20 local nephrology centres in Norway and then referred to one national transplant centre for final approval and TX.

This one transplant centre, which handles all types of transplantations, covers the needs of 5 million Norwegians making it the largest centre of its kind in Scandinavia. All organ harvesting is also performed by the surgeons in this centre. Simple logistics lead to reduced costs and the second shortest average cold ischemia time in Scandinavia, despite long distances that need to be travelled for both organ retrieval and for patients coming to Oslo to receive their transplant.

Norway is a member and one of the founders of Scandiatransplant, which serves as a centralized computer system for all of Scandinavia and also controls the organ exchange within Scandinavia according to an agreed set of rules. This system gives supranational preference to children, patients with especially complicating antibodies and has also introduced a permissible mismatch program. Initially, the rate of exchange of organs among Scandinavian countries was approximately 25 %, giving special preference to HLA matching. Within recent years, the rate of exchange has been reduced to between 5–10 %. Less emphasis has been put on HLA matching and more on short cold ischemia time, which results in more organs being used locally and further acts as a motivating factor for the transplant teams. These guidelines are available on the Scandiatransplant homepage. In that some Scandinavian countries have a higher transplantation rate than others and while recipient wait lists also vary, a system to avoid an imbalance within Scandiatransplant has been developed, in which organs of comparable quality have to be *returned* to the donor country within half a year. Before this system was introduced, Norway was losing a significant amount of organs each year.

25.3 Number of Living Donors Has Not Kept up with the Increase of Uremic Patients in Norway

As can be seen in Fig. 25.3, there was an initial increase of LDs after the introduction of calcinurin inhibitor (CNI) in 1983–1984, but only marginal further increase in the years to follow, despite a steady increase in uremic patients in the same period (Fig. 25.4).

This problem has been discussed repeatedly with local nephrologists and in 2007 our transplant centre introduced a LD coordinator that streamlines the process of finding suitable LDs for patients. From a surgical point of view, the introduction of laparoscopic donor nephrectomy in 1998, modified with hand assistance in 2005, should improve the LD situation further. It has led to less operative trauma, no intercostal nerve injuries, and faster postoperative recovery.[3] The highest number of LDs was 104 registered in 2009 (incidence: 21.55 pmp), which proceeded to drop again so that LDs now only constitute 24 % of the total number of transplants

[3] Mjøen et al. (2010).

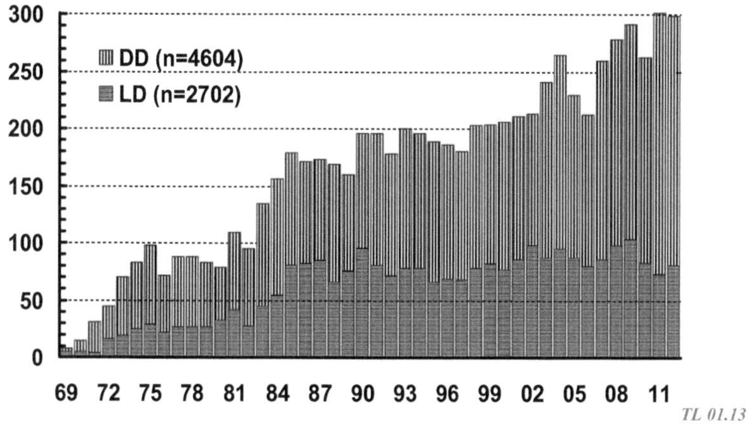

Fig. 25.3 Kidney transplantation in Norway with all available organ sources since the start of the national program. Data are given in number of patients per year from 1969–2012. In brackets: total number of patients. *DD* deceased donor, *LD* living donor. (Data taken from: Norwegian Renal Registry 2013)

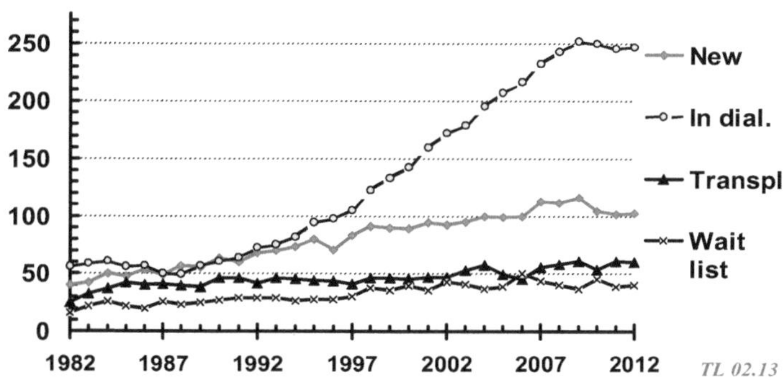

Fig. 25.4 Patients with end-stage uraemia in Norway and treatment modalities since 1982. Data per million inhabitants. (Data taken from the Norwegian Renal Registry 2013)

(incidence in 2011: 14.7 pmp). The relatively low percentage of live donation at present is also caused by an increase in DDs, as will be discussed later.

25.4 Live Donation Is Not Practised Uniformly in Norway

The use of LDs in the different regions in Norway varies with up to 50 % pmp, which could not readily be explained by demographic differences. The attitude of nephrologists and their centres towards live donation, the workload they are exposed to, or lack of systematic programs for the evaluation and processing of whole families are some probable explanations.

Thus in 2011, the Norwegian Directorate for Health appointed an expert group that developed a set of guidelines called: "Kidney Donation from Living Donor. Selection and Follow up of the Donor" (Nyredonasjon fra levende giver 2012).

A few of these guidelines are mentioned below and partially reflect already well-established routines:

- Transplantation with a kidney from a LD should be the first choice for patients with end-stage renal failure and preferably be performed pre-emptively, if the patient is eligible.
- Evaluation programs should be developed for both the registry of patients and potential donors in order to streamline the process.
- The patients' nephrologist is responsible for initiating this process, but should not be responsible for the evaluation of potential LDs.
- If the patient permits, the donor's doctor will actively approach first-degree family members for possible donation. Distant family members will only be considered if presented spontaneously and long-term friends will only be considered after the evaluation by a committee.
- There should be a system of full compensation for the expenses the LD has had in connection with the donation process.
- Life-long follow-up of LDs and a national registry of donor data should be continued and anonymous data contributed to a common Scandinavian living donor database at Scandiatransplant.
- Rikshospitalet, Oslo University hospital, should initiate regional courses to motivate and educate centres about the process of live donation.

These courses commenced in Fall 2013.

25.5 Deceased Donation in Norway

Parallel to live donation, deceased donation has existed since before the start of the official program, the first DD transplant taking place in 1956. Compared to some other countries, organ retrieval from DDs has only been moderately successful throughout the years. With the success of the Spanish DD program, similar systems were introduced in Norway, but to a lesser extent, especially in terms of economic support. It has been a relatively slow process, starting in 2002 with the introduction of doctors specifically responsible for the donors in 28 donor hospitals. In 2007 economic compensation and defined time for donor-related activity was integrated, but limited to the university hospitals. In 2008, DRG (Diagnosis-Related Group) compensation for additional expenses in connection with the DD process also had a positive effect on the DD rate. Since 2007, a pre-existing Intensive Care Registry (NIR) that records mortality in the intensive care units started registering potential DDs and whether deceased donation had been properly evaluated in each case.

Even though Rikshospitalet is the hub in the national transplant program, the local nephrology centres are responsible for the eligibility process prior to referring patients to the Rikshospitalet for transplantation and also later for the follow-up. The coordination of this national program is achieved through yearly meetings with the nephrologists. The system is further strengthened by The Norwegian Resource Group for Organ Donation (NOROD) from 1992, which offers regional courses about deceased donation at least four times per year. In 2005, a national coordinator for deceased donation was introduced to The Norwegian Directorate of Health, which from 2009 onwards was supported by the initiation of a National Council for Transplantation. In 1997, The Foundation for Organ Donation was formed by patient organisations and has been very active toward the government and polititions, as well as the press and the public in general. The response has been very positive with practically no negative coverage in the press. In that there is only one transplant centre, there has been no public discussion between university institutions, which has been the case in some of our neighboring countries. End-stage uraemia has increased at a rate of 5–15 % per year over the last decade, which is caused by an aging population and lifestyle-related diseases like obesity, hypertension, diabetes, and increased arteriosclerosis. There is also a general demand in the population for more active medical treatment of older age groups. The medical community has therefore repeatedly warned about the consequences this will have on the need for treatment of uremic patients, with transplantation being the cheapest and best treatment for the majority of patients.

In 2007, the government set down a bold but necessary set of goals for future transplantation activity:

- Renal transplantation with LD should be maintained at 40 %.
- The DD rate should be increased to 30 pmp.

In 2011, the government issued an "Action Plan for Prevention and Treatment of Chronic Renal Disease" that laid down rules for preventive measures, early detection, and treatment of renal disease and transplantation when indicated (Handlingsplan 2011). This plan also states that the access to transplantation should be evenly distributed and of high quality, independent of geographical location, individual economy, ethnic background, and social status. This reflects the basic philosophy of our universal health care system.

With multiple measures and a recent increased emphasis on extended criteria for DD, the DD rate has increased by 50 % over the last 10 years to 23.27 pmp in 2012. The conversion rate for deceased donation (proportion of possible DDs that become actual DDs) was 80 % in 2012 and family refusal of donation only 17 %, which is the lowest recorded. In 2011, a total of 38 % of DDs were older than 60, with the oldest being 86. We have previously shown that this source of organs performs quite well.[4] The selection of marginal donors is done through clinical evaluation. Histological results from renal biopsies are not available preoperatively and we do not use extra-corporal perfusion machines. Despite this, the DD

[4] Foss et al. (2009).

grafts showed primary functions in approximately 85 % of cases in 2012. With the combined efforts of LD and DD, the DD wait list is now stable (Fig. 25.4).

The mean waiting time for a DD graft is 8 months. Mean waiting time for a first renal graft is 6 months (79 % of the patients on the wait list) and 65 months for those waiting for their fourth graft (1 % of the patients). This relatively short waiting time for the large majority of patients is, however, a problem when arguing with the nephrologists, the patients, and the potential donors for a LD. In some centres the evaluation of family members for live donation may take up to 8 months.

25.6 Arguments for Live Donation

Advantages for the recipients:

- Better graft and recipient survival.
- Only 1–2 months waiting time after a suitable LD has been found.
- Increased likelihood of pre-emptive transplantation and planned surgery. Especially important in paediatric or diabetic patients.
- Pre-treatment of patients who have donor-specific HLA antibodies.
- Pre-treatment of patients with living donors that have incompatible blood groups.

Few disadvantages for the donor:

- There has been no operative mortality in our LD program.
- The pre- and postoperative morbidity is rather low with further improvement through modern operative techniques.
- Post donation life expectancy and life quality exceeds that of the general population.
- Living donor satisfaction has been high.

Westlie et al. evaluated the LD satisfaction among Norwegian donors in 485 patients post donation, by asking the question: If you had the chance to do it again, would you consent to donating your kidney? He found that 83.3 % answered that they would definitely and 10.7 % said they would probably have donated again, and even in cases where the recipient died 89 % of the donors said they would definitely or probably have donated again. A typical response in this category of LDs was that they felt that they had at least done everything that was possible to save the patient. Only 4.3% said they would definitely not do it again.[5]

In a recent study by Mjøen et al. 1984 kidney donors from the period 1963–2007 were contacted by the Norwegian Renal Registry, of whome 76 % responded.[6] All of them received the Short-Form-36 (SF-36) and a questionnaire specifically designed for kidney donors.

[5] Westlie et al. (1993).

[6] Mjøen et al. (2011b).

Table 25.1 Short Form-36. Quality of the scores in kidney donors and controls. (Table adapted from Mjøen et al. 2011b)

Health status scales	Kidney donors (n=1414)	Controls (n=6800)	P-value
Physical function	89.3 (17.5)	87.5 (18.7)	<0.001
Role physical	82.9 (34.0)	80.4 (35.2)	<0.001
Bodily pain	78.5 (26.1)	74.3 (26.8)	<0.001
General health	81.1 (21.0)	76.8 (21.6)	<0.001
Vitality	64.5 (21.1)	62.0 (21.0)	<0.001
Social function	89.7 (19.5)	88.1 (20.2)	<0.001
Role emotional	89.9 (26.8)	87.8 (28.2)	<0.001
Mental health	83.6 (15.1)	81.4 (15.4)	<0.001
Physical component summary scale	51.3 (9.5)	50.1 (9.9)	<0.001
Mental component summary scale	54.0 (8.4)	53.1 (9.0)	<0.046

As can be seen in Table 25.1, kidney donors scored significantly higher than the general population sample on all eight subscales of the SF-36 after adjusting for age, gender, and education.

Mjøen et al. also show that the overall and cardiovascular mortality of living donors was lower than for a selected control group with a health status which hypothetically would allow for donation, even though age-stratified death rates were found to be elevated for LDs who were 70–79 years of age at the time of donation.[7]

An important argument for live donation for doctors and health authorities is that our generally fortunate situation is caused by the fact that we have had an active policy towards live donation, which has eased the pressure on the DD wait list. This positive situation could easily slip if we lose focus. We still have not reached the goals proposed by our health care authorities and an increase in the number of patients with terminal renal failure is to be expected, despite emerging strategies to improve preventive measures.

References

Council of Europe. 1997. Convention on human rights and biomedicine (Oviedo). http://conventions.coe.int/treaty/EN/Treaties/Html/164.htm.

Directive 2010/53/EU of the European Parliament and the Council of 7 July 2010 on: Standards of quality and safety of human organs intended for transplantation. http://www.ec.europa.eu/health/bloodtissuesorgans/organs/indexen.htm.

Foss, A., K. Heldal, H. Scott, et al. 2009. Kidneys from deceased donors more than 75 years perform acceptably after transplantation. *Transplantation* 87 (10): 1437–1441.

[7] Mjøen et al. (2011a).

Handlingsplan for forebygging og behandling av kronisk nyresykdom (2011–2015). Helsedirektoratet, red. 2011. IS-1884. http://www.helsedirektoratet.no/publikasjoner/rapporter/handlingsplanforforebyggingogbehandlingavkronisknyresykdom20112015815204.

Lovdata. 1973. Lov om transplantasjon, obduksjon, avgivelse av lik med mer. http://www.lovdata.no/all/nl-19730209-006.html.

Mjøen, G., H. Holdaas, P. Pfeffer, et al. 2010. Minimally invasive living donor nephrectomy—Introduction of hand-assistance. *Transplant International: Official Journal of the European Society for Organ Transplantation* 23 (10): 1008–1014.

Mjøen, G., A. Reisaeter, S. Hallan, et al. 2011a. Overall and cardiovascular mortality in Norwegian kidney donors compared to the background population. *Nephrology, Dialysis, Transplantation: Official Publication of the European Dialysis and Transplant Association—European Renal Association* 27 (1): 443–447. doi:10.1093/ndt/gfr303.

Mjøen, G., K. Stavem, L. Westlie, et al. 2011b. Quality of life in kidney donors. *American Jornal of Transplantation* 11:1315–1319.

Newsletter Transplant. 2012. http://www.edqm.eu/site/newsletter_transplant_vol_17_no_1_sept_2012pdf-en-31013-2.html.

Norwegian Renal Registry. 2010/2013. http://www.nephro.no.

Nyredonasjon fra levende giver. 2012. Utvelgelse og oppfølging av giver. Helsedirektoratet IS-2003. http://www.helsedirektoratet.no.

Pfeffer, P., and D. Albrechtsen, eds. 2011. *En gave for livet. Historien om transplantasjon i Norge.* Oslo: UNIPUB.

Scandiatransplant homepage. http://www.scandiatransplant.org.

Westlie, L., P. Fauchald, T. Talseth, et al. 1993. Quality of life in Norwegian kidney donors. *Nephrology, Dialysis, Transplantation: Official Publication of the European Dialysis and Transplant Association—European Renal Association* 8:1146–1150.

Per Pfeffer MD, PhD Retired since 2012. Per was previously a board member for Scandiatransplant, President of the Scandinavian Transplantation Society, council member for ESOT, Chairman of the European Committee on Organ Transplantation, Council of Europe, fellow of the European Board of Surgery, UEMS, and the Head of Transplant Surgical Section, Oslo University Hospital. Scientific publications: *Transplant Immunology and Clinical Transplantation.*

Chapter 26
The Spanish Model of Organ Donation and Transplantation

Rafael Matesanz and Beatriz Domínguez-Gil

26.1 Introduction

Solid organ transplantation saves the lives or improves the quality of life of about 100,000 patients worldwide every year.[1] The consolidation of transplantation therapies derives from the excellent results achieved by the transplantation of virtually all types of organs, something which was made possible in a relatively short period of time, seeing as the first successful kidney transplant between humans was carried out back in 1954.[2] Organ transplantation is different from other medical services because its practice does not rely solely on technical development or professional expertise. The success of transplantation also depends on the availability of an organ from a willing and suitable living or deceased donor. A shortage of organs is a universal obstacle that precludes the full expansion of transplantation therapies, determining the death and clinical deterioration of patients on the waiting list for an organ transplant. In addition to and as a result of the unequal distribution of wealth in the world, organ shortage is also the root cause for unethical practices such as organ trafficking and transplant tourism, practices that violate fundamental human rights, like those of human dignity and integrity, and erode the image of the donation and transplantation systems, perpetuating shortage.[3]

Through *Resolution WHA 63.22*, the World Health Assembly urged Member States "to strengthen national and multinational authorities and/or capacities to

[1] Global Observatory on organ donation and transplantation.

[2] Murray (2005).

[3] Joint Council of Europe/United Nations Study.

R. Matesanz (✉) · B. Domínguez-Gil
National Transplant Organization, Madrid, Spain
e-mail: rmatesanz@msssi.es

B. Domínguez-Gil
e-mail: bdominguez@msps.es, bdominguez@msssi.es

R. J. Jox et al. (eds.), *Organ Transplantation in Times of Donor Shortage*,
International Library of Ethics, Law, and the New Medicine 59,
DOI 10.1007/978-3-319-16441-0_26

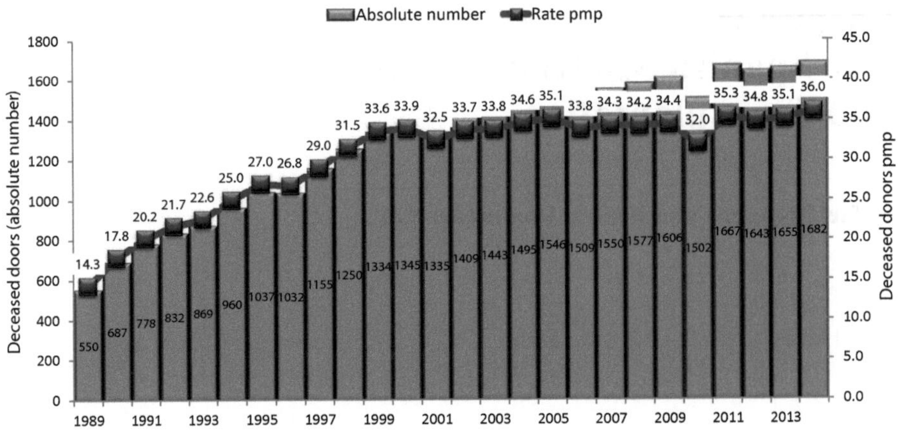

Fig. 26.1 Evolution of transplantation activities in Spain, in terms of number of solid organ transplant procedures (absolute numbers). Between the years 1989–2014.

provide oversight, organization and coordination of donation and transplantation activities, with special attention to maximizing donation from deceased donors and to protect the welfare of living donors with appropriate health-care services and long-term follow-up" (Sixty third World Health Assembly). The Resolution was adopted two months after participants at the *3rd World Health Organization(WHO) Global Consultation on Organ Donation and Transplantation* called on governments for accountability in the pursuit of self-sufficiency in transplantation (Madrid Resolution). In other words, to cover the transplantation needs of their patients by using resources within their own patient population and through both decreasing the burden of chronic diseases leading to the need of a transplant and increasing the availability of human organs.[4] Initiatives in this regard are to have a solid ethical basis by respecting international ethical standards, such as the *WHO Guiding Principles on Human Cell, Tissue and Organ Transplantation.*[5]

The call to address the transplantation needs of a particular population is to be highlighted in a diverse global landscape where huge disparities exist between countries in terms of transplantation activities, mainly due to differences in deceased donation rates. Deceased donation ranges from its non-existence in many countries throughout the world to rates of more than 30 donors per million population (pmp).[6] In this global scenario, Spain occupies a privileged position, with the highest deceased donation rates ever described for a large country and maintained at 33–35 donors pmp within the last years, leading to transplantation rates close to 90 transplant procedures pmp in 2012 (Figs. 26.1 and 26.2). With about 14 donors pmp at the end of the eighties, the activity in Spain was at a mid-low position when

[4] The Madrid Resolution on Organ Donation and Transplantation (2011).

[5] WHO Guiding Principles on Human Cell, Tissue and Organ Transplantation

[6] Global Observatory on organ donation and transplantation.

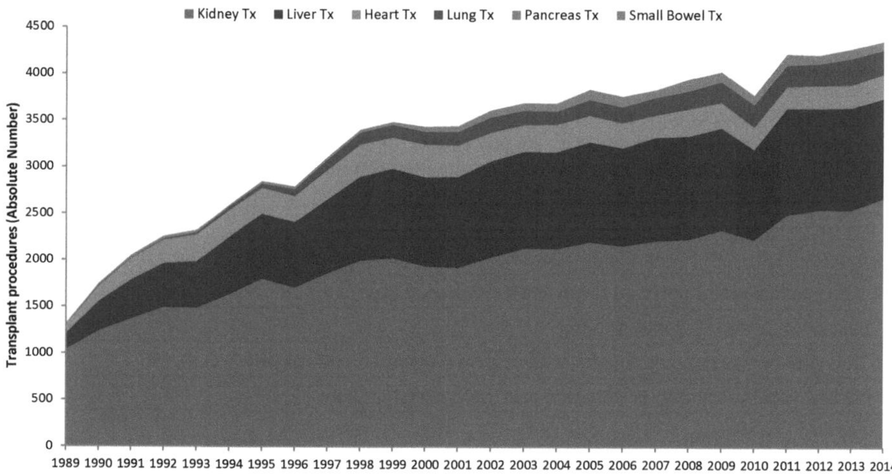

Fig. 26.2 Evolution of transplantation activities in Spain, in terms of number of solid organ transplant procedures (absolute numbers). Between the years 1989–2014.

compared to other European and non-European countries. The increase in deceased donation, and consequently in the number of solid organ transplants, has been the result of the implementation of a set of measures, mainly of an organizational nature, collectively and internationally named the *Spanish Model on Organ Donation and Transplantation*—hereafter, the *Spanish Model*. This manuscript aims at reviewing the elements of this system, a global reference in the pursuit of the self-sufficiency paradigm.

26.2 The Spanish Model on Organ Donation and Transplantation

The measures composing the *Spanish Model* were adopted after the *Spanish National Transplant Organization* (Organización Nacional de Trasplantes—ONT) was created in 1989. ONT was conceived as a technical agency dependent on the Ministry of Health and in charge of the oversight of all donation and transplantation activities in the country. Dependency on the Ministry of Health was representative of transplantation being placed on the political agenda—an anticipated response to the call for national accountability that the WHO would launch almost 20 years later. Results of the *Spanish Model* derive from the basic principle of having an appropriate organization centered around the process of deceased donation, particularly around the process of donation after brain death (DBD), representing 90–95 % of the deceased donation activity in the country as a whole.

Measures implemented in Spain were based on an appropriate background from the health-care, technical and legal point of view. The Spanish health-care system is

Table 26.1 Main elements of the Spanish model of organ donation and transplantation

Transplant coordination network on three levels: National—ONT-, regional, hospital
Special profile of transplant coordinators • In-house professionals, part of the hospital staff • Medical doctors, mainly critical care physicians, supported by nurses • Part-time dedication to the transplant coordination activities • Independence from the transplant teams. Appointed by and reporting to the hospitals' medical director
Central office—ONT—as a supporting agency. Not just an organ sharing-allocation agency
Quality assurance program in the deceased donation process
Great effort in professional training
Close attention to the mass media with a special communication policy
Hospital reimbursement for donation and transplantation activities

a public one with universal coverage for the population, entailing that transplantation is included in the public health-care portfolio and every citizen will have access to that therapy if needed. Technically, the country was able to count on extraordinarily prepared, enthusiastic, innovative and motivated transplant teams from the very beginning. The Spanish Transplantation Law was first enacted in 1979, containing the basic elements of any occidental transplantation law.[7] An opting-out system for consent to donation has been in place since then in Spain. It is quite frequent that the Spanish success is attributed to this legal system of consent. However, the presumed consent policy is not strictly applied in practice; relatives are always approached and have the final veto.[8] From a political point of view, the Spanish donation and transplantation system had to accommodate to the reality of political competencies having been transferred to the 17 different autonomous regions of Spain: any national initiative in the field ought to be reached by inter-regional consensus. The main elements of the *Spanish Model* are listed in Table 26.1 and are described in detail below.[9]

26.2.1 Transplant Coordination Network on Three Levels

The coordination of donation activities has been conceived and structured on three different, but interrelated levels: national, regional and hospital. The national level is represented by ONT and the regional level by 17 regional transplant coordination offices, one per autonomous region. These first two levels, both being dependent on the national and regional health-care authorities respectively, act as an interface between the technical and the political strata and in full support of the effective

[7] Matesanz (1998).

[8] Matesanz and Domínguez-Gil (2009).

[9] Matesanz and Miranda (2002); Matesanz and Domínguez-Gil (2009); Matesanz et al. (2011).

realization of the process of donation from the deceased. Any national decision on donation and transplantation activities is made in agreement with the *National Transplant Committee of the Health Interterritorial Council*, composed of ONT as chair and the 17 regional coordinators. The hospital level of coordination is represented by a network of hospitals officially authorized for handling procurement activities, in direct charge of developing the deceased donation process in an efficient way. This network evolved from less than 20 hospitals in 1989 to 118 in 1992, a rapid evolution which reflects the important efforts performed by the system and the political support received already in its very first years. The network has kept increasing with 181 hospitals being involved in 2012.

26.2.2 In-Hospital Transplant Coordination Teams

A transplant coordination team is appointed at each procurement hospital, constituting a team that is responsible for developing a proactive donor detection program and effectively converting potential into actual donors. The transplant coordinators (TCs) in Spain, particularly the leaders of the transplant coordination teams, have a unique profile conceived to facilitate the early identification and referral of possible or potential organ donors, the critical phase of the process of deceased donation. TCs are *in-house professionals*, part of the staff of the procurement hospital that is involved, rather than having professionals that are located outside of the hospitals and that would have to be contacted upon the identification of a potential donor. TCs are *nominated by and report to the medical board* of the hospital, hence not being dependent on the head of the transplantation teams. Most of the TCs are *part-time dedicated* to donation activities, which allows them to be appointed even at hospitals with a low deceased donor potential. The part-time dedication also permits these professionals to leave the coordination tasks and return to and be fully dedicated to their original activities when appropriate. Notably, the majority of the leaders of the transplant coordination teams in Spain are *critical care physicians*. TCs thus develop their daily activity directly at those units where 12.4 % of deaths occur in persons with a clinical condition consistent with brain death.[10]

26.2.3 Central Office—ONT—as a Supporting Agency

ONT acts as a supporting agency to the network of procurement hospitals in addition to being in charge of organ sharing and allocation in the country, according to predefined and agreed-upon medical criteria. ONT's support and that provided by some regional offices is especially important for small hospitals, which frequently do not have the capability of developing the whole process of deceased donation on their own.

[10] De la Rosa et al. (2012).

26.2.4 Quality Assurance Program in the Deceased Donation Process

The *Quality Assurance Program in the Deceased Donation Process* has become an essential tool in the consolidation of the system.[11] So far focused on DBD, the program aims at assessing and monitoring the potential of deceased organ donation, evaluating performance and identifying key areas for improvement in the realization of the deceased donation process. Already in place for more than 10 years, the program is based on a continuous and systematic review of the clinical charts of all patients dying at critical care units in the procurement hospitals. The program includes an internal audit performed by TCs locally that allows the building up of specific performance reference indicators. This activity is complemented by external audits carried out by expert TCs belonging to a region different to the one to which the evaluated hospital belongs. External audits are performed under the request of regional TCs and provide a unique opportunity for sharing practices and experiences and thus identifying possible actions for improvement in the form of recommendations targeted at the transplant coordination team and the hospital managers.

26.2.5 Great Efforts in Professional Training

Training is an essential component of the *Spanish Model*. Regular courses focused on the entire process of deceased donation and some of its particular phases have been targeted to all professionals directly or indirectly involved in the process—TCs, along with intensive care doctors during their residency period, professionals from intensive care, the emergency department and the stroke units. Since 1991, more than 14,000 professionals in Spain have been trained through these courses, which have now been implemented in many other countries.[12]

A particular reference should be made to courses of communicating in critical situations that have been provided regularly by ONT in an attempt to cover this training gap for most professionals in charge of critically ill patients. In a survey performed in 2006 to a representative sample of the Spanish population, 67.4% of the interviewed stated their willingness to become organ donors after death. Although public support for donation in Spain can be considered to be high, the aforementioned percentage was similar to those obtained in previous surveys performed back in 1993 and 1999.[13] Moreover, support towards donation after death in Spain is in a mid-position compared to other European countries, according to a recent Eurobarometer analysis.[14] Therefore, it cannot be concluded that the general support towards donation is the only reason for the high consent—and donation—rate

---

[11] De la Rosa et al. (2012).

[12] Páez et al. (2009).

[13] Domínguez-Gil et al. (2010).

[14] Organ donation and transplantation. Special Eurobarometer.

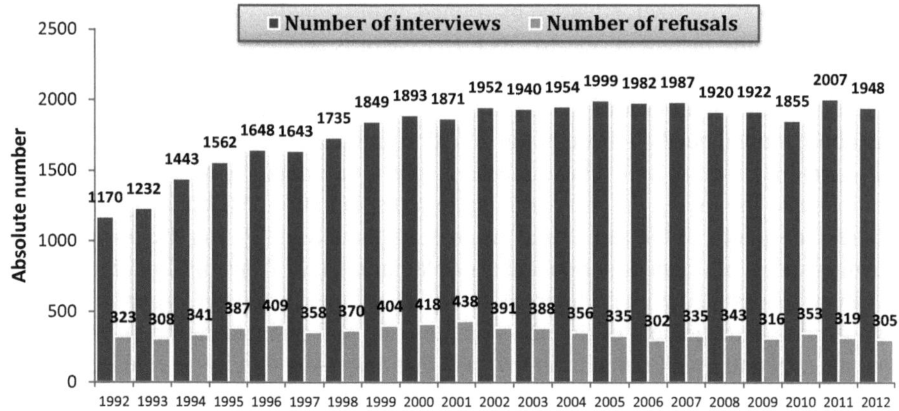

Fig. 26.3 Evolution of number of families approached and refusals to deceased organ donation in Spain. Between the years 1989–2012

observed in the Spanish setting (Fig. 26.3). A plausible explanation is the progressive improvement in the way professionals approach the relatives and provide dedicated care at the moment of mourning, which is a direct result of the training efforts mentioned above.

26.2.6 Close Attention to the Media

Constructing a positive social climate towards donation and generating the trust of the society in the system have not been attempted to be reached through the adoption of what have been considered *classical* measures to face organ shortage, such as direct promotional campaigns or the development and promotion of specific tools to facilitate the recording of wishes concerning donation during lifetime. On the contrary, support for donation and public trust in the system has been gained through the *close attention that the donation and transplantation system has been paying to the mass media.*[15]While direct publicity campaigns have proven to have little if any effect on public support towards donation and on donation rates, this is not the case for the lay media. Negative and positive news may greatly influence public opinion—and that of professionals—and have an impact on consent and donation rates, a phenomenon known as the *Panorama effect.*[16] This basic observation has driven the development of a specific communication policy by ONT and its network, devoted to accurately and correctly informing the media on issues related to donation and transplantation, which is the best way of reaching the general public.

This strategy is based on four basic principles: (i) A 24-hour transplantation hotline is available for consultation for the lay public, professionals and the media. One

[15] Matesanz and Miranda (1996); Matesanz (1996).

[16] Matesanz (1996).

single telephone number, attended by trained professionals, is provided to the entire country yielding instant access to ONT. (ii) There is an easy and permanent access to the media. Professionals at ONT can be reached continuously for consultation. (iii) Connection with journalists is built through dedicated meetings aimed at learning about mutual needs—those of the donation and transplantation system and those of journalists themselves. These meetings are a pragmatic approach to influence and educate the media on issues related to transplantation. Misconceptions can be addressed openly, at the same time emphasizing and highlighting the positive life-saving aspects of organ donation and transplantation. (iv) Transmission of messages is always performed with no intermediaries. These measures have brought about an appropriate management of the news on donation and transplantation by the media and an easy and quick reaction in the case that adverse publicity be released at any time. Finally, both transplant professionals and individuals responsible for health-care have been aware of the fact that it is necessary to stick to a reliable and homogeneous system of information in which the public can have full confidence. This can only be achieved if the messages are clear, well defined, positive and essentially shared by all those involved in the process of organ donation and transplantation.

26.2.7 Hospital Reimbursement for Donation and Transplantation Activities

Finally, *procurement hospitals are reimbursed for their activities*, including both human and material resources.[17] Donation is considered a medical activity, which is to be properly funded like any other medical activity. The corresponding regional health authorities allocate a specific budget to cover the resources needed for the effective development of these activities at every hospital. Generally speaking, the transplant coordination structure represents approximately 5 % of all the costs related to donation, procurement and solid organ transplantation in the country. However, thanks to the number of patients who receive a kidney transplant and are thus removed from dialysis therapy, this organizational approach ends up saving the national health-care system twice the cost of all donation, procurement and transplantation activities every year.

26.3 Conclusion

In conclusion, the *Spanish Model* is an example of continuous and dedicated efforts in the pursuit of self-sufficiency in transplantation, in absolute compliance with the *WHO Guiding Principles on Human Cell, Tissue and Organ Transplantation*. It is the essence of maximizing donation from the deceased, as promulgated by

[17] Matesanz (2001).

the *World Health Assembly Resolution 63.22* and the *Madrid Resolution.* System improvements through the development of a properly trained and devoted network of transplant coordination teams, led by intensive care physicians and supported by regional authorities and the ONT, have been the key feature. Social acceptance of donation by the Spanish population may also be seen as a component of this success, which results from the close cooperation with the mass media, but overall from the response of society to the creation of a solid system on organ donation and transplantation, which has been sustainable over time.

References

De la Rosa, G., B. Domínguez-Gil, R. Matesanz, S. Ramón, J. Alonso-Álvarez, and J. Araiz, et al. 2012. Continuously evaluating performance in deceased donation: The Spanish quality assurance program. *American Journal of Transplantation* 12 (9): 2507–2513.

Domínguez-Gil, B., M. J. Martín, M. O. Valentín, B. Scandroglio, E. Coll, and J. S. López, et al. 2010. Decrease in refusals to donate in Spain despite no substantial change in the population's attitude towards donation. *Organs, Tissues and Cells* 13:17–24.

Global Observatory on organ donation and transplantation. Global observatory on donation and transplantation website. http://www.transplant-observatory.org. Accessed July 2013.

Joint Council of Europe/United Nations Study. On trafficking in organs, tissues and cells and trafficking in human beings for the purpose of the removal of organs. Council of Europe website. http://www.coe.int/t/dghl/monitoring/trafficking/default_en.asp. Accessed July 2013.

Matesanz, R. 1996. The panorama effect on altruistic organ donation. *Transplantation* 62:1700–1701.

Matesanz, R. 1998. Cadaveric organ donation: Comparison of legislation in various countries of Europe. *Nephrology Dialysis Transplantation* 13:1632–1635.

Matesanz, R. 2001. Trasplantes de órganos, gestión y sistemas sanitarios. *Nefrología* 21 (Suppl 4): 3–12.

Matesanz, R., and B. Domínguez-Gil. 2007. Strategies to optimize deceased organ donation. *Transplantation Reviews* 21:177–188.

Matesanz, R., and B. Domínguez-Gil. 2009. Pros and cons of a regulated market in organs. *Lancet* 374 (9707): 2049.

Matesanz, R., and B. Miranda. 1996. Organ donation—the role of the media and public opinion. *Nephrology Dialysis Transplantation* 11:2127–2128.

Matesanz, R., and B. Miranda. 2002. A decade of continuous improvement in cadaveric organ. *Journal Nephrology* 15 (1): 22–28.

Matesanz, R., B. Domínguez-Gil, E. Coll, G. de la Rosa, and R. Marazuela. 2011. Spanish experience as a leading country: What kind of measures were taken? *Transplant International* 24 (4): 333–343.

Murray, J. E. 2005. The 50th anniversary of the first successful human organ. *Revista de investigacion clinica* (Mar-Apr) 57 (2): 118–9.

Organ donation and transplantation. Special Eurobarometer 333a. European Commission websiste. http://ec.europa.eu/public_opinion/archives/ebs/ebs_333a_en.pdf. Accessed July 2013.

Páez, G., R. Valero, and M. Manyalich. 2009. Training of health care students and professionals: A pivotal element in the process of optimal organ donation awareness and professionalization. *Transplantation Proceedings* 41 (6): 2025–2029.

Sixty third World Health Assembly. Resolution 63.22 on human organ and tissue transplantation. Global observatory on donation and transplantation website. http://www.transplant-observatory.org/Contents/Library/Documents%20and%20guidelines/Documents0/Documents%20and%20Guidelines/WHO%20Resolutions/WHA63recen.pdf. Accessed July 2013.

The Madrid Resolution on Organ Donation and Transplantation. 2011. National responsibilities in meeting the needs of patients, guided by the WHO principles. *Transplantation* 91 (11S): S29–S31.

WHO Guiding Principles on Human Cell, Tissue and Organ Transplantation. WHO website. http://www.who.int/transplantation/Guiding_PrinciplesTransplantation_WHA63.22en.pdf. Accessed July 2013.

Rafael Matesanz MD, PhD is the Director of the National Transplant Organization in Spain. After its foundation in 1989, the National Transplant Organization contributed to increase the organ donation rate in Spain from 14 donors per million population (pmp) to over 35 donors pmp in 2011. Dr. Matesanz is the President of the Iberoamerican Network/Council of Donation and Transplantation and former Chair of the European Committee on Organ Transplantation of the Council of Europe. He contributed to developing the new transplant law (2010) in Spain.

Beatriz Domínguez-Gil is a medical doctor, PhD in internal medicine, and specializes in Nephrology. After several years working as a nephrologist in the clinical setting as well as a clinical researcher in the field of nephrology and organ transplantation, she joined the Spanish National Transplant Organization (ONT) in November 2006. ONT is a collaborative center of the World Health Organization (WHO) and hosted the Third WHO Global Consultation in donation and transplantation in Madrid in March 2010. Beatriz Domínguez-Gil is also Chair of the European Donation and Transplant Coordination Organization (EDTCO), a section of the European Society of Organ Transplantation (ESOT) bringing forward high professional and ethical standards for transplant coordinators in the European setting.

Chapter 27
The Business of Saving Lives. Organ Donation at OneLegacy in Southern California

Thomas Mone

27.1 Introduction

The LMU Center for Advanced Studies in Munich has chosen to investigate the challenge of the shortage of organ donors for life-saving transplants in Germany and world-wide; a topic that is ideal for a multi-disciplinary program since it requires an understanding of the roles of biology, medicine, psychology, sociology, communication, ethics, economics and organizational management. Transplantation is also a very timely topic due to immediate challenges taking place in the German transplant community that have resulted in decreases in donation and subsequent increase in waiting time and deaths on German waitlists. This review of the challenges, successes, principles, and interventions employed to dramatically improve donation in Southern California will ideally provide models of organization and operation that transcend political and cultural variances and can help improve donation and transplantation in Germany and elsewhere.

OneLegacy is the *Organ Procurement Organization* (OPO) whose staff of 300 personnel serves Southern California and its population of 19.5 million people, 215 Hospitals, 11 Transplant Centers, and seven Medical Examiner offices. As such, OneLegacy is the largest of the 58 OPOs in the US, which serve populations that range from 1 to 19.5 million. All of these OPOs grew out of recovery programs that began 50 years ago as components of the fledgling transplant programs (Mone 2006; Shafer 2006). The OPO regions reflect to this day the geo-politics of their start-up centers and in large part, organs recovered are allocated to the OPOs' local communities first and shared more broadly when no recipient is nearby. And while perfect-match kidneys may travel across the country and the sickest liver recipient in a broader region may receive the next organ, *local-first* remains the basis of organ sharing (Graham 2006). A problematic consequence of this historic allocation sys-

T. Mone (✉)
OneLegacy, Los Angeles, CA, USA
e-mail: tdmone@onelegacy.org

R. J. Jox et al. (eds.), *Organ Transplantation in Times of Donor Shortage*,
International Library of Ethics, Law, and the New Medicine 59,
DOI 10.1007/978-3-319-16441-0_27

tem is that potential organ donors are not uniformly distributed across the US, with the some regions having 40–50 % higher potential and concordant 40–50 % shorter waiting times for transplant (Sheehy et al. 2012).

This geo-political/medical reality creates a need for extraordinary performance in more challenged areas with lower donor potential and has resulted in concerted efforts at OPOs like OneLegacy. The results of this effort can be seen in the graphs of Donor Authorization Rate, Donors, Transplants, and Donors per Million Population (normalized for varying international death rates) (Mone 2013). All four graphs demonstrate significant growth over the last decade and given OneLegacy's very high proportion of foreign-born and first and second-generation immigrants (approximately 50 %) (Reibel 2013; US Census QuickFacts 2010; US Organ Procurement and Transplant Network 2013) and the disparity of potential donation rates and actual donation rates across Europe suggest that the interventions employed at OneLegacy may have value in Germany and other regions of the world.

27.2 Principles of Organ Donation Success

Studies of successful donation programs (Mone 2002, 2012; Matesanz 2011b) have identified eight management and organizational principles that are followed by successful programs:

- Ethics-based Regulation & Oversight for public trust
- Separation of donation from transplant
- Communication of the value of donation to the public
- Allocation rules to ensure fairness
- Professionalization/Role Specialization for expertise
- Collaboration of OPOs, Hospitals and Transplant Ctrs
- Transparency with the public
- Innovation in the science of donation

Context Applying these principles requires an understanding of the healthcare system of each country. In the US, where healthcare is largely supplied and paid for by private organizations, the OPOs act as a *vendor* or *supplier* to transplant programs (Mone 2002). However in Spain where healthcare is routinely provided by governmentally funded institutions, OPOs are often a budgeted department or service of a hospital (Matesanz 2011b; Manyalich 2011). These and other culturally-determined variations will affect *how* these eight principles are applied, but they do not change the fact that all eight must be present to improve organ donation.

Ethics-based Regulation and Oversight In the US, the ethical underpinnings of donation and transplant are incorporated in the Uniform Anatomical Gift Act (CAH & SC 2012) which recognizes the autonomy of the donor to make the decision to donate, independent of family or institutions. The law also recognizes the family or legal agent's right to decide when the individual has not. The UAGA clearly dismisses the notion of state-authorized recovery of organs. *Presumed Consent*, which is often discussed as a solution to the organ shortage but in fact has never been shown to be applied in practice and has never resulted in increased donation (Boyarsky et al. 2011; Matesanz 2011b; Rithalia et al. 2009).

Separation from Transplantation This may be one of the more controversial of the eight Principles, as many countries continue to operate their recovery programs from within transplant centers. However, the highest performing OPOs in the US, Spain and elsewhere separate these functions first and foremost to ensure adequate and consistent funding of donation, to remove incentives for the misallocation of organs to the center's lower-ranked recipients, and to motivate the maximum utilization of organs across a broader sharing region.

Communication Organ donation education has ranged from being weak and understated and fearful of associating with the specter of death to being factual and respectful but still private quiet, to an intentional effort to *inspire* people to donate by celebrating the life that is saved through transplant and the legacy of the life that was cut short but fulfilled through donation. OneLegacy and successful OPOs throughout the world have opted to engage in public and proactive donation education programs. This more public approach is grounded in the recognition that organ donation is not about death; rather organ donation is about the choices people make once death has occurred (Stadtler 2005; Cameron et al. 2013). This is a fundamental principle and practice of successful donation programs and while it is always respectful of the deceased donor, it accepts that the death has happened, is an independent event, that families ultimately must and do look forward, and recognizes the opportunity to help them do so by choosing to create a legacy of life through organ donation.

Allocation Given the reality in which the availability of organs is such that there will always be scarcity (even if everyone who could donate upon death did so, which is only 0.5 % of all deaths (Sheehy et al. 2012)), it is essential to ensure that all of those who can donate do so. To accomplish this it is essential that all who may be asked to donate believe that if they need a transplant they will have an equal opportunity to receive one. Thus the allocation of these scarce organs must be perceived as fair. Of course *fair* has a number of possible interpretations, so organ allocation systems are in a constant state of evolution. In the US this evolution has migrated from first-come-first served, regardless of economic factors to a more refined balance with identifying those with the most immediate need and greatest likelihood to successfully survive with a transplant (Graham 2006; Yeh 2011).

Professionalization/Specialization While organ donation practice began as a task of transplant center nurses, with the separation of duties to OPOs the unique needs of donor management and organ resuscitation medicine took precedence in the hiring and training of OPO personnel. As OPOs have grown, the duties and processes of organ donation have evolved to create at least seven specific skill set/specialty needs (Mone 2002). Thus, additional roles, training, and formal and informal certification of these roles and personnel have developed. Applying such specialization remains a challenge in smaller OPOs, but where the workload affords it, specialization has resulted in higher donation performance and lower costs; especially in a healthcare world in which critical care nurses and MDs are in short supply.

Collaboration While Separation and Specialization bring clear benefits to donation, they create the potential for isolation and can inhibit critical cross-communication; commonly known as a "Silo Effect" (Hotaran 2009). Thus, OPOs, Donor Hospitals, Transplant Centers, and the staff within each institution must establish formal and informal means of and reasons for regular communication. This starts with identifying common goals, sharing consequential events and problems in the search of systemic solutions, and speaking with one voice of the benefits, safety, and opportunity of donation. And, as technology advances, sharing real-time information on donors, donor management goals, and donor condition, and allocation status is essential to ensure short and long-term collaboration on the common end goal of saving lives through donation and transplant (Staes et al. 2005).

Transparency All efforts at removing the myths and misconceptions associated with donation which have been rather successful in western countries can easily become undone if rare problematic events occur and worse if they are ignored or covered up. Straightforward medical errors like inadequate brain death testing that allowed a child to be prepared for organ donation while conscious but temporarily paralyzed *could* have decimated donation if not corrected at the time, procedurally for the future, and honestly communicated with the public. (Associated Press 2008) However, the facts and rarity of the case were openly discussed in the media, and it was noted that if his family had *not* opted for donation he might have been extubated and never have recovered. Thus, a potentially horrendous mistake was shown to be an inadvertent blessing and the public discussion furthered the cause of donation rather than harmed it. Public relations specialists have long-advocated absolute transparency in such circumstance to limit the opportunity for speculation that is caused by a vacuum of information. Because donation begins upon death, the primal and visceral fears of death that we are born with rapidly rise, but can easily be quelled with clear, direct information and *transparency* in response to inquiry, such as when a liver mis-allocation bypassed some 50 patients in Southern California, but donation actually rose due to full public disclosure (Ornstein 2005).

Of course, a commitment to transparency can be tested when errors of omission or commission occur. It is for this reason that successful OPOs and donation systems support and include robust systems of organizational and process audit. In the US OPOs it is common to have two or three departments of government (CMS, HRSA, FDA), the federally contracted UNOS and transplant centers, and multiple tissue processors, conduct audits of OPO data and practices. Additionally, US OPOs participate in independent accreditation by their peers (AOPO 2012); all in the effort to ensure that public trust is maintained by making sure the process and results are monitored and tracked and communicated.

Innovation This principle may end up being a catch-all for the many developments yet to come in successful organ donation, but for now it is focused on the aggressive use of latest generation donor-testing, electronic donor records, to capture, transmit and analyze donor information, the development of new organ resuscitative pumping devices, allocation algorithms to maximize the matches and life-years gained form transplantation. And of course donation and transplant *innovation* must include means to enhance, clone, print, genetically modify and mechanically replace organs that will one day put the donation community out of business by enabling the transplant of all who are waiting. Innovations like NAT testing have added new levels of safety (Nowicki et al. 2006), Electronic Donor Records enable Intensivist and Surgeon consults and informed decision making based on the complete medical record rather than a telephonic summary, and lung pumps are resuscitating previously untransplantable lungs and enabling them to remain viable for 5 times longer than only 3 years ago (Cypel 2011)

27.3 Donation Process

With these fundamental principles in place, OneLegacy and successful OPOs employ a systematic process of delineating the tasks, recruiting and training specialists and developing programs, policies and procedures to accomplish donation:

- *Donation Development* to Educate and Inspire the General and Healthcare Professional Communities (35 % of OneLegacy's 170 Organ Recovery staff; marketing and communication skilled individuals)
- *Potential Donor Referral*response and assessment (10 %; Call Center personnel)
- *Donor Evaluation for Clinical Suitability* (10 %; primarily clinical first responders, like paramedics)
- *Family Support and Authorization for Donation* (12 %; multi-lingual, grief-trained counselors)
- *Donor Management, Testing, Organ Resuscitation* (24 %; Critical Care RNs with Intensivist MD consultant)
- *Organ Placement and Recovery* (6 %; Surgical Technicians and specially trained organ placement personnel)
- *Aftercare* (3 %; social workers and grief specialists)

Donation Development At OneLegacy, more than other OPOs, it is essential to communicate this message in languages, media and venues that are accessible to the 70 % of the population that is non-white/non-English speaking/immigrant (US Census QuickFacts 2010). In creating these materials the task is more complex than simply transplanting language, as individuals from other cultures inevitably arrive with spiritual, ancestral, death and healthcare beliefs and understanding that are very different than multi-generation white English-speaking American. Thus, OneLegacy employs communication strategies that cross cultural boundaries such as the annual Rose Parade that is seen by 84 million viewers (ToR 2013). This typr of event, whose audience assembles and watches for purely celebratory reasons having nothing to do with organ donation, are presented with donors and recipients from every cultural and ethnic group of the region and religious and community leaders who proclaim their religions and communities' support for organ donation; which is often not known by their own community members.

OneLegacy also seeks to utilize public statements from political, cultural, and institutional leaders to demonstrate that donation is both the right and natural thing to do and that it is a safe thing to do (to overcome unfounded fears that "doctors may not try to save my life because they want my organs"). Among the leaders who have been very public in their support have been Steve Jobs, following his liver transplant, Governor and actor Arnold Schwarzenegger, hospital leaders and television stars like Alex O'Loughlin. And to amplify this effort, OneLegacy created Donate Life Hollywood; an initiative to help television and movie writers tell accurate and still dramatic stories of donation and transplant and to celebrate and promote in the media those producers and shows that have helped remove fears and promote donation; much like Pedro Almodovar has done in Spain (Stenner and Moreno 2013).

Professional education at OneLegacy is focused on the continuing responsibility to educate new hospital staff RNs, MDs and support staff on the facts of donation, the opportunity to make donation a part of end-of-life care for families, and to celebrate the decision to donate through such acts as flying a Donate Life flag at the hospital every time there is a donor. These actions collaborate to share a message that donation is not a topic to avoid; rather it is an event to celebrate and thereby honor the donor, the donor family and the life of the recipients who have been saved.

Donor Referral and Evaluation These two process steps have always been a part of donation and the one innovation that OneLegacy can share is the separation of the roles and processes; done primarily to reduce dependence and workload on the most highly educated and expensive staff, Critical Care RNs. Currently the first phase of referral is performed by a dedicated Call Center team of staff with minimal prior clinical training, but focused orientation and a rigid electronic donor referral system that ensures the capture and communication of critical information. The ultimate evaluation of donor potential is enabled by *first-responder* paramedics who capture critical clinical information on-site in the donor hospital and communicate this via the electronic donor record system to the highly experienced Organ Team Lead, a Critical Care Nurse Procurement Coordinator who may also bring in the Intensivist Consultant to determine suitability for donation (USDHHS ACOT 2003).

Donor Authorization At OneLegacy, Authorization moved from being the RN Procurement Coordinator's task to the Family Care Specialist's (FCS) in large part because of the unique language and cultural needs of our highly diverse communities. This transition quickly demonstrated a significant secondary result: our FCSs had more time to spend with families, could help them understand their sudden loss and answer their many questions, and simultaneously earn their trust so that when the donation opportunity was presented, it was done from a position of mutual understanding. The transition also allowed OneLegacy to recruit and hire staff with the verbal skills, grief training, and personality traits that improved the donation authorization experience and since the FCS role was established OneLegacy has seen a 67 % increase in donation (Ebadat 2014).

Donor Management, Testing, and Medical Examiner Clearance Ten years ago the primary goal of donor management was to stabilize the donor, place the organs with transplant centers, and recover them in OR, ideally within 4–8 h. Underlying this thought was the presumption that organs would only deteriorate in the donor and should be removed as quickly as possible. In more recent years it has become clear that the donor can continue to serve the organs by enabling the treatment to offset the clinical consequences of brain death and its hormonal surge and reduced circulation. Thus, the role of the Procurement Coordinator has evolved and the technology of pharmacology management, ventilator management and interventional medicine to assess and improve organ function has stretched the average case time form 6–8 h to 36–48 h. The result of this longer management time has been an increase in organs transplanted per donor of at least 10–20 %, thereby enabling thousands of additional life-saving transplants. Today, we are also seeing the development of powerful *external* resuscitative devices and pumps designed to extend the time until an organ can be transplanted and in the best scenarios, such as recent advance in lung pumps, improving lung function and allowing the transplant of previously unusable lungs (McKeown 2012).

As critical as clinical management is the testing of donors to limit the transmission of contagious diseases. Serology tests that look for the antibodies of an infectious agent have long been the standard of practice, but since 2004 OneLegacy has been supplementing these tests with TMA-Nucleic Acid Testing that looks for the HIV and Hepatitis viruses. This testing was added in attempts to reduce the *window period* of time from infection to antibody production and thereby enhance surgeon and recipient confidence in the safety of the organs. While still in debate across the field, currently 70 % of US OPOs test all of their donors and the remainder test high-risk donors with NAT testing (Aswad et al. 2005).

Medical Examiner clearance deserves mentioning because in cases of deaths of unknown or possibly criminal cause coroners historically prevented the recovery of organs in 10 % of authorized organ donation cases, quite often in the very rare pediatric cases. Fortunately, collaboration between the US National Association of Medical Examiners (NAME), local law enforcement and transplant and donation programs, has shown that donation has never hampered a prosecution nor interfered with the determination of cause of death. Since NAME published this position statement, Medical Examiner declines have dropped to fewer than 1 % of cases in the US.

Organ Placement In the US, this process has been driven by the national system of organ allocation overseen by UNOS (The United Network for Organ Sharing) since 1984, with UNOS computers generating the current waiting list for each organ of each donor and routinely identifying recipients first in the local OPO recovery area. Until 2008 this list prompted a series of telephonic conversation between OPO and transplant teams that were lengthy and made it very difficult to work very far down a list. With the establishment of UNOD Donor-Net (that was modeled on OneLegacy's web-based organ offer system used in Los Angeles since 2002) organ offers are now made via a web-based system that allows offers in parallel and enables more offers across the country. The most critical aspect of organ allocation however, is the ability for real-time and retrospective audit of offers to ensure that they meet the UNOS allocation criteria and that the waitlist was followed which is essential to maintain transplant center and public trust (Gerber et al. 2010).

Aftercare While OneLegacy and our colleague OPOs position donation as not about death but about the choices one makes to save lives once death has occurred, the fact is that donor families are in a state of shock and grief in the days and months following their loss. Aftercare is designed to provide them referral to community resources as well as trained ears to listen to their stories and concerns; a service we provide for up to a year. At OneLegacy we also use this time to acquaint donor families with opportunities to participate with OneLegacy in volunteer *Ambassador* roles to help us promote donation in their communities *and* to share and celebrate their donation in the media and very public activities like the Tournament of Roses Donate Life Float, our Donate Life Run Walk and public and private speaking engagements. Thus, aftercare both serves the personal need of families and reassures them that the OPO cares about them and not simply their donor organs, but it also enables the donor families to speak to skeptical and inexperienced communities of people from a first-hand experience that demonstrates the highly personal and valuable result of organ donation (Maloney and Wolfelt 2010).

27.4 OneLegacy's Unique Applications of the Principles and Processes of Donation

Ethnic, cultural, and linguistic diversity are the most significant drivers of OneLegacy's implementation of the principles and process of successful organ donation. While the US population is 63 % white and 89 % native-born, OneLegacy's community is only 34 % white and 30 % foreign-born. Thus, OneLegacy has a unique need to tailor our messaging and education and staffing to meet the needs of a community that can be determined to have far less exposure and comfort with organ donation than our peer OPOs. Thus, public education programs are focused in consulates, foreign language churches and cultural fairs. Further, we have worked with the State of California to have Organ Donation education introduced into the school health curriculum in order to speak to children about to obtain their first driver license about the value of organs donation; a discussion that is unlikely to happen in the home.

The focus on drivers is motivated because the US has a strong history of organ donor registration via the driver license. In fact, 110 million Americans including 10 million Californians are registered donors, and per our legal and ethical support of autonomy, these registered donors' decisions to donate are honored, without asking for permission for the family (and I should report that families of registered donors are supportive 99 % of the time).

At present, OneLegacy is engaged in the most detailed *drill-down* ethnic study ever performed in organ donation that is attempting to correlate demographic factors, such as ethnicity, language, income level, educational attainment, by postal zip code (neighborhood) with donation rates by neighborhood, donor registration and donation rates by hospital. We anticipate that this analysis will enable us to fine-tune our public messages focused on specific neighborhoods and ethnic sub-group. For instance, we have learned that while Hispanic donation rates are relatively high, they are highest in Mexican immigrant communities, nearly as high in Guatemalan communities, but a good deal lower in El Salvadoran communities. We have also learned a good deal about the cultural *differences* between these communities of immigrants. Thus we will now focus our messaging where we can have the greatest impact in increasing donation.

Among the factors OneLegacy tracks to better understand our diverse communities are:

- Race
- Culture
- Language
- Gender
- Nationality
- Income
- Generation
- Age
- Lifestyle
- Profession
- Education
- Politics
- Religion
- Neighborhood
- Community
- Spirituality
- Driving Habits

In summary, OneLegacy, like all successful OPOs in the US and worldwide, has applied management and clinical science to analyze and structure the organ donation process in the attempts of continuing to improve donation and save lives through transplantation. OneLegacy has seen dramatic success in increasing donation, but the need for organs continues to grow as our communities age and medical science allows those suffering chronic organ failure to survive longer waiting for an organ transplant. Only by ensuring that the identified principles and processes of Organ Donation are implemented and continually monitored for adherence and improvement can OneLegacy or any organ donation and transplantation program anticipate accomplishing our ultimate goal of ending deaths on the waitlists.

References

Aita, K. 2011. New organ transplant policies in Japan, including the family-oriented priority donation clause. *Transplantation* 91 (5): 489–491.

AOPO. 2012. Accreditation. http://www.aopo.org/accreditation-a18. Accessed 27 Jan 2012.

Associated Press. 2008. Oklahoma man who was declared dead says he feels 'pretty good'. http://www.nydailynews.com/news/world/oklahoma-man-declared-dead-feels-pretty-good-article-1.286113. Accessed 17 Oct 2014.

Aswad, S., T. Mone, et al. 2005. Role of nucleic acid testing in cadaver organ donor screening: Detection of hepatitis C virus RNA in seropositive and seronegative donors. *Journal of Viral Hepatitis* 12:627–634.

Boyarsky, B., et al. 2011. Potential limitations of presumed consent legislation. *Transplantation* XX (X).

CAH & SC (California Health and Safety Code). 2012. Health and Safety Code section 7150-7156.5. http://www.legaltips.org/california/california_health_and_safety_code/7150-7156.5.aspx. Accessed 30 Jan 2012.

Cameron, A., et al. 2013. Social media and organ donor registration: The facebook effect. *American Journal of Transplantation* 13:2059–2065.

Carlson, N. 2010. How Steve Jobs got sick, got better, and decided to save some lives—Forbes. http://www.forbes.com/sites/velocity/2010/04/20/how-steve-jobs-got-sick-got-better-and-decided-to-save-some-lives/print/. Accessed 23 Jan 2012.

Chapman, J., et al. 2008. National Clinical Taskforce on Organ and Tissue Donation; Supporting Evidence: Final Report—2008, Canberra, Department of Health and Aging: Australian Government.

Costa, N., et al. 2011. 2010 International Donation and Transplantation Activity, Organs Tissue & Cells. European Transplant Coordinators Organization Bologna: Editrice Compositori.

Costa, N., L. Noel, et al. 2011. NOTIFY exploring Vigilence notification for organs, tissues, and cells. Centro Nazionale Trapianti, World Health Organization, SOHO V&S (Vigilance and Surveillance of Substances of Human Origin) Project Bologna: Editrice Compositori.

Cunningham, A. 2008. Australian Transplant Coordinators Association National Guidelines for Organ and Tissue Donation. http://www.atca.org.au/. Accessed 18 Jan 2012.

Cypel. 2011. Normothermic ex vivo lung perfusion in clinical lung transplantation. *New England Journal of Medicine* 364:1431–1440.

de Groot, Y. J., et al. 2011. Remarkable changes in the choice of timing to discuss organ donation with the relatives of a patient: A study in 228 organ donations in 20 years. *Critical Care* 15:R235.

DLA (Donate Life America)/Astellas poll conducted by Survey Sampling International. 2010. http://www.donatelife.net/pdfs/DLA_Report_Card_2010_FINAL.pdf. Accessed 31 March 2011.

DLA. 2011. National Donor Designation Report Card. www.donatelife.net/wp-content/uploads/2011/04/DLA-Report-BKLT-30733-2.pdf. Accessed 29 Jan 2012.

Donate Life America. 2010. US National Donor Designation Report Card. http://www.donatelife.net/pdfs/DLA_Report_Card_2010_FINAL.pdf. Accessed 31 March 2011.

Ebadat, A., et al. 2014. Improving organ donation rates by modifying the family approach process. *The Journal of Trauma and Acute Care Surgery* 76 (6): 1473–1475. doi:10.1097/TA.0b013e318265cdb9.

Etzioni, A. 2003. Organ donation: A communitarian approach. *Kennedy Institute of Ethics Journal* 13 (1): 1–18.

Garcia, K., et al. 2006. *Multi-cultural considerations in organ donation and transplantation in a clinician's guide to donation and transplant,* 351–358. Lenexa: Applied Measurement Professionals, Inc.

Gerber, D. A., et al. 2010. DonorNet and the potential effects on organ utilization. *The American Journal of Transplantation* 10 (Part 2): 1081–1089.

Graham, W., et al. 2006. *Organ allocation in a clinician's guide to donation and transplant,* 321. Lenexa: Applied Measurement Professionals, Inc.

Harmon, W., and F. Delmonico. 2006. Payment for kidneys: A government-regulated system is not ethically achievable. *Clinical Journal of the American Society of Nephrology* 1:1146–1147.
HODS. 2012. Halachic aspects of Organ Donation. http://www.hods.org/English/h-issues/faq-halachic.asp. Accessed 30 Jan 2012.
Hornby, K., et al. 2010. A systematic review of autoresuscitation after cardiac arrest. *Critical Care Medicine* 38 (5): 1246–1253.
Hotaran, Ilinca. 2009. Silo effect vs. supply chain effect. *Review of International Comparative Management* 216 (Special Number 1/2009).
IDRD (International Death Rate Data). 2011. CIA World Factbook at. https://www.cia.gov/library/publications/the-world-factbook/. Accessed 31 March 2011.
IRCOS (Islamic Religious Council of Singapore). 2007. Islamic Rulings on Organ Transplant and Organ Donation. http://www.muis.gov.sg/cms/index.aspx. Accessed 30 Jan 2012.
IRODAT. 2011. European Transplant Coordinators Organization IRODAT. http://www.european-transplantcoordinators.org/clinical-resources/irodat/. Accessed 4 April 2011.
Kirste, G. 2011. *Guide to the safety and quality assurance for the transplantation of organs, tissues and cells*. 4th ed. Strasbourg: Council of Europe.
Maloney, R., and A. Wolfelt. 2010. *Caring for donor families before, during and after*. Fort Collins: Companion Press.
Manyalich, M. 2010. Organ donation quality managers training in the European Training Program for Organ Donation (Etpod) project for an efficient management of transplant procurement offices. *Supplement to Transplantation* 90 (2): 567.
Manyalich, M. 2011. Organ procurement: Spanish transplant procurement management. *Asian Cardiovascular & Thoracic Annals* 19 (3/4): 268–278.
Matas, A. 2006. Why we should develop a regulated system of kidney sales: A call for action! *Clinical Journal of the American Society of Nephrology* 1:1129–1132.
Matesanz, R. et al. 2011b. Spanish experience as a leading country: What kind of measures were taken? *Transplant International* 24:333–343.
McKeown, D. W. 2012. Management of the heartbeating brain-dead organ donor. *British Journal of Anaesthesia* 108 (S1): i96–i107.
Mendeloff, J., et al. 2004. Procuring organ donors as a health investment: How much should we be willing to spend? *Transplantation* 78 (12): 1704–1710.
Menza, R., and P. J. Geraghty. 2006. *Evaluation and assessment of donors in a clinician's guide to donation and transplant,* 805–818. Lenexa: Applied Measurement Professionals, Inc.
Moers, C., et al. 2009. The influence of deceased donor age and old-for-old allocation on kidney transplant outcome. *Transplantation* 88:542–552.
Monaco, A. P., and P. J. Morris. 2004. How much is a year of quality life worth? *Transplantation* 78 (12): 1703.
Mone, T. 2002. The business of organ procurement. *Current Opinion in Organ Transplantation* 7:60–64.
Mone, T. 2008. Reimbursement and the Changing Nature of the Donor Pool: USDHHS Advisory Committee on Organ Transplantation.
Mone, T. 2010. Donate Life California Presumed Consent White Paper. http://www.onelegacy.org/site/site/docs/DLC_WhitePaper_PresumedConsent_0911.pdf. Accessed 29 Jan 2012.
Mone, T. 2012. *Oxford textbook of clinical nephrology*. 4th ed. publication pending 2014.
Mone, T. 2013. OneLegacy ten-year performance.
Morgan, S. E., et al. 2008. In their own words: The reasons why people will (not) sign an organ donor card. *Health Communication* 23:23–33.
Morgan, S. E., et al. 2009. The power of narratives: The effect of entertainment television organ donation storylines on the attitudes, knowledge, and behaviours of donors and nondonors. *Journal of Communication* 59:135–151.
Nakagawa, T. 2008. Pediatric Donor Management and Dosing Guidelines: NATCO. www.natco1.org. Accessed 26 Jan 2012.
NCCUSL. 2006. US Uniform Anatomical Gift Act. http://www.nccusl.org/Act.aspx?title=Anatomical%20Gift%20Act%20(2006). Accessed 30 Jan 2012.

Neuberger, J., and G. Thomas. 2011. When the law meets organ transplantation: The experience from the United Kingdom. *Transplantation* 92 (3): 262–264.

NHS. 2010. Donation after Cardiac Death, Adult—Assessment: Map of Medicine Limited. www.uktransplant.org.uk. Accessed 26 Jan 2012.

NHS. 2011a. Organ Donation for Transplantation Improving Donor Identification and Consent Rates for Deceased Organ Donation: British National Health Service. http://www.bts.org.uk/EasySiteWeb/getresource.axd?AssetID=1033&type=full&servicetype=Attachment. Accessed 25 Jan 2012.

NHS. 2011b. Organ Allocation. http://www.uktransplant.org.uk/ukt/about_transplants/organ_allocation/organ_allocation.jsp. Accessed 26 Jan 2012.

NHS UK Transplant. 2006. Standards of Practice for Donor Transplant Co-ordinators. http://www.uktransplant.org.uk/ukt/about_transplants/donor_care/donor_care.jsp. Accessed 18 Jan 2012.

North American Transplant Coordinators Organization (NATCO). 2009. Core Competencies for the Procurement Transplant Coordinator. http://natco1.org/prof_development/core_competencies.html. Accessed 18 Jan 2012.

Nowicki, M., et al. 2006. Prevalence of antibodies to Trypanosoma cruzi among solid organ donors in Southern California: A population at risk *Transplantation* 81:477–479.

OPTN/UNOS. 2011. Organ Procurement and transplant Network/United Network for Organ Sharing Policies. http://optn.transplant.hrsa.gov/policiesAndBylaws/policies.asp. Accessed 29 Jan 2012.

Ornstein, Charles. 2005. Hospital Halts Organ Program: LA Times. http://www.latimes.com/news/la-me-newtransplant27sep27-story.html#page=1. Accessed 17 Oct 2014.

PalmSource, Inc. 2004. Palm Powered Smartphones Help Expedite Organ Transplants—Saving Lives and Creating Business Efficiency. http://www.onelegacy.org/site/professionals/library/publications.html. Accessed 29 Jan 2012.

Pelligrino, E. 2008. Controversies in the Determination of Death: Washington DC USA President's Council on Bioethics.

Peterson, T., et al. 2006. *Surgical recovery of organs in a clinician's guide to donation and transplant,* 857–866. Lenexa: Applied Measurement Professionals, Inc.

Post, M. 2011. Continuum of Care/What Happens Next?/Aftercare: OneLegacy. http://www.onelegacy.org/site/professionals/20111011_odtsymposium.html. Accessed 26 Jan 2012.

Powner, D., and K. O'Conner. 2006. *Adult clinical donor care in a clinician's guide to donation and transplant,* 819–838. Lenexa: Applied Measurement Professionals, Inc.

Price, D. P. T. 2012. Legal framework governing deceased organ donation in the UK. *British Journal of Anaesthesia* 108 (S1): i68–i72.

Pugliese, M. R., et al. 2003. Improving donor identification with the Donor Action Programme. *Transplantation International* 16:21–25.

Reibel, M. 2013. Final Report—OneLegacy Donor Potential.

Report of the Madrid Consultation. 2011. Part 1: European and universal challenges in organ donation and transplantation, searching for global solutions. *Transplantation* 91 (11): S39–S91.

Rithalia, A., et al. 2009. Impact of presumed consent on donation rates: A systematic review. *British Medical Journal* 338:a3162.

Rosenblum, A. M. 2011. The authority of next-of-kin in explicit and presumed consent systems for deceased organ donation: An analysis of 54 nations. *Nephrology Dialysis Transplantation* 0:1–14.

Rudow, D., L. Ohler, and T. Shafer. 2006. *A clinician's guide to donation and transplantation.* Lenexa: NATCO,/Applied Measurement Professional, Inc.

Sarwal, M. M., et al. 2011. Transplantomics and biomarkers in organ transplantation: A report from the first international conference. *Transplantation* 91 (4): 379–382.

Shafer, T. 2006. *The history of the transplant coordinator in a clinician's guide to donation and transplant,* 7–320. Lenexa: Applied Measurement Professionals, Inc.

Sheehy, E., et al. 2003. Estimating the number of potential organ donors in the United States. *New England Journal of Medicine* 349:667–674.

Sheehy, E., et al. 2012. Investigating geographic variation in mortality in the context of organ donation. *American Journal of Transplantation* (Pending Publication).

Sheth, K., et al. 2012. Autoresuscitation after asystole in patients being considered for organ donation. *Critical Care Medicine* 40 (1): 158–161.
Siu, W. G., et al. 2011. Successful organ donation from brain dead donors in a Chinese organ transplantation center. *The American Journal of Transplantation* 11 (10): 2247–2249.
Stadtler, M. 2005. The donate life rose parade float: How an innovative, integrated public awareness campaign effectively reaches a worldwide audience. *Organs and Tissues* (3): 169–172.
Stadtler, M. 2007. European Overview & Challenges in Donation After Cardiac Death NATCO. www.natco1.org/members/documents/130-145Stadtler.pdf. Accessed 26 Jan 2012.
Staes, Catherine J., et al. 2005. Development of an information model for storing organ donor data within an electronic medical record. *Journal of the American Medical Informatics Association* 12 (3): 357–363.
Stenner, Paul, and Eduardo Moreno. 2013. Liminality and affectivity: The case of deceased organ donation. *Subjectivity* 6 (3): 229–253.
The State of Play in EU States. 2009. European Hospital. http://www.european-hospital.com/en/article/6126.html. Accessed 31 March 2011.
ToR, Tournament of Roses. 2013. http://www.tournamentofroses.com/Portals/0/2013_Media_Recap.pdf. Accessed 17 Oct 2014.
Tuttle-Newhall, J. E., et al. 2009. Organ donation and utilization in the United States: 1998–2007. *American Journal of Transplantation* 9 (Part 2): 879–893.
Tzu Chi (2011) *The useless vs. the great use*. Hualien: Tzu Chi Foundation.
USDHHS ACOT. 2003. Advisory Committee on Organ Transplantation Recommendations 29–35. http://organdonor.gov/legislation/acotrecs2935.html.
USDHHS. 2012. Selected Statutory and Regulatory History of Organ Transplantation. www.organdonor.gov. Accessed 30 Jan 2012.
U.S. Renal Data System Annual Data Report. 2005. http://www.kidney.org/news/newsroom/fs_new/esrdinUS.cfm. Accessed 31 March 2011.
US Census. 2010. http://quickfacts.census.gov/qfd/states/00000.html. Accessed 24 Jan 2013.
US CMS. 2006. Federal Register/Vol. 71, No. 104.
US Organ Procurement and Transplant Network Data. 2010. http://optn.transplant.hrsa.gov/latestData/rptData.asp. Accessed 24 Jan 2012.
US Organ Procurement and Transplant Network Data (USOPTN). 2012. http://optn.transplant.hrsa.gov/latestData/rptData.asp. Accessed 1 Oct 2013.
US Organ Procurement and Transplant Network DSA Dash Board. 2011. AOPO. http://www.aopo.org/related-links-data-organ-donation-transplantation-a40. Accessed 24 Jan 2012.
US Organ Procurement Transplant Network National Waiting List Data. 2011. http://optn.transplant.hrsa.gov/latestData/rptData.asp. Accessed 31 March 2011.
Veatch Robert, M. 2000. *Transplantation ethics*. Washington, DC: Georgetown University Press.
Wood, K., et al. 2004. Care of the potential organ donor. *New England Journal of Medicine* 351:2730–2739.
Yeh, H., et al. 2011. Geographic inequity in access to livers for transplantation. *Transplantation* 91:479–486.

Thomas Mone is the Chief Executive Officer of OneLegacy, the Organ and Tissue Recovery organization serving Southern California that recovers 1400+ organs and 100,000 tissues for transplant each year while serving the most demographically and culturally diverse population in the U.S. and perhaps the world. Prior to working in transplantation, Mr. Mone directed hospitals for 20 years and he started his career as a health finance analyst in the US Department of Health and Human Services. His research and publications have been focused on increasing organ donation rates across multicultural communities and improving the utilization and safety of organ transplantation via advances in donor testing.

[illegible]

[illegible] Accessed 14 March 2013.

[illegible] 2014 [illegible] 2013 [illegible]

[illegible] World [illegible]

[illegible]

Chapter 28
The Ethics of Controlled Donation After Cardiac Death

Sohaila Bastami

28.1 Background

Organ donation is a widely accepted method of combating organ failure and could determine between life and death for many patients with end-stage organ failure. However, in Switzerland (Swisstransplant 2012), as well as in other parts of the world (United Network for Organ Sharing 2013; National Health Services 2013), there is a lower amount of transplantable organs than there are persons who need them. How could one address this shortage? Demand may be reduced by improving preventive measures, and supply increased by expanding organ donation (Bastami et al. 2013). In the past few years, the incidence of brain death has decreased in several developed countries (Baxter 2001; Snell et al. 2004): "A balance has been reached between improved efficiency in recognizing suitable donors and improved prevention and management of the medical conditions that result in brain death (i.e. vehicle and cerebrovascular accidents) and organ donation (Snell et al. 2004)." One possibility of augmenting deceased donation is using more donors after cardiac death—i.e. utilizing the organs of persons who died after suffering cardiorespiratory arrest. Physicians wait a pre-determined time period (75 s (Boucek et al. 2008) to 20 min (Geraci and Sepe 2011)) after cardiac arrest and then proceed to remove the organs. The use of these particular organs is estimated to increase the availability of organs by over 20 % (Doig and Rocker 2003). At the University Hospital Zurich, a pioneering institution in Switzerland, donation after cardiac death (DCD) was re-introduced in October 2011 after it was stopped for a few years which was, among other things, due to uncertainty pertaining to the wording of the Transplantation Act (Schweizerische Eidgenossenschaft 2004) that was introduced in 2007. Namely, Article 8 § 2 states, "If no documented consent or refusal by the deceased person is

S. Bastami (✉)
Institute for Biomedical Ethics and History of Medicine, University of Zurich, Zurich, Switzerland
e-mail: bastami@ethik.uzh.ch

R. J. Jox et al. (eds.), *Organ Transplantation in Times of Donor Shortage*,
International Library of Ethics, Law, and the New Medicine 59,
DOI 10.1007/978-3-319-16441-0_28

Table 28.1 Maastricht categories, modified from (Kootstra 1997)

Uncontrolled vs. controlled	Maastricht category	Description
Uncontrolled	Maastricht 1	Dead on arrival at hospital
	Maastricht 2	Cannot be successfully resuscitated
	Maastricht 4	Brain dead with consecutive cardiac arrest
Controlled	Maastricht 3	Terminally ill, expected to die of cardiocirculatory arrest after termination of life support

available, the next of kin must be asked whether they are aware of the person having declared an intention to donate." This implies that the next-of-kin should only be asked about donation after the potential donor has died. In cDCD however, the next-of-kin must be asked about the donation wish of the potential donor after the decision to withdraw therapy has been made, albeit before therapy is withdrawn, so that the donation process may be carefully planned. Therefore, controlled DCD seemed to be incompatible with the Act. Furthermore, there were contradictions between the medical ethical guidelines of the Swiss Academy of Medical Sciences from 2005 pertaining to the diagnosis of death in organ transplantation (Schweizerische Akademie der Medizinischen Wissenschaften 2005) and the Transplantation Act. In 2010, a legal opinion (Guillod Olivier and Mélanie Mader 2010) was published which stated that cDCD was compatible with the Transplantation Act. In 2011, the Swiss Academy of Medical Sciences published revised medical-ethical guidelines concerning organ donation and including DCD (Schweizerische Akademie der Medizinischen Wissenschaften 2011).

In Switzerland, physicians wait 10 min without resuscitative measures after cardiac arrest and then clinically diagnose brain death secondary to cardiac arrest. This is due to the fact that the death of a human being is defined as brain death in the Transplantation Act (Art. 9 TxG, (Schweizerische Eidgenossenschaft 2004)). After diagnosing brain death, organs may be retrieved. DCD in Switzerland always means donation after cardiocirculatory arrest with secondary brain death.

DCD can be separated into uncontrolled and controlled donation, see Table 28.1.

The deceased donation alternative to DCD is donation after brain death (DBD). Brain dead patients fulfill the Harvard Criteria for brain death that were set forth for the first time by the Ad Hoc Committee of the Harvard Medical School in 1968. One of the self-proclaimed reasons for this committee's work was that "[o]bsolete criteria for the definition of death can lead to controversy in obtaining organs for transplantation" (Ad Hoc Committee of the Harvard Medical School 1968). However, controversies on whether patients are actually dead surround the subject of brain death (Bernat 1992; Miller and Truog 2008; Jonas 1987). DCD is not free of controversies, either. The controversies differ depending on whether donation is

Table 28.2 Ethical challenges in cDCD

1st challenge: Appropriate form of consent from surrogate decision makers for cDCD
2nd challenge: Potential conflict of interest
3rd challenge: Location of death with according strain on family and medical personnel
4th challenge: Pre-mortem measures for the good of the recipient and adequate form of consent
5th challenge: Impact on medical care at end of life
6th challenge: Dead donor rule—adequate hands-off period after asystole (Certainty of death)

performed in a controlled or in an uncontrolled fashion. We[1] focus on controlled DCD (cDCD), seeing as that is the only form of DCD that is performed at the University Hospital Zurich.

Controlled DCD patients are terminally ill and depend on life support for life-sustaining cardiac activity. After the termination of life support, the patients die of cardiocirculatory arrest. As explained above, physicians wait a pre-determined period of time after the occurrence of asystole (see above) and then retrieve the organs. This differs from DBD in that the decision to donate is made while the patient is still alive, albeit usually after the decision is made that life-sustaining therapy will be discontinued. This has major ethical implications, which will be explored below.

28.2 Ethical Challenges in cDCD

In order to detect the ethical problems innate to DCD, the author conducted a narrative review of the literature in PubMed. Search terms were "donation cardiac death ethics" and snowballing was used as an ancillary search strategy. PubMed was searched on November 26th, 2011, from inception. The literature review revealed six recurring ethical challenges that arise in cDCD, see Table 28.2. The challenges do not appear in any particular order and are explored in detail in the subchapter "*Relationship between ethical challenges and research questions*".

28.3 The Study

28.3.1 Aims of the Study

After having set forth the challenges innate to DCD, we conducted a study of family members of DCD donors that aims at illustrating their experiences pertaining

[1] This research was undertaken as part of the author's PhD project, which was supervised by Prof. Dr. med. Dr. phil. Nikola Biller-Andorno (Director, Institute of Biomedical Ethics, University of Zurich), PD Dr. med. Dipl. soz. Tanja Krones (Clinical Ethicist, Zurich University Hospital) and Prof. Dr. med. Markus Weber (Head of the Department of Operative Disciplines, Chief of the Clinic for Visceral, Thorax and Vascular Surgery, Triemli Hospital, Zurich).

to the first four of the six challenges. The rationale behind limiting ourselves to the first four questions is explained below. To our knowledge, there is no data on the experiences of families of DCD donors, except in the pediatric setting (Hoover et al. 2014). Our study endeavors to illustrate how these families experience donation. In order to discover this, we planned a study of the donation experiences of both types of donor families, to contrast the two types of donation in order to find out what is distinctive about DCD. Our ultimate research question is, "under which circumstances is cDCD an ethically acceptable option to increase donation in Switzerland."

28.3.2 Relevance of Empirical Data

One might ask what the relevance of the empirical data is to the ethical debate? While a normative analysis can tell us something about what ought to be done, the empirical analysis tells us something about what is currently being done or perhaps about people's attitudes towards certain things. How are these two analyses related? While a full discussion of the role of empirical data in ethical discussions goes beyond the scope of this book chapter, we will attempt to give a short answer to this question. Normative analyses may be based on descriptive assumptions, e.g. slippery slope arguments of the empirical kind. In such situations, empirical work can expose false assumptions and thus strengthen or weaken arguments. Alternately, empirical research can analyze whether ethically relevant interventions have the intended results ((Vollmann and Schildmann 2011), p. 18). In order for moral rules to have practical relevance, they should connect with pre-existing moral convictions ((Vollmann and Schildmann 2011), p. 19). Empirical studies may illustrate such convictions, again underlining the importance of the connection between the normative and the empirical. "Detailed and systematic analyses of stakeholders' moral experiences and attitudes […] contribute to a context-sensitive insight into certain moral practices in health care (Salloch et al. 2012)."

28.3.3 Methodology

The data, which we wanted to study, was how donation-related procedures and donation itself were experienced by next-of-kin.

We obtained the data by means of qualitative semi-structured focused interviews (Merton et al. 1990). We used a qualitative approach to the data because we were interested in the research participants' subjective experiences and opinions. The focused interview is used to interview persons who "are known to have been involved in *a particular situation:* they have seen a film, heard a radio program, […] taken part in a psychological experiment or in an uncontrolled, but observed, social situation" ((Merton et al. 1990), p. 3). The interview aims to fathom the experience and personal perception of the situation ((Przyborski and Wohlrab-Sahr 2009), p. 147).

The first part of the interview guide we created was narrative in order to open the field to the participants. Our aim was to foster *retrospection* as defined in Merton et al., so that the participants recall their immediate reactions to the situations rather than re-considering the stimulus situation and reporting their present reactions to it ((Merton et al. 1990), p. 24).

Data was obtained with the help of the transplant coordinators at the University Hospital Zurich. They contacted the donor families who donated between 1995–2005 and 2011–2012 in a letter with information about our study. These cohorts were chosen in order to retrospectively illustrate donation experiences according to the old protocols, but also to include donor families who donated according to the new protocol. The rationale behind using the transplant coordinators as mediators was that they have access to potential research participants'addresses. In the letter, donor families were asked for their consent to participate in our research. If they wanted to participate, they could contact the author over the phone, e-mail or via post. DCD donor families were contacted before DBD donor families were. Of the 57 DCD donor families, 36 addresses were found. 7 interviews were able to be performed. Of the 118 DBD donor families, 48 addresses were found and 11 interviews were able to take place. The sample we obtained does not claim to be representative for donation-related experiences at University Hospital Zurich. Rather, it is a self-selected sample.

28.4 Relationship Between Ethical Challenges and Research Questions

As explained above, our study aims at illustrating the Zurich experiences with the first four of the six ethical challenges that were identified in the literature review and described in Table 28.2. The relationship between the ethical challenges and the research questions in the study of DCD donor families is identified in this chapter:

The procedures for cDCD differ greatly from the procedures inherent to DBD. DBD is the more common form of donation. It is important that donors or, in case of their inability to consent, their surrogate decision makers understand what they are consenting to (1st challenge). For this reason, the new Swiss Donor Card comes with an information brochure that explains the difference between a DCD and a DBD donor and the major differences in the donation processes in simple terms. However, if someone filled in an old version of the donor card, it cannot be assumed that they knew about DCD donation. In order to ensure that donors participating in DCD and their families are well-informed, every donor or, where applicable, every surrogate decision maker, regardless of how old the donor card is, should be thoroughly informed about the donation process. This should be done until knowledge about DCD is common enough for transplant requestors to be able to safely assume that donors who signed a donor card were aware of what DCD donation means. Thus, donor autonomy may be respected. Our study aims at illustrating whether donor families felt they had enough information about the donation process. Also, next-of-kins' narrations give us insight into whether they were aware of the donor's donation form and whether they understood the need for certain DCD-specific practices, such as the reason for urgency after the advent of cardiac arrest. Our findings show that DCD donor families were not specifically aware (except in one case) that their loved one had donated after cardiac death. It is unclear whether this is because they were not informed, or the information was too complex, or they were unable to retain the information due to the massive stress they were in, or because they did not find the distinction important.

A commonly shared fear in the general population is that of being declared dead too soon if one is in possession of a donor card (Hessing and Elffers 1986) (2nd challenge). The danger of warm ischemia mainly exists in DCD donors, so that time is a much more important factor in these donors than in DBD donors. The organs of a DCD donor become unusable for donation if asystole does not occur quickly enough after extubation. In such cases, physicians have to take care not to feel pressured to hasten the donor's death in order to ensure that donation can take place (2nd challenge). One way to prevent conflicts of interest is to separate health care providers caring for the donor from those caring for the recipient, and to completely separate the decision to end life-sustaining therapy from the decision to donate. In our study, we ask about the latter separation and whether the family members think that the concern about donor care being compromised for the good of the recipient is realistic. We found that the donor families in general had a very high level of trust in the health care system in general and the doctors specifically.

Another problem in cDCD is that the family must either say their goodbyes from their loved one while he is still alive or do so after his death in a limited time frame. In Switzerland, according to the old protocols preceding the new Transplantation Act from the year 2007, only kidneys were transplanted from DCD donors. Nowadays, other organs are transplanted as well. Livers and lungs have less tolerance for ischemia than kidneys and must therefore be removed and transplanted faster. For that reason, experts have suggested moving the location of withdrawal of care from the intensive care unit to the operating room (3rd challenge). Concerns exist that the patient will die a "high tech death," "[…] beneath operating room lights, amidst masked, gowned, and gloved strangers, who have prepared his (her) body for the eviscerating surgery that will follow" (Fox 1993). We are warned about reducing humans to an "ensemble of […] interchangeable […] spare parts," i.e. to a "useful precadaver" (Ramsey 1970). The patient's high-tech, low-touch death in the operating room may affect the atmosphere in which the family says its goodbye. Medical personnel may also be adversely influenced by the fact that the operating room is no longer a place of life, but also a place where therapy may be withdrawn and therefore a place of death (Fox 1993). Certainly, if the family chooses to remain with the donor until death is declared, they will have to rush out of the operating room or intensive care unit after asystole so that organ procurement can ensue. The hectic atmosphere surrounding their loved one's death may adversely influence the family's goodbye, making their outcome with donation worse than their outcome without donation. Our study asks about the atmosphere surrounding the dying patient and how the location of death affected the family's goodbye. The interviewee is also asked to comment on possibly changing the location of death to the operating room. These problems do not arise in DBD, as those donors are declared dead before measures for transplantation are taken. Their medical care at the end of life is not affected. In the context of cDCD, the moral question arises whether the lack of organs should be given enough importance for it to impact how we deal with the dying. Family members opinions diverged on whether a good-bye in the operating room would be acceptable. All donor relatives had said their good-byes in the intensive care unit.

After cardiac arrest in controlled donors, it would be best to perform certain organ-protective measures before death occurs. For example, heparin may be administered intravenously before asystole, in that this permits a systemic distribution of the drug via the cardiocirculatory system. Also, femoral catheters may be placed before death, in order to minimize warm ischemia after asystole. By placing the catheters before death, physicians can perform a cold flush and perhaps extracorporeal membrane oxygenation of the organs right after the declaration of death, as opposed to having to place the catheters then. An important question is whether patients who decide to participate in DCD, or their surrogate decision makers, would take part in DCD if they knew that their agreement to participate could lead to additional medical measures being taken before their death and that perhaps there would be a trade-off between optimal palliative care and the measures explained above that aim at retrieving the organs in an optimal state (4th and 5th challenge). Such measures are done for the good of the recipient, but can compromise the medical care that the donor receives before dying (Campbell and Weber 1995; Edwards et al. 1999). Our study does not ask about the impact of donation on medical care at the end of life, in that we believe this is a matter that families would not know about. However, a study of medical personnel's experiences who were involved in donation could shed light on this matter

Pre-mortem organ-protective measures bear the risk of using the patient as a mere means, because the interventions are performed for the good of the recipient and are not physically beneficial to the donor. This would clash with the Kantian imperative that human beings ought always to be ends in themselves (The Humanity Formula, in (Johnson 2010)). If the donor gives his informed consent to the interventions, he makes their goals his own and is no longer used as a mere means. It is therefore important to get the donor's or his surrogate decision maker's informed consent (Bastami et al. 2012). This requirement is incorporated in the Transplantation Act (TxG (Schweizerische Eidgenossenschaft 2004)). Our study uses hypothetical scenarios to ask donor families how they would feel about such procedures and what form of consent they would find agreeable, if any. Family members' opinions diverged on the subject of organ-preserving measures.

Some experts discuss using the organs of the dying (after obtaining informed consent) as supplementary to using organs from the dead. From a principlist perspective, the leading principles would be "autonomy" and "non-maleficence" (Verheijde et al. 2007). The dying patient, on the one hand, could autonomously agree to donating his organs while he is dying. Physicians who would refuse such patients could be accused of paternalism. At the same time, physicians have the obligation to "do no harm", and it remains to be seen how that obligation could be respected if vital organs are donated by the dying.

In Switzerland, as explained above, DCD is always secondary to brain death (Art. 9 TxG, (Schweizerische Eidgenossenschaft 2004)). In other countries, the waiting period between asystole and retrieval ranges from 75 s (Boucek et al. 2008) to 20 min (Geraci and Sepe 2011). If the waiting period is short, the heart may begin to beat after the occurrence of seemingly irreversible asystole (Murphy et al. 2008) and partial neurological function of the patient may reappear (Maleck et al. 1998). Some physicians purposefully suppress this type of a "reanimation" (Dejohn and Zwischenberger 2006; DuBois 1999; Rady et al. 2007). Under such conditions, the question arises whether such donors are dead after the corresponding waiting period, or whether organ retrieval is what kills them (6th challenge, see (Menikoff 2002; Potts and Evans 2005; Youngner et al. 1999)). Killing patients through organ retrieval would clash with the dead donor rule which states that organ donation may not be the cause of death of patients (Robertson 1999).

The definitive findings of our study will be published in a journal article. As of now, the following tentative conclusions can be drawn: It was seen that the similarities between the experiences of both types of donors outweighed the differences. Both DCD and DBD relatives were forced to take responsibility for discontinuing life-support and ultimately, donation. They tried to presume the patient's will, i.e. figure out what the patient would have wanted. The patient's future quality of life played an important role in the decision-making process, also in the case of DBD donors, which shows the difficulties relatives had with the concept. In retrospection, the relatives oscillated between viewing donation as giving meaning, and being burdened with a sense of guilt for having donated their loved one's organs and possibly being to blame for their loved one's death. Our findings coincided with the findings in the literature on DBD donor families.

28.5 Conclusion

cDCD has been reintroduced in Switzerland as an important measure to combat the shortage of organs. However, this form of donation brings with it specific ethical challenges. Our research identified and analyzed these challenges, as well as mapped our research questions on the experiences of DCD donor families in relation to these challenges. In order to advance the cause of donation in a responsible fashion, accompanying research on its impact on families is necessary, especially pertaining to DCD as very little research exists on family member's relevant experiences. Our planned study is a part of this effort.

References

Ad Hoc Committee of the Harvard Medical School. 1968. A definition of irreversible coma. Report of the Ad Hoc Committee of the Harvard Medical School to Examine the Definition of Brain Death. *JAMA* 205 (6): 337–340.

Bastami, Sohaila, Tanja Krones, and Nikola Biller-Andorno. 2012. Whose consent matters? Controlled donationafter cardiac death and premortem organ-preserving measures. *Transplantation* 93 (10): 965–969.

Bastami, Sohaila, Oliver Matthes, Tanja Krones, and Nikola Biller-Andorno. 2013. Systematic review of attitudes toward donation after cardiac death among healthcare providers and the general public. *Critical Care Medicine* 41 (3): 897–905.

Baxter, David. 2001. *The urban futures institute report 51. Beyond comparison: Canada's organ donation rates in an international context.* Vancouver: The Urban Futures Institute.

Bernat, James. 1992. How much of the brain must die in brain death? *Journal of Clinical Ethics* 3 (1): 21–26.

Guillod Olivier and Mélanie Mader. 2010. Vorbereitende medizinische Massnahmen im Hinblick auf eine Organentnahme—Rechtsgutachten zu verschiedenen Fragen im Zusammenhang mit dem Transplantationsgesetz.

Boucek, Mark M., Christine Mashburn, Susan M. Dunn, Rebecca Frizell, Leah Edwards, Biagio Pietra, and David Campbell. 2008. Pediatric heart transplantation after declaration of cardiocirculatory death. *The New England Journal of Medicine* 359 (7): 709–714. doi:10.1056/NEJMoa0800660.

Campbell, Margaret L., and Leonard J. Weber. 1995. Procuring organs from a non-heart-beating cadaver: Commentary on a case report. *Kennedy Institute of Ethics Journal* 5 (1): 35–42; discussion 43–39.

Dejohn, Carla, and Joseph B. Zwischenberger. 2006. Ethical implications of extracorporeal interval support for organ retrieval (EISOR). *ASAIO Journal* 52 (2): 119–122. doi:10.1097/01.mat.0000206486.80829.58 [doi] 00002480-200603000-00001 [pii].

Doig, C. J., and G. Rocker. 2003. Retrieving organs from non-heart-beating organ donors: A review of medical and ethical issues. *Canadian Journal of Anesthesia* 50 (10): 1069–1076. doi:10.1007/bf03018376.

DuBois, J. 1999. Non-heart-beating organ donation: A defense of the required determination of death. *The Journal of Law, Medicine & Ethics* 27 (2): 126–136.

Edwards, John M., Richard D. Hasz, and Virginia M. Robertson. 1999. Non heart beating organ donation: Process and review. *AACN Clinical Issues* 10 (2): 293–300.

Fox, Renée C. 1993. "An ignoble form of cannibalism": Reflections on the Pittsburgh protocol for procuring organs from non-heart-beating cadavers. *Kennedy Institute of Ethics Journal* 3 (2): 231–239.

Geraci, Paolo M., and Vincenzo Sepe. 2011. Non-heart-beating organ donation in Italy. *Minerva Anestesiologica* 77 (6): 613–623.

Hessing, Dick J., and Henk Elffers. 1986. Attitude toward death, fear of being declared dead too soon, and donation of organs after death. *Omega (Westport)* 17 (2): 115–126.

Hoover, Stephanie M., Susan L. Bratton, Elizabeth Roach, and Lenora M. Olsen. 2014. Parental experiences and recommendations in donation after circulatory determination of death. *Pediatric Critical Care Medicine* 15 (2): 105–111.

Johnson, Robert. 2010. Kant's moral philosophy. The stanford encyclopedia of philosophy. http://plato.stanford.edu/archives/sum2010/entries/kant-moral/. Accessed 6 Oct 2011.

Jonas, Hans. 1987. Gehirntod und menschliche Organbank: Zur pragmatischen Umdefinierung des Todes. In *Technik, Medizin und Ethik—Praxis des Prinzips Verantwortung*, ed. Hans Jonas, 222. Frankfurt a. M: Insel Verlag.

Kootstra, Gauke. 1997. The asystolic, or non-heartbeating, donor. *Transplantation* 63 (7): 917–921.

Maleck, Wolfgang H., Swen N. Piper, Johannes Triem, Joachim Boldt, and Franz U. Zittel. 1998. Unexpected return of spontaneous circulation after cessation of resuscitation (Lazarus phenomenon). *Resuscitation* 39 (1–2): 125–128. doi:S0300-9572(98)00119-1 [pii].

Schweizerische Akademie der Medizinischen Wissenschaften. 2005. *Feststelung des Todes mit Bezug auf Organtransplantation*—Medizinisch-Ethische Richtlinien der SAMW. Basel: SAMW.

Menikoff, Jerry. 2002. The importance of being dead: Non-heart-beating organ donation. *Issues in Law & Medicine* 18 (1): 3–20.

Merton, Robert K., Marjorie Fiske, and Patricia L. Kendall. 1990. *The focused interview—A manual of problems and procedures*, 2nd edn. New York: The Free Press.
Miller, Franklin G., and Robert D. Truog. 2008. Rethinking the ethics of vital organ donation. *The Hastings Center Report* 38 (6): 38–46.
Murphy, Paul, Alexander Manara, Dominic Bell, and Martin Smith. 2008. Controlled non-heart beating organ donation: neither the whole solution nor a step too far. *Anaesthesia* 63 (5): 526–530. doi:ANA5397 [pii] 10.1111/j.1365–2044.2007.05397.x [doi].
National Health Services. 2013. NHS Home Page. http://www.organdonation.nhs.uk. Accessed 2 Jan 2013.
Potts, Michael, and David W. Evans. 2005. Does it matter that organ donors are not dead? Ethical and policy implications. *Journal of Medical Ethics* 31 (7): 406–409. doi:31/7/406 [pii] 10.1136/jme.2004.010298 [doi].
Przyborski, Aglaja, and Monika Wohlrab-Sahr. 2009. *Qualitative Sozialforschung—Ein Arbeitsbuch*, 2nd edn. München: Oldenbourg Wissenschaftsverlag GmbH.
Rady, Mohamed Y., Joseph L. Verheijde, and Joan McGregor. 2007. "Non-heart-beating," or "cardiac death," organ donation: Why we should care. *Journal of Hospital Medicine* 2 (5): 324–334. doi:10.1002/jhm.204 [doi].
Ramsey, Paul. 1970. *The patient as person: Explorations in medical ethics*. New Haven: Yale University Press.
Robertson, John A. 1999. The dead donor rule. *The Hastings Center Report* 29 (6): 6–14.
Salloch, Sabine, Jan Schildmann, and Jochen Vollmann. 2012. Empirical research in medical ethics: How conceptual accounts on normative-empirical collaboration may improve research practice. *BMC Medical Ethics* 13 (5): 4. doi:D-NLM: PMC3355047 EDAT-2012/04/17 06:00 MHDA-2012/07/17 06:00 CRDT-2012/04/17 06:00 PHST-2011/08/05 [received] PHST-2012/04/13 [accepted] PHST-2012/04/13 [aheadofprint] AID-1472-6939-13-5 [pii] AID-10.1186/1472-6939-13-5 [doi] PST-epublish.
Schweizerische Akademie der Medizinischen Wissenschaften. 2011. *Feststellung des Todes mit Bezug auf Organtransplantationen—Medizinisch-Ethische Richtlinien der SAMW*. Basel: SAMW.
Schweizerische Eidgenossenschaft. 2004. Bundesgesetz über die Transplantation von Organen, Geweben und Zellen. http://www.admin.ch/ch/d/sr/810_21/index.html. Accessed 2 Jan 2013.
Snell, Gregory I., Bronwyn J. Levvey, and Trevor J. Williams. 2004. Non-heart beating organ donation. *Internal Medicine Journal* 34 (8): 501–503. doi:10.1111/j.1444-0903.2004.00663.x [doi] IMJ663 [pii].
Swisstransplant. 2012. Kennzahlen zur Organtransplantation in der Schweiz. http://www.swisstransplant.org/pdf/Quartalszahlen-Q3-deutsch-final-1.pdf. Accessed 2 Jan 2013.
United Network for Organ Sharing. 2013. UNOS Home Page. http://www.unos.org. Accessed 2 Jan 2013.
Verheijde, J. L., Rady, M. Y., & McGregor, J. (2007). Recovery of transplantable organs after cardiac or circulatory death: Transforming the paradigm for the ethics of organ donation. *Philosophy, Ethics, and Humanities in Medicine, 2, 8.*
Vollmann, Jochen, and Jan Schildmann. 2011. *Empirische Medizinethik—Konzepte, Methoden und Ergebnisse*. Berlin: LIT.
Youngner, Stuart J., Robert M. Arnold, and Michael A. DeVita. 1999. When is "dead"? *The Hastings Center Report* 29 (6): 14–21.

Sohaila Bastami is a senior teaching and research associate at the Institute for Biomedical Ethics and History of Medicine, University of Zurich, as well as a resident in Clinical Ethics at the University Hospital Zurich. Dr. Bastami has a medical degree from the University of Zurich and has a medical degree as well as a PhD in Biomedical Ethics from the University of Zurich a PhD in Biomedical Ethics. She has also completed a fellowship at the Division of Medical Ethics, Harvard University, USA. Dr. S. Bastami was the recipient of the MD PhD Scholarship of the Swiss National Science Foundation as well as a scholarship from the Swiss Study Foundation. Her research focus lies on clinical ethics at the end of life, specifically palliative care and organ transplantation.

Chapter 29
Protocols for Uncontrolled Donation After Circulatory Death. The Thin Red Line Between Life (Resuscitation Attempts) and Death (Organ Retrieval After Circulatory Death)

Iván Ortega-Deballon, David Rodríguez-Arias and Maxwell J. Smith

29.1 Introduction

In the 1990s, the ever-increasing demand for organs led Spain, and later also France as well as other European countries, to authorise uncontrolled donation after circulatory death (uDCD). More recently, NYC developed its own uDCD protocol.

DCD is a form of organ donation that takes place after the cessation of circulatory function, but not of all brain function. Controlled DCD occurs in a hospital when life support is removed. In turn, uDCD is initiated following an unexpected, mostly although not always, out-of-hospital cardiac arrest (OHCA), where, after resuscitation attempts are judged futile and the patient is declared dead, interventions are restarted to preserve his or her organs. Following legislation and policy adoption in Spain and France, uDCD is also beginning to be considered and implemented in the United States.

Since its inception, uDCD has generated both excitement and concern. On the one hand, these protocols potentially increase organ donation rates by making potential donors out of individuals who suffer OHCAs. On the other hand, uDCD raises a number of ethical concerns regarding the truthfulness of the information provided to donor relatives, and the possibility that organ donation could compromise treatment for some patients in refractory cardiac arrest.

Between July 2007 and September 2010, government officials, subject experts, and community participants collaborated *to derive a clinically appropriate and ethi-*

I. Ortega-Deballon (✉)
Division of Critical Care Medicine, Montreal Children's Hospital (MCH), Montreal, Canada
e-mail: iviortega@gmail.com

D. Rodríguez-Arias
Departamento de Filosofia I. Facultad de Filosofia, Universidad de Granada, Granada, Spain

M. J. Smith
Joint Centre for Bioethics, university of Toronto, Ontario, Canada

R. J. Jox et al. (eds.), *Organ Transplantation in Times of Donor Shortage*,
International Library of Ethics, Law, and the New Medicine 59,
DOI 10.1007/978-3-319-16441-0_29

cally sound uDCD protocol for NYC. Although this protocol addresses some ethical issues that have been raised in response to European uDCD protocols, new ethical issues have also emerged from the NYC protocol. In this chapter, we will discuss the strengths and possible ethical challenges of the NYC uDCD protocol by comparing it to current Spanish and French protocols. By highlighting and elucidating ethical concerns with existing uDCD protocols, it is our goal to affect positive policy change in those protocols and others that are likely to be developed worldwide.

29.2 Spanish and French uDCD Protocols

In both France and Spain, when an OHCA is reported by emergency medical services (EMS), an ambulance or a helicopter staffed by a physician, an emergency nurse, and emergency medical technicians is commissioned to the scene. After ordinary life support attempts—i.e. 30 min of advanced cardiopulmonary resuscitation—by the medical team are judged futile, the individual is transferred to a hospital with continued mechanical chest compression and ventilation to preserve the individual's organs. The individual is declared dead at the hospital following a 5-min *no-touch* period of asystole. Then, normothermic extracorporeal membrane oxygenation (nECMO) is initiated to preserve organs until authorization for donation is obtained from the individual's family (Rodriguez-Arias et al 2013 HCR).

29.3 NYC uDCD Protocol*

In contrast, the New York City (NYC) (Wall et al 2011, AJT) protocol commissions a dedicated organ preservation unit (OPU) to the scene, which is staffed with a family services specialist, two organ preservation technicians, and an emergency medicine physician seeking to preserve the organs of individuals who have suffered an OHCA. Once resuscitation maneuvers are judged unsuccessful, according to termination of resuscitation (TOR) EMS policies, the individual is declared dead. Unlike European protocols, the death of the potential donor is declared before he or she arrives at the hospital (Matesanz et al 2012, ONT). Organ preservation techniques are implemented immediately. The OPU staff arrives at the OHCA location in an organ preservation vehicle (OPV) within 2 min of TOR and determines whether there is evidence of prior first person consent for organ donation. The OPU conducts pre-hospital screening examinations including clinical brain stem assessment and, if the OHCA victim is eligible for organ procurement, starts organ preservation in the OPV. Mechanical ventilation and chest compressions are used and an intravenous dose of heparin and/or a tissue plasminogen activator (t-PA) is administered. At the hospital, nECMO is established to preserve the organs. The next of kin is approached to confirm prior consent.

(*) So far, the NYC protocol has not obtained any solid organ despite of enrolling several potential donors from the prehospital setting (Note from the authors, updated when writting this chapter)

29.4 Ethical Issues in uDCD Protocols: Spanish and French vs NYC Protocols

29.4.1 Policy and Decision-Making Process Transparency

Some authors have claimed that Spanish and French policies on uDCD have been introduced without previous societal consensus and without transparency (Rodriguez-Arias 2010, Lancet; Rodriguez-Arias 2013, HCR). In Spain, uDCD was performed for 4 years before a law explicitly authorized its use, while in France in 2006, and in Spain in 2000, laws were quietly passed without previous debate by experts or groups designated to represent each respective society's values and interests (Adnet et al 2009; Agence de la biomédecine 2008; Tenaillon 2009). In contrast, the NYC uDCD protocol has been a pioneer in this respect by involving the active participation of stakeholders (Wall SP et al. 2011, AJT).

29.4.2 Place and Timing of Death Determination and its Communication to the Family

In Spanish and French uDCD protocols, the potential donor's death is certified at the hospital, even though a pre-hospital emergency physician authorized to declare death is always part of the EMS unit and could therefore declare death at that point. In fact, if the individual is not a suitable candidate for organ procurement, death is declared *in situ*. The individual will only be transported to the hospital, where a formal death declaration takes place, if organ retrieval is planned (Matesanz et al 2012, ONT; Rodirguez-Arias et al 2013, HCR; Agence de la biomédecine 2008; Antoine C et al 2007; Tenaillon 2009).

This differs significantly from the NYC protocol (Wall et al 2011, AJT), where a declaration of death is always signed at the OHCA scene. In Spain and France this choice is strategic (Rodriguez-Arias et al 2013, HCR); it avoids having to inform the next of kin that the victim is being transported to the hospital merely as a potential organ donor. In both countries, a soft opt-out model for organ retrieval exists, implying that the absence of explicit individual refusal automatically makes an individual a potential donor, but requires that an individual's possible refusal to donate should be sought by checking their belongings and consulting with proxy decision makers. However, in practice, organ procurement is not undertaken if the family refuses donation. In Spain, this policy is commonly interpreted to support the placement of a cannula for nECMO without exploring the family's opinion, even though this is not supported by law (Matesanz et al 2012 ONT; Roriguez-Arias et al 2013, HCR; Real 2070/1999; Ley 41/2002; Rodriguez-Arias et al 2010, Lancet). By contrast, in the NYC protocol the donor's next of kin is informed about the fact that the only reason his or her relative is being transported to the hospital is the possibility of him or her becoming an organ donor. As such, preservation techniques are initiated only after a relative's authorization. The first person consent in the NYC protocol justifies being transferred to the hospital with the OPU, which makes it possible to honor the individual's known wishes about organ donation.

In Spain, some EMS professionals have questioned whether relatives of potential donors should be made aware of the actual reasons why individuals are transferred to the hospital (Rodriguez-Arias et al 2013, HCR; Rodriguez-Arias et al 2012, Lancet; Matesanz et al 2012, ONT). The official protocol recommends that "the family should only be told that the patient has been transferred to the hospital." This recommendation contradicts the Spanish Law on Patient Autonomy, health professionals' codes of ethics, and several recommendations for DCD in Europe and in the US (Committee on non-heart beating transplantation, IOM 2000; Ley 41/2002 de 14 de Noviembre; Quigley et al 2008 JME; (Real 2070/1999; Rodriguez-Arias et al 2010, Lancet; Rodriguez-Arias et al 2013 HCR). In most cases, this information is not provided to the next of kin, even though there are shortcomings among professionals in their ability to communicate bad news in these countries, as well. In France, the Agence de la Biomédecine took a positive step when discussing the opportunity to inform relatives about the real reason for transporting patients to the hospital as potential organ donors. However, the final recommendation of this official institution still includes the use of unclear language regarding the status of the patient and deceptive expressions about the purpose of administering organ preservation techniques, which are explicitly referred to as "therapeutic measures" (Agence de la biomédecine 2008).

Compared to Spanish and French uDCD protocols, the NYC protocol is clearly more transparent and more consistent with the clauses of the 1999 Maastricht Conference on transparency, the Institute of Medicine (Committee on non-heart-beating trnasplantation, IOM 2000), and recommendations of the Society of Critical Care Medicine. This is apparent in the need for next of kin to consent prior to transportation to the hospital and thus protects not only individual autonomy, but also public trust for organ donation procedures in general, and uDCD in particular. Furthermore, it avoids investing important resources in organ preservation techniques, in that there is no certainty that the family will consent to organ retrieval (Adnet et al 2009; Rodriguez-Arias et al 2013, HCR; Tenaillon et al 2009).

29.4.3 Allocation of Resources and Opportunity Costs

In Spain and France, an ethical issue of distributive justice arises because scarce and expensive resources are used for an individual who has not officially been declared dead. In fact, while the emergency medical unit is conveying a potential uDCD donor, patients who could benefit from these means may be neglected (Rodriguez-Arias et al 2013 HCR). In this respect, the NYC uDCD protocol entails an improvement, since a different vehicle (OPV), rather than an EMS unit whose usual role is to save lives, is used to transport the deceased individual to the hospital (Wall et al 2011 AJT). Still, criticism has been directed at the NYC protocol with regard to involving two specialized health providers, one of them a physician, to preserve organs in the OPV, but not involving them for the purpose of saving the lives of critically ill patients in EMS units (Rodriguez-Arias et al 2013, HCR).

In any case, the *opportunity cost*, defined as the inherent value of the best alternatives not chosen, is greater in Spanish and French uDCD protocols than in the NYC protocol, in that specialized emergency medical resources are not available for any potential emergency calls during that period (usually no less than 90 min) (Rodriguez-Arias et al 2013 HCR).

29.4.4 The Question of Whether the Individual is Dead

With uDCD protocols, it is unclear whether potentially recoverable patients are given all available therapeutic options, whether the protocol itself diminishes patients' chances of survival, and, ultimately, whether and when uDCD donors can be considered dead (Bracco et al 2007 Intensive Care Medicine; Doig et al 2008; Joffe et al 2011; Manara 2010; Marquis 2010).

29.4.4.1 Do Potentially Recoverable Patients Receive all Available Therapeutic Options?

The medical capacity to recover patients suffering from an OHCA is increasing in some places as a result of the development of non-conventional resuscitation procedures (NCRPs) (Doig et al 2008; Lederer et al 2004, Resuscitation; Lee et al 2008, Lancet; Morimura et al 2011, Resuscitation; (Nagao et al 2010, Circulation Journal; Rodriguez-Arias et al 2012, Lancet). In fact, international guidelines insist on the necessity to carry out a minimally interrupted resuscitation. The most recent guidelines on resuscitation endorse high-quality CPR guided by the suspected or known cause of cardiac arrest, permanent monitoring, and support by devices to transport the patient to the hospital (or within the hospital) without discontinuing resuscitation efforts (Nolan et al 2010, Resuscitation; Vanden Hoek et al 2010, Circulation).

In the hospital setting, at least in some regions of Europe, the United States and Asia, NCRPs are now available (Chen-Lu et al 2011, AJEM; Lederer et al 2004, Resuscitation; Lee 2008, Lancet; Morimura et al 2011, Resuscitation; Nagao et al 2010, Circ Journal; Sunde et al 2008, Crit Care Med). As such, EMSs play the role of a bridge between the OHCA setting and the beforementioned in-hospital therapeutic interventions. Importantly, only a particular profile of patients suffering OHCAs would benefit from NCRPs, and many efforts are being undertaken to define which patients should be candidates for NCRPs (Peek 2011, Resuscitation; Rodriguez-Arias et al 2012, Lancet). Current increasing evidence suggests that the updated possibilities of treatment for refractory OHCA can conflict with current uDCD protocols (Bracco 2007, Intensive Care Medicine; Doig et al 2008; Manara 2010, Resuscitation; Rodriguez-Arias et al 2012 Lancet). Some authors have warned that uDCD protocols continue to grow in number, while a desirable parallel development of NCRPs is not taking place.

Thus, some potentially recoverable patients may not receive all available therapeutic options. During the transport of uDCD candidates to the hospital, interventions are strictly intended to preserve organs. With the Spanish and French uDCD protocols, an individual who has not yet been declared dead does not receive available therapeutic options that are required for high-quality CPR. In other words, despite potential donors not being officially declared dead, they are treated as such (Ortega-Deballon et al 2014 HLV; Rodriguez-Arias et al 2012, Lancet; Rodriguez-Arias et al 2013, HCR). With the NYC protocol, donors may be prematurely declared dead, and this diagnosis is assumed to justify not attempting to administer life-saving measures (Bernat et al 2010, Crit Care Med; Bracco et al 2007, Int Care Med; Doig et al 2008; Joffe et al 2011).

29.4.4.2 How do the European and NYC Protocols Deal with this Conflict?

No adequate reflection on the coexistence of NCRP and uDCD protocols has been made until recently (Bracco et al 2007, Int Care Med); Doig et al 2008; Joffe et al 2011; Rodriguez-Arias et al 2012, Lancet). While uDCD protocols are implemented in six different regions of Spain, none have developed NCRP programs. In contrast, in France where some cities have both programs, health professionals have been pioneers in acknowledging the ethical, legal, and health policy concerns associated with this situation (Adnet et al 2009; Nau 2008; Tenaillon 2009). In Japan and in central and northern European countries, there has been pioneering research on NCRPs, but uDCD protocols are very rare in these regions. Finally, promoters of the NYC protocol offer a generic opinion on NCRPs that are inconsistent with current international guidelines by saying that these interventions "are unproven to restore any meaningful brain circulation, given the timing of restoration and other unique circumstances inherent to out-of-hospital uDCD." According to Wall et al., patients do not *wake up* after prolonged cardiac arrest without the return of spontaneous circulation.[1] However, there is contradicting evidence suggesting the exact opposite (Bracco et al 2007; Doig et al 2008; Joffe et al 2011; Morimura et al 2011; Rodriguez-Arias et al 2012, Lancet).

29.4.4.3 When are uDCD Donors Really Dead?

Neither the European nor the NYC uDCD protocols rule out the possibility that the individual who is being transported to the hospital as a potential organ donor may recover vital functions (i.e. circulatory and/or neurologic functions). In the following, we will first explore whether uDCD donors are dead under circulatory criteria, and then discuss whether they can be considered dead according to neurologic criteria.

[1] Wall et al. (2011).

Do Uncontrolled DCD Protocols Rule out the Possibility of the Return of Spontaneous Circulation (ROSC)? In some cases, individuals transported to the hospital as potential donors with ongoing CPR had ROSC on arrival (Manara 2010; Marquis 2010 HCR; Mateos-Rodriguez et al 2010, Resuscitation). This is troubling as it raises the question of how spontaneous circulation can return in a patient for whom standard resuscitative efforts have been considered unsuccessful. In fact, restoration of spontaneous circulation has been reported to occur anywhere from a few seconds to 33 min after failed CPR (Hornby et al 2010, Crit Care Med). Mechanical chest compression and ventilation *in itinere* can maintain high-quality circulatory function. The likelihood of ROSC is potentially increased by the presence of residual vasoactive drugs used during CPR. Certainly, ROSC does not necessarily involve a recovery of neurologic function; however, it is important to note that circulatory criteria are sufficient for legally declaring the death of these individuals. These criteria, first and foremost, are not present in individuals with ROSC. The question that remains is whether they fulfill neurologic criteria (Bernat et al 2010; Doig et al 2008; Joffe et al 2011; Marquis 2010; Nau JY 2008).

Do Uncontrolled DCD Protocols Rule out the Possibility of Neurologic Recovery? In some rare cases, 6% in some series, patients being transported to the hospital as potential donors have not only recovered a pulse, but also regained consciousness. In some cases, patients have recovered completely with a good quality of life. Mateos *et al.* claim that, "[i]f these individuals had not been included in the [non-heart-beating donation] protocol, resuscitation would have stopped after 30 min and the patients would not have survived" (Mateos-Rodríguez et al. 2010). However, what would the outcome have been like for these survivors and other patients who did become donors if they had benefited from NCRP programs as opposed to just techniques strictly intended to preserve their organs? (Bracco et al 2007; Doig et al 2008; Joffe et al 2011; Manara 2010; Rodriguez-Arias et al 2012, Lancet; Rodriguez-Arias et al 2013, HCR).

These cases, albeit that they are probably exceptions, can certainly threaten the image of organ transplantation. In France, a case of cognitive recovery from a DCD donor was published in *Le Monde* in 2008.[2] In Spain, at least three potential donors have been discharged from the hospital, one of them with complete neurologic recovery (Mateos-Rodriguez et al 2010, Resuscitation).

29.4.4.4 Do uDCD Protocols Diminish Patients' Chances of Survival?

Many authors, including a Health Resources and Services Administration (HSRA) panel of experts, have warned that restoring brain blood flow through ECMO can retroactively negate the cause of death of (Bernat 2010; Bracco et al 2007; Doig

[2] Nau (2008).

et al 2008; Joffe 2011; Manara 2010; Motta 2005) (already declared dead) uDCD donors and can even result in their suffering. Spanish and French authorities have not explicitly acknowledged this risk, although the strategy to block the aorta with a balloon obturator is also used in these countries (Agence de la biomédecine 2008; Matesanz et al 2012, ONT). The NYC protocol echoes this concern and requires a bedside brain stem assessment to clinically evaluate consciousness, but explicitly justifies the insertion of the aortic balloon occlusion catheter to avoid brain blood flow (Wall et al 2011, AJT; Rodirguez-Arias et al 2013, HCR). The implication here is that if ECMO is used for the preservation of organs of potential organ donors this can lead to a recovery of circulatory function and even cerebral function of the individual. Interestingly, stakeholders of the NYC protocol decided to accept uDCD even though it was explicitly acknowledged that both circulatory and neurologic functions could be restored. This ought to raise concerns about the fulfillment of the dead donor rule in those cases (Bernat 2010; Marquis 2010; Rodriguez-Arias et al 2013, HCR).

The NYC protocol is not different from European protocols in prioritizing organ preservation over resuscitation of at least some selected OHCA patients who could survive if resuscitation was pursued with the same enthusiasm as organ procurement is.

The administration of heparin is a further intervention strictly intended to preserve the organs that, when used, might decrease an individual's chances of survival (Motta 2005). In the NYC protocol, 30,000 IU of intravenous heparin or/and 100 mg of t-PA are administered to the donor on site or during the transport to the hospital (Wall et al 2011, AJT). In Spain and France, heparin cannot be administered to donors until they arrive at the hospital, after death has been declared.

Only in the case of an OHCA caused by thromboembolic disease could heparin administration be beneficial to the individual (Nolan et al 2010 Resuscitation; Vanden Hoek et al 2010 Circulation). Uncontrolled DCD proponents in the US argue that such interventions contribute to preserving the organs of individuals. However, the question remains whether or not these individuals should have been declared dead already. The question is more pressing in that some donors have regained consciousness despite the fact that all interventions they received were strictly intended to preserve their organs and not their lives (Mateos-Rodriguez et al 2010, Resuscitation; Nau 2008 Le Monde).

29.5 Conclusions and Final Thoughts

Uncontrolled and controlled DCD protocols bring excellent results. However, a number of ethical concerns threaten the long-term outcomes of these programs. In particular, ethical concerns arise in environments where uDCD exists but where NCRPs, which require analogous technical and human resources, are not offered.

Scientific, technical, and ethical criteria to differentiate patients from potential donors among the victims of OHCA should be clear and transparent. In centers where, nowadays, only one option is available, i.e., uDCD or NCRP, a conflict arises among health care professionals: do we try to save lives or should we preserve the organs of potential donors? Furthermore, a social perception of suspicion and distrust could result from the possibility that the prospect of a donation would compromise the optimal quality of health care.

We believe that uDCD protocols and NCRP programs can and should coexist, although the former should be subjected to the failure of the latter. Thus, only after every scientifically directed and ethically justifiable effort available to save a patient's life has been put forth without success should an OHCA victim be considered a potential organ donor, as agreed upon and published by international consensus on DCD (Ortega-Deballon et al 2014 HLV; Rodriguez-Arias et al 2012, Lancet). With some important objections, the NYC uDCD protocol has proven to be a laudable effort in this direction. However, it is important to identify the aspects of uDCD protocols that need improvement as a result of the cumulative scientific evidence in the management of cardiac arrest before giving up resuscitative attempts. Both European protocols and the NYC uDCD protocol should be evaluated with this in mind.

The ultimate goal is to achieve an increase in organ donation rates. However, not all paths should be considered acceptable to achieve this goal. To be consistent with current knowledge in both the medical and scientific communities, but also ethics standards, the issues discussed in this chapter are significant enough to call for a comprehensive review of uDCD protocols as a whole. Transplant policy makers should care just as much about *what* they are trying to achieve, as about *how* to get there.

Conflicts of Interest and Financial Disclosures None to report

References

Adnet, F., R. Dufau, F. Roussin, and F. Lapostolle. 2009. Prélèvements sur donneurs décédés après arrêt cardiaque: l'expérience des urgentistes. *Le Courrier de la Transplantation* 9:48–49.

Agence de la biomédecine. 2008. Protocole versión du 13 avril 2008 définissant "les conditions à respecter pour réaliser des prélèvements de reins sur donneurs décédés après arrêt cardiaque dans les établissements de santé autorisés aux prélèvements d'organes".

Antoine, C., and A. Tenaillon. 2007. Conditions à respecter pour réaliser des prélèvements de reins sur des donneurs à coeur arrêté dans un établissement de santé autorisé aux prélèvements d'organes. Agence de la Biomédecine (ABM). Prélèvement reins sur donneur à coeur arrêté.

Bernat, J. L., A. M. Capron, T. P. Bleck, S. Blosser, S. L. Bratton, J. F. Childress, et al. 2010. The circulatory-respiratory determination of death in organ donation. *Critical Care Medicine* 38:963–970.

Bracco, D., N. Noiseux, and T. M. Hemmerling. 2007. The thin line between life and death. *Intensive Care Medicine* 33:751–754.

Chen-Lu, Y., J. Wen, L. You-Ping, and Y. K. Shi. 2011. Cardiocerebral resuscitation vs cardiopulmonary resuscitation for cardiac arrest: A systematic review published online ahead of print April 25, 2011. *American Journal of Emergency Medicine*. doi:10.1016/j.ajem.2011.02.035.

Committee on Non-Heart-Beating Transplantation II, Institute of Medicine. 2000. *Non-heart-beating organ transplantation: Practice and protocols*. Washington, DC: National Academy of Sciences.

Doig, C. J., and D. A. Zygun. 2008. (Uncontrolled) Donation after cardiac determination of death: A note of caution. *The Journal of Law, Medicine & Ethics* 36:760–765.

Hornby, K., L. Hornby, and S. D. Shemie. 2010. A systematic review of autoresuscitation after cardiac arrest. *Critical Care Medicine* 38:1246–1253.

Joffe, A. R., J. Carcillo, N. Anton, A. deCaen, Y. Y. Han, M. J. Bell, et al. 2011. Donation after cardiocirculatory death: A call for a moratorium pending full public disclosure and fully informed consent. *Philosophy, Ethics, and Humanities in Medicine* 6:17.

Lederer, W., C. Lichtenberger, C. Pechlaner, J. Kinzl, G. Kroesen, and M. Baubin. 2004. Long-term survival and neurological outcome of patients who received recombinant tissue plasminogen activator during out-of-hospital cardiac arrest. *Resuscitation* 61:123–129.

Lee, S. W., and Y. S. Hong. 2008. Extracorporeal life-support in patients requiring CPR. Lancet. Comment to Cardiopulmonary resuscitation with assisted extracorporeal life support versus conventional cardiopulmonary resuscitation in adults with in-hospital cardiac arrest: An observational study and propensity analysis. Lancet 2008; published online July 7. doi:10.1016/S0140-6736(08)60958-7.

Ley. 41/2002 de 14 de noviembre. básica reguladora de la autonomía del paciente y de derechos y obligaciones en materia de información y documentación clínica. BOE 274. 40126–40132.

Manara, A. R., and I. Thomas. 2010. The use of circulatory criteria to diagnose death after unsuccessful cardiopulmonary resuscitation. *Resuscitation* 81:781–783.

Marquis, D. 2010. Are DCD donors dead? *The Hastings Center Report* 40 (3): 24–31.

Mateos-Rodríguez, A., L. Pardillos-Ferrer, J. M. Navalpotro-Pascual, C. Barba-Alonso, M. E. Martin-Maldonado, and A. Andrés-Belmonte. 2010. Kidney transplant function using organs from non-heart-beating donors maintained by mechanical chest compressions. *Resuscitation* 81:904–907.

Matesanz, R., E. Coll Torres, B. Dominguez-Gil Gonzalez, and L. Perojo Vega. 2012. *Donación en asistolia en España: Situación actual y recomendaciones*. Madrid: ONT.

Morimura, N., T. Sakamoto, K. Nagao, Y. Asai, H. Yokota, Y. Tahara, et al. 2011. Extracorporeal cardiopulmonary resuscitation for out-of-hospital cardiac arrest: A review of the Japanese literature. *Resuscitation* 82:10–14.

Motta, E. D. 2005. The ethics of heparin administration to the potential non-heart-beating organ donor. *Journal of Professional Nursing* 21:97–102.

Nagao, K., K. Kikushima, K. Watanabe, E. Tachibana, Y. Tominaga, K. Tada, et al. 2010. Early induction of hypothermia during cardiac arrest improves neurological outcomes in patients with out-of-hospital cardiac arrest who undergo emergency cardiopulmonary bypass and percutaneous coronary intervention. *Circulation Journal* 74:77–85.

Nau, J. Y. 2008. Le donneur d'organes n'était pas mort. Le monde.

Nolan, J. P., J. Soar, D. A. Zideman, D. Biarent, L. L. Bossaert, C. Deakin, et al. 2010. European resuscitation council guidelines for resuscitation 2010 section 1. Executive summary. *Resuscitation* 81:1219–1276.

Ortega-Deballon I., and E. De la Plaza-Horche. 2014. A comprehensive approach to refractory cardiac arrest: Saving more lives one way or another. Heart, Lung and Vessels. Invited Editorial. In press.

Peek, G. J. 2011. Community extracorporeal life support for cardiac arrest. When should it be used? *Resuscitation* 82:1117.

Quigley, M., M. Brazier, R. Chadwick, M. N. Michel, and D. Paredes 2008. The organs crisis and the Spanish model: Theoretical versus pragmatic considerations. *Journal of Medical Ethics* 34:223–224.

Real Decreto 2070/1999, del 30 de diciembre, por el que se regulan las actividades de obtención y utilización clínica de órganos humanos y la coordinación territorial en materia de donación y trasplante de órganos y tejidos.

Rodríguez-Arias, D., and I. O. Deballon. 2012. Protocols for uncontrolled donation after circulatory death. *Lancet* 379:1275–1276.

Rodríguez-Arias, D., L. Wright, and D. Paredes. 2010. Success factors and ethical challenges of the Spanish model of organ donation. *Lancet* 376:1109–1112.

Rodríguez-Arias, D., I. Ortega-Deballon, M. J. Smith, and S. J. Youngner. 2013. Casting light and doubt on uncontrolled DCDD protocols. *The Hastings Center Report* 43 (1): 27–30.

Sunde, K. 2008. Experimental and clinical use of ongoing mechanical cardiopulmonary resuscitation during angiography and percutaneous coronary intervention. *Critical Care Medicine* 36:405–408.

Tenaillon, A. 2009. Aspects éthiques des prélèvements d'organes sur donneurs décédés après arrêt cardiaque. *Le Courrier de la Transplantation* 9:50–58.

Vanden Hoek, T. L., L. J. Morrison, M. Shuster, M. Donnino, E. Sinz, E. J. Lavonas, et al. 2010. Part 12: Cardiac arrest in special situations. American Heart Association Guidelines for cardiopulmonary resuscitation and emergency cardiovascular care. *Circulation* 122:829–861.

Wall, S. P., B. J. Kaufman, A. J. Gilbert, Y. Yushkov, M. Goldstein, and J. E. Rivera, et al. 2011. Derivation of the uncontrolled donation after circulatory determination of death protocol for New York City. *American Journal of Transplantation* 11:1417–1426.

Iván Ortega-Deballon is a research associate at the Division of Critical Care Medicine, Montreal Children's Hospital (MCH). He is working within the Deceased Organ Donation research program at MCH and the Loeb Chair and Research Consortium at the University of Ottawa. He is interested in working on the complex intersection of pre-mortem life-saving versus post-mortem organ-preserving interventions such as high quality Resuscitation and ECMO. He is also involved with health policy development relevant to deceased donation with Canadian Blood Services and Canadian National Transplant Research Program. Ivan is a specialist in law and medical ethics and an associate professor at the University. He is also a Flight Emergency Nurse Practitioner and has worked in the Helicopter Emergency Medical Services and ground Mobile Intensive Care Units in Spain, France and Denmark. In Madrid, he was responsible for the care of potential organ donors during transport after cardiac arrest and for the approach to the next-of-kin of the potential donor.

David Rodríguez-Arias PhD, is Investigador Ramón y Cajal at the Departamento de Filosofía I, Facultad de Filosofía, Universidad de Granada, Spain. He also belongs to the Group of Excellence G-41 on Applied Ethics of the University of Salamanca. His doctoral research included a broad international survey on the concept of death employed by 600 professionals in France, the US and Spain (INCONFUSE study). In 2009, his PhD dissertation received a research distinction (best dissertation defended in the Philosophy Department) and the National Bioethics Prize by the Víctor Grífols i Lucas Foundation. He has been a visiting fellow at Case Western Reserve University, the University of Toronto Joint Center for Bioethics and the Hastings Center. His research is mainly devoted to the ethical and international aspects of organ transplantation, with a focus on the determination of death.

Maxwell J. Smith is a PhD candidate in Public Health Sciences and Bioethics at the Dalla Lana School of Public Health and Joint Centre for Bioethics at the University of Toronto, where he is studying the concept and role of justice in public health emergency preparedness and response. He is also a Canadian Institute's of Health Research (CIHR) fellow in Public Health Policy, a CIHR Frederick Banting and Charles Best Canada Graduate Scholar, and a research associate with the University of Toronto Munk School of Global Affairs' Comparative Program on Health and Society. In 2012, Max was awarded the CIHR Douglas Kinsella Doctoral Award for Research in Bioethics, the Peter A. Singer Graduate Award in Bioethics, and the Mervis-Simon Family Award in Bioethics. He recently completed a residency as a visiting researcher at the Brocher Foundation (2013).

Index

R. J. Jox et al. (eds.), *Organ Transplantation in Times of Donor Shortage*,
International Library of Ethics, Law, and the New Medicine 59,
DOI 10.1007/978-3-319-16441-0

MIX
Papier aus verantwortungsvollen Quellen
Paper from responsible sources
FSC® C105338

If you have any concerns about our products,
you can contact us on
ProductSafety@springernature.com

In case Publisher is established outside the EU,
the EU authorized representative is:
Springer Nature Customer Service Center GmbH
Europaplatz 3, 69115 Heidelberg, Germany

Printed by Libri Plureos GmbH
in Hamburg, Germany